Thoracic Imaging
A Core Review

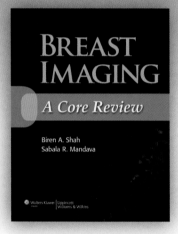
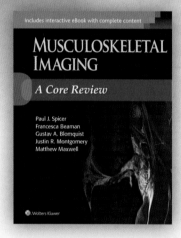
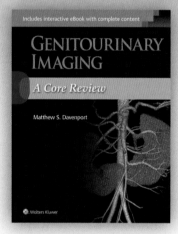
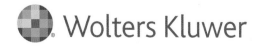

Thoracic Imaging

A Core Review

EDITORS

Stephen B. Hobbs, MD

Assistant Professor
Department of Radiology
Division of Cardiovascular and Thoracic Radiology
Medical Director, Radiology Informatics and Information Technology
University of Kentucky
Lexington, Kentucky

Christian W. Cox, MD

Assistant Professor
Department of Radiology
Division of Thoracic Radiology
Mayo Clinic
Rochester, Minnesota

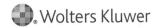

Philadelphia • Baltimore • New York • London
Buenos Aires • Hong Kong • Sydney • Tokyo

Acquisitions Editor: Ryan Shaw
Product Development Editor: Lauren Pecarich
Production Product Manager: David Saltzberg
Senior Manufacturing Coordinator: Beth Welsh
Design Coordinator: Stephen Druding
Prepress Vendor: SPi Global

© 2016 by Wolters Kluwer

Two Commerce Square
2001 Market Street
Philadelphia, PA 19103 USA
LWW.com

Printed in China

Library of Congress Cataloging-in-Publication Data
Thoracic imaging (Hobbs)
  Thoracic imaging : a core review / editors, Stephen B. Hobbs, Christian W. Cox.
      p. ; cm.
  Includes bibliographical references and index.
  ISBN 978-1-4698-9883-4 (alk. paper)
  I. Hobbs, Stephen B., editor. II. Cox, Christian W., editor. III. Title.
  [DNLM: 1. Thoracic Diseases—diagnosis—Examination Questions. 2. Diagnostic Imaging—Examination Questions.   WF 18.2]
  RC734.I43
  616.2'40754—dc23
                                                                    2015016162

To my wife, Fareesh, the love of my life. Without your support, this book would not have been possible.

STEPHEN B. HOBBS

To my wife, Sarah. You are my love.

To my children, Elizabeth, Catherine and Benjamin. You are my joy.

CHRISTIAN W. COX

CONTRIBUTORS

CHAPTER FOUR - INTENSIVE CARE UNIT

Dipti Nevrekar, MD

Staff Radiologist
Department of Radiology
National Jewish Health
StatRad
Denver, Colorado

CHAPTER FIVE - PULMONARY PATHOLOGY

Infectious Pneumonia

Michael Winkler, MD, FSCCT, FICA

Assistant Professor
Department of Radiology
Division of Cardiovascular and Thoracic Radiology
University of Kentucky
Lexington, KY

Diffuse Lung Disease

Marianna Zagurovskaya, MD

Assistant Professor
Department of Radiology
University of Kentucky
Lexington, Kentucky

Diffuse Alveolar Disease and Inflammatory Conditions Airways Disease

Carlos A Rojas, MD

Assistant Professor
Department of Radiology
Associate Director, Diagnostic Radiology Residency Program
University of South Florida
Tampa, Florida

Thoracic Manifestations of Systemic Disease

David Lynch, MB

Professor
Department of Radiology
National Jewish Health
Denver, Colorado

Atelectasis and Collapse

Christopher M. Walker, MD

Assistant Professor
Department of Radiology
Saint Luke's Hospital of Kansas City
University of Missouri - Kansas City
Kansas City, Missouri

Pulmonary Physiology

Angel Coz-Yataco, MD, FCCP

Assistant Professor
Department of Internal Medicine
Division of Pulmonary, Critical Care and Sleep Medicine
Associate Fellowship Program Director, Pulmonary and Critical Care
University of Kentucky
Lexington, Kentucky

CHAPTER SIX - DISEASES OF THE PLEURA, CHEST WALL, AND DIAPHRAGM

Jonathan A. Phelan, DO

Instructor of Radiology
Senior Clinical Associate
Division of Cardiothoracic Radiology
Mayo Clinic
Jacksonville, Florida

CHAPTER NINE - LUNG CANCER

Michael A Brooks, MD

Associate Professor
Departments of Radiology and Medicine
Vice Chair of Radiology
Division Chief, Cardiovascular and Thoracic Imaging
University of Kentucky
Lexington, Kentucky

CHAPTER TEN - TRAUMA

James Lee, MD

Assistant Professor
Department of Radiology
Division of Emergency Radiology and Abdominal Radiology
University of Kentucky
Lexington, Kentucky

David Nickels, MD

Assistant Professor
Department of Radiology
Division Chief, Emergency Radiology
University of Kentucky
Lexington, Kentucky

CHAPTER ELEVEN - CONGENITAL DISEASE
(ADULT PRESENTATIONS)

Anne-Marie Sykes, MD, FRCP

Assistant Professor
Department of Radiology
Division of Thoracic Radiology
Mayo Clinic
Rochester, Minnesota

CHAPTER TWELVE - POSTOPERATIVE THORAX

Jeremiah Martin, MB, BCH, FRCSI, FACS

Assistant Professor
Department of Surgery
Division of Cardiothoracic Surgery
Surgical Director, Markey Cancer Center Multidisciplinary
    Lung Cancer Clinic
University of Kentucky
Lexington, Kentucky

Thoracic Imaging: A Core Review is the fourth book added to the *Core Review Series*. This book covers the most important aspects of thoracic imaging in a manner that I am confident will serve as a useful guide for residents to assess their knowledge and review the material in a question style format that is similar to the ABR Core examination.

Dr. Stephen Hobbs and Dr. Christian Cox have succeeded in producing a book that exemplifies the philosophy and goals of the *Core Review Series*. They have done an excellent job in covering key topics and providing quality images. The multiple-choice questions have been divided logically into chapters so as to make it easy for learners to work on particular topics as needed. Each question has a corresponding answer with an explanation of not only why a particular option is correct but also why the other options are incorrect. There are also references provided for each question for those who want to delve more deeply into a specific subject. This format is also useful for radiologists preparing for Maintenance of Certification (MOC).

The intent of the *Core Review Series* is to provide the resident, fellow, or practicing physician a review of the important conceptual, factual, and practical aspects of a subject by providing approximately 300 multiple-choice questions, in a format similar to the ABR Core examination. The *Core Review Series* is not intended to be exhaustive but to provide material likely to be tested on the ABR Core exam and that would be required in clinical practice.

As Series Editor of the *Core Review Series*, I have had the pleasure to work with many outstanding individuals across the country who contributed to the series. This series represents countless hours of work and involvement by many and it would not have come together without their participation.

Dr. Stephen Hobbs, Dr. Christian Cox, and their contributors are to be congratulated on doing an outstanding job. I believe *Thoracic Imaging: A Core Review* will serve as an excellent resource for residents during their board preparation and a valuable reference for fellows and practicing radiologists.

Biren A. Shah, MD, FACR
Series Editor

SERIES FOREWORD

PREFACE

With the relatively recent changes to the American Board of Radiology (ABR) examination process, the preparation residents undergo must adapt. Gone are the days spent honing skills specifically for an oral exam. The new examination emphasizes a more comprehensive understanding of disease processes and integration of imaging into overall patient care. There remains a paucity of study material specifically geared toward this new style.

Accordingly, this book serves as a guide for residents to assess their knowledge and review material in a format similar to the new board style. The questions are divided into different sections directly adapted from the ABR study syllabus to make it easy for the readers to work on particular topics. Explanations are concise but thorough with references provided for each question for those that want to delve more deeply into a specific subject. Radiologists preparing for their Maintenance of Certification (MOC) exam are also likely to find this format helpful.

There are multiple individuals (past fellows, current colleagues, and senior mentors) who contributed to this publication. This book could not have been finished without the efforts of all these people, each of whom took time from their busy lives to research, write, and submit content in a timely manner. Our heartfelt thanks to all of them.

Many thanks to the staff at Wolters Kluwer Health for giving us this opportunity.

Last, but not least, we are incredibly grateful to our families, who have endured our long hours of work and encouraged us throughout the process.

We hope that this book will serve as a useful tool for residents on their road to becoming Board-certified radiologists and that it will continue to be a reference in their future careers.

Stephen B. Hobbs
Christian W. Cox

ACKNOWLEDGMENTS

We would like to specifically acknowledge Dr. Peter Sachs, University of Colorado, who provided a number of the cases included in this book.

CONTENTS

1 Basics of Imaging

QUESTIONS

1 An obese female patient undergoing CT pulmonary angiography experiences pain with injection of 40 mL IV iodinated contrast, which quickly resolves. On physical exam 10 minutes later, the injection site appears as below, and the patient complains of mild increasing pain. What is the best course of action?

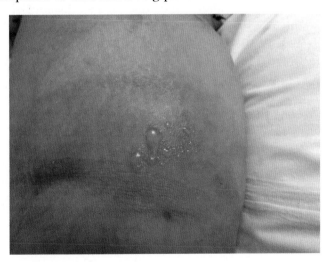

   A. No action necessary.
   B. Keep the patient for observation.
   C. Administer 50 mg IV Benadryl.
   D. Surgical consultation.

2 Which of the following measurements of CT radiation dose takes into account the anatomic region and tissue being scanned?

   A. CT dose index (CTDI)
   B. Volumetric CT dose index (CTDI$_{vol}$)
   C. Dose–length product (DLP)
   D. Effective dose

3a Explain the appearance of the CT pulmonary angiogram below.

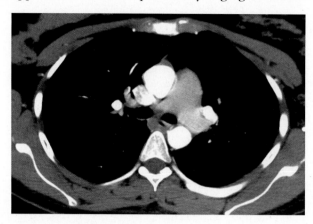

    A. Imaging delayed relative to contrast bolus
    B. Transient interruption of contrast
    C. Imaging early relative to contrast bolus
    D. Contrast bolus interrupted by extravasation

3b What physiologic process explains the phenomenon of transient interruption of contrast?

    A. Unopacified IVC blood filling atrium due to deep inspiration
    B. Flexion in the extremity at the IV site blocking the contrast bolus
    C. Cardiac arrhythmia changing flow rates of the bolus
    D. Transient decrease in blood pressure slowing bolus progression

4a Apart from red bone marrow, what is the most radiosensitive organ in the chest of a male patient?

    A. Lungs
    B. Breasts
    C. Thyroid
    D. Esophagus

4b Apart from red bone marrow, what is the most radiosensitive organ in the chest of a young female patient?

    A. Heart
    B. Breasts
    C. Thyroid
    D. Esophagus

5a In addition to chest x-ray, which of the following examinations has the highest rating for initial evaluation of high-energy blunt thoracic trauma according to the ACR Appropriateness criteria?

    A. CTA of the chest
    B. CT chest without contrast
    C. MRI/MRA chest with and without contrast
    D. Ultrasound of the chest

5b Which of the following examinations has the highest rating for evaluation of suspected cardiac injury after initial radiographs and clinical evaluation?

    A. Transthoracic echocardiography
    B. CTA coronary arteries
    C. Transesophageal echocardiography
    D. Cardiac MRI

6a What magnetic resonance artifact is identified by the arrow overlying a known foregut duplication cyst?

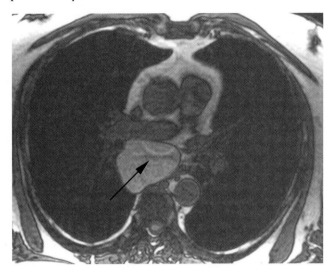

A. Aliasing
B. Pulsation
C. Truncation
D. Chemical shift

6b In which direction is pulsation artifact?

A. Anterior to posterior
B. Parallel to the greatest magnetic field
C. Z-axis
D. Phase-encoded axis

7a What is the primary CT finding?

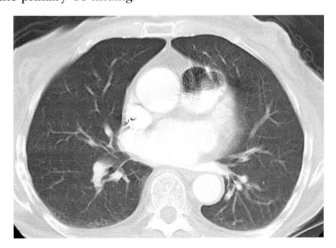

A. Normal chest CT through pulmonary artery
B. Pulmonary artery air embolism
C. Pulmonary artery fat embolism
D. Pulmonary artery foreign body

7b Give the best recommendation for this asymptomatic patient.

A. Oblique left lateral decubitus position until resorption

B. Emergent surgical consult

C. Call code and begin basic life support.

D. No intervention, patient may leave department

8 Based on the Fleischner Society recommendations for follow-up of subsolid nodules, what is the initial follow-up recommendation for a pure ground-glass nodule found on CT measuring greater than 5 mm?

A. 3 months

B. 6 months

C. 12 months

D. 24 months

9 On evaluating interval growth of a rounded (spherical) nodule, approximately what percentage increase in diameter correlates with a doubling of tissue volume?

A. 10%

B. 25%

C. 50%

D. 100%

10 Which of the following would exclude a patient from lung cancer screening with low-dose CT of the chest based on the US Preventive Services Task Force (USPSTF) recommendations?

A. 50-year-old patient

B. Greater than 30-pack-year smoking history

C. Coronary artery disease without angina

D. Smoking cessation 10 years prior

11 What is the most common iodinated intravenous contrast complication in myasthenia gravis?

A. Progressive muscle extremity weakness

B. Anaphylaxis

C. New or progressive acute respiratory compromise

D. No specific complications are associated with iodinated IV contrast.

12 Using the ACR Appropriateness Criteria, which of the following clinical conditions has the highest indication for a preoperative chest x-ray?

A. Chronic cardiopulmonary disease in a 60-year-old patient

B. Acute cardiopulmonary disease in a 60-year-old patient

C. Asymptomatic 80-year-old patients

D. Chronic cardiopulmonary disease in an 80-year-old patient

13 What is the cause of ring artifact on CT?

A. Volume averaging

B. Photon starvation

C. Faulty detector

D. Beam hardening

14 What is the approximate conversion factor value for calculating effective radiation dose from the reported dose–length product in a chest CT?

   A. 0 µSv/mGy
   B. 2 µSv/mGy
   C. 5 µSv/mGy
   D. 18 µSv/mGy

15 Which CT imaging parameter change will result in the greatest radiation dose reduction?

   A. Decreasing the mAs by 20%
   B. Decreasing the z-axis by 20%
   C. Decreasing the kV by 20%
   D. Decreasing the noise index by 20%

ANSWERS AND EXPLANATIONS

1 **Answer D.** In the setting of IV iodinated contrast extravasation, immediate surgical consultation or transfer to emergency care is recommended if the patient demonstrates any of the following: "progressive swelling or pain, altered tissue perfusion as evidenced by decreased capillary refill at any time after the extravasation has occurred, change in sensation in the affected limb, and skin ulceration or blistering." The most common severe complication of IV iodinated contrast extravasation is compartment syndrome, with likelihood increasing as the quantity of extravasated contrast increases, but small volumes have also been reported to cause compartment syndrome.

If any noticeable amount of extravasation occurs at the injection site, the patient will at least need observation for several hours. Severity and prognosis of IV iodinated contrast extravasation is difficult, and close follow-up is recommended to exclude delayed development of signs and symptoms. Only after the radiologist is comfortable that the patient's signs and symptoms are resolving and no new complaints are arising, can the patient be discharged. Treatment for extravasations not requiring surgical consultation is variable but generally includes elevation of the affected limb and application of a hot or cold compress.

Reference: ACR Manual on Contrast Media, (v. 9) 2013.

2 **Answer D.** Both CTDI and DLP are terms related to absorbed dose which describes the energy from ionizing radiation absorbed per unit mass. The units are expressed in grays (Gy) for absorbed dose. The $CTDI_{vol}$ is simply the most commonly used descriptor for CTDI and is expressed as the average dose over the scanned volume, typically expressed in mGy. Multiplying this $CTDI_{vol}$ value by the scan length results in the DLP (units of mGy * cm). The effective dose (measured in sieverts, Sv) takes into account the tissue being scanned and its relative radiosensitivity. It takes into account both sex and an age-averaged reference person. Because of the age-averaged reference person, the applicability of effective dose for an individual scan and patient is limited. Effective dose was designed for estimating radiation exposure of entire populations.

Reference: Huda W, Mettler FA. Volume CT dose index and dose–length product displayed during CT: what good are they? *Radiology* 2011;258:236–242.

3a **Answer B.**

3b **Answer A.** As the contrast bolus migrates from the superior vena cava (SVC) to the right atrium during a CT pulmonary angiogram, unopacified blood from the inferior vena cava (IVC) is mixing with the contrast-dense blood in the right atrium. If the patient performs deep inspiration during the contrast administration, low thoracic pressure draws an increased volume of unopacified blood from the IVC creating a transient column of low contrast density blood passing through the pulmonary vasculature. Consequently, the CT pulmonary angiogram demonstrates high contrast density in the SVC and aorta while the pulmonary artery appears suboptimally contrast filled. To support the mechanism of the "abdominal–thoracic pump," Wittram and Yoo measured average Hounsfield units (HU) in the right atrium and right ventricle compared to the average HUs in the SVC and IVC to calculate the approximate contributions of the SVC and IVC. Since imaging of the chest takes a variable amount of time, the effect of transient interruption of contrast may not be evenly distributed throughout the lungs as the contrast interruption passes before the imaging is complete. Additionally, these transient breaks in contrast may be mistaken for pulmonary embolism.

Recommendations to minimize transient interruption of contrast focus on limiting deep inspiration immediately prior to imaging. Medical imaging facilities may accomplish this in various ways. For instance, some institutions may perform CT pulmonary angiography at "suspended respiration" rather than full inspiration while others may work on coaching of patients on proper inspiratory technique with slow gradual deep inspiration.

References: Gosselin MV, Rassner UA, Thieszen SL, et al. Contrast dynamics during CT pulmonary angiogram. *J Thorac Imaging* 2004;19:1–7.

Wittram C, Yoo AJ. Transient interruption of contrast on CT pulmonary angiography: proof of mechanism. *J Thorac Imaging* 2007;22:125–129.

4a **Answer A.**

4b **Answer B.**   The most radiosensitive organs are the red bone marrow, colon, lung, and stomach. In a female patient, the breast is also one of the most radiosensitive (tied with lung). The thyroid is radiosensitive but to a lesser degree than the lung or breast. The esophagus and heart are the least radiosensitive of those listed.

Reference: ICRP. The 2007 recommendations of the International Commission on Radiological Protection. ICRP Publication 103. *Ann ICRP* 2007;37(2-4).

5a **Answer A.**

5b **Answer A.**   The ACR Appropriateness Criteria designate scores from a range of 1 to 9 for currently available imaging techniques in specific clinical scenarios. These criteria are readily accessible and are useful for guiding clinician imaging requests. A score of 1 to 3 generally corresponds with an exam that is "usually not appropriate." A score of 4 to 6 "may be appropriate," and a score of 7 to 9 is "usually appropriate."

Based on these criteria, chest radiographs and contrast-enhanced chest CT are considered complementary in the setting of blunt trauma and almost always indicated (score of 9). The chest CT should be performed using CTA technique to enhance evaluation for traumatic aortic injury if possible. Noncontrast CT and ultrasound are only sometimes indicated (score of 5). Contrast chest MRI is usually not appropriate (score of 2).

In the setting of suspected cardiac injury after initial evaluation, the highest rating is for transthoracic echocardiography (score of 8). This can exclude cardiac chamber rupture and acute valvular injury. Coronary CTA would only be advised in the setting of suspected coronary injury (score of 5). Transesophageal echo is generally not required unless there is a need to clarify findings on transthoracic echo (score of 5). Cardiac MRI may take 45 minutes to 1 hour and is generally not possible or advisable for patients with significant acute blunt force trauma (score of 4). It may be useful as a problem-solving tool for isolated and specific questions that are not answerable with echocardiography alone.

Reference: Chung JH, Cox CW, Mohammed TL, et al. ACR appropriateness criteria blunt chest trauma. *J Am Coll Radiol* 2014;11(4):345–351.

6a **Answer B.**

6b **Answer A.**   Regular or sporadic motion during MR imaging creates motion artifact, which improperly assigns signal to alternative locations greatest in the phase-encoded direction. Regular motion can be macroscopic as in cardiac or respiratory motion or microscopic as in pulsation artifact. In this case, the blood flow within the aorta is sinusoidal creating repetitive artifacts in the phase-encoded axis. The distance between artifacts is proportional to the frequency of the pulsatile flow. Other potential MR artifacts do not create this type of repetitive artifact. In aliasing, the field of view excludes a portion of anatomy that then wraps to the opposite side of the image. Truncation artifact occurs from data lost from fine anatomic detail due to a finite number of spectral components in digital image reconstruction. Finally, chemical shift artifact occurs in well-demarcated borders between fat and water, where the slight difference in proton precession frequency between fat and water creates signal void or overlap at the border in the frequency-encoded direction.

Reference: Arena L, Morehouse HT, Safir J. MR imaging artifacts that simulate disease: how to recognize and eliminate them. *Radiographics* 1995;15:1373–1394.

7a **Answer B.**

7b **Answer A.**   Not uncommonly, some small air emboli occur with contrast injection during CT imaging. The small amounts of air are trapped and resorbed in the pulmonary arterioles if not before and the patient remains asymptomatic. These smaller air collections are of greater concern in the setting of a right-to-left shunt where air can transfer to the systemic arterial system and create a vapor lock thereby blocking blood flow in critical small vessels such as the coronary or carotid arteries. In the pulmonary arterial system, a larger amount of air is required before a large enough vessel is blocked to be clinically significant and if large enough, can block cardiac output. In this case, the air injected is greater than average, and if still on the table, the patient may benefit from oblique left lateral decubitus positioning and administration of 100% O_2 until the air collection resorbs.

Reference: ACR Manual on Contrast Media, (v. 9) 2013.

8 **Answer A.**   Based on current recommendations, initial follow-up should be a repeat low-dose CT of the chest in 3 months. The rationale is that many ground-glass nodules will resolve over this time period due to their infectious or inflammatory cause. Lesions that persist will generally require longer annual follow-up for a minimum of 3 years until growth is identified or a solid component develops. Familiarity with the Fleischner Society recommendations is very useful in daily clinical practice and for communication with referring clinicians about best practice for nodule surveillance.

Reference: Naidich DP, Bankier AA, MacMahon H, et al. Recommendations for the management of subsolid pulmonary nodules detected at CT: a statement from the Fleischner Society. *Radiology* 2013;266(1):304–317.

9 **Answer B.**   Assuming that a nodule is spherical, as many small pulmonary nodules are, the volume calculation is $4/3\pi r^3$. As such, a doubling time of volume correlates with a 26% increase in diameter. Realize that when doubling time is discussed, it is most frequently in relation to volume, not diameter, so this distinction is important for determining follow-up growth patterns.

Reference: Truong MT, Ko JP, Rossi SE, et al. Update in the evaluation of the solitary pulmonary nodule. *Radiographics* 2014;34(6):1658–1679.

10 **Answer A.** THE USPSFT recommends annual screening for lung cancer for those patients (1) who are between 55 and 80 years old, (2) who have at least a 30-pack-year smoking history, (3) who have smoked within the last 15 years, (4) who are willing to undergo treatment if a lesion is discovered, and (5) who do not have a health problem that would otherwise severely limit their life expectancy. Of the choices provided, the 50-year-old patient would be excluded on the basis of age regardless of his or her smoking history. Coronary artery disease without angina would not be expected to severely limit life expectancy to the degree that screening would be unindicated.

Reference: Recommendation Summary. U.S. Preventive Services Task Force. September 2014. http://www.uspreventiveservicestaskforce.org/Page/Topic/recommendation-summary/lung-cancer-screening

11 **Answer C.** Comparing 112 myasthenia gravis patients receiving low osmolar iodinated intravenous contrast media (LOCM) during CT to 155 myasthenia gravis patients imaged without contrast demonstrated a statistically significant increase in symptoms with LOCM administration. The most common exacerbation was "new or progressive acute respiratory compromise."

Reference: Somashekar DK, Davenport MS, Cohan RH, et al. Effect of intravenous low-osmolality iodinated contrast media on patients with myasthenia gravis. *Radiology* 2013;267(3):727–734.

12 **Answer B.** As explained above in the answer for question 5, the ACR Appropriateness Criteria designate scores from a range of 1 to 9 for currently available imaging techniques in specific clinical scenarios.

Obtaining chest x-rays prior to a surgical procedure has become routine for many facilities; however, there is only limited value for this in many cases. Of the reasons listed here, the highest recommendation is for acute cardiopulmonary disease in any age patient (score of 9). The next highest recommendation would be for an elderly patient (>70 years old) with chronic cardiopulmonary disease (score of 8 if no recent radiograph and score of 6 if recent radiograph is already available within the last 6 months). Evaluation of chronic cardiopulmonary disease in a nonelderly patient does not receive a discrete score recommendation but would likely fall just above the asymptomatic patient of any age (score of 2).

Reference: Mohammed TL, Kirsch J, Amorosa JK, et al. ACR Appropriateness Criteria routine admission and preop chest radiography. Available at https://acsearch.acr.org/docs/69451/Narrative/American College of Radiology. Accessed December 29, 2014.

13 **Answer C.** A ring defect on CT is indicative of a miscalibration of one or more CT detectors. Solid-state detectors, which function independently, are at increased risk for ring artifact. While ring artifacts may not be mistaken for pathology, they can degrade image quality. None of the other choices produce discrete ring defects on CT imaging. Volume averaging decreases contrast resolution by averaging the values of two small adjacent objects of differing densities. Photon starvation generally results in streaking artifact manifesting as darkened bands, particularly at the level of the shoulders on chest CT although can produce round defects in the upper abdomen on reduced dose CT imaging of the chest. Finally, beam-hardening artifacts result from attenuation of low-energy photons causing cupping and streak artifacts.

Reference: Barrett JF, Keat N. Artifacts in CT: recognition and avoidance. *Radiographics* 2004;24:1679–1691.

14 **Answer D.** Established conversion factors have been determined for converting dose–length product to effective dose dependent on the type

CT examination. For head, body (to include chest), and cervical spine CT examinations, the conversion factors are 2.2, 18, and 5.4 µSv/mGy, respectively. The low conversion factor for head CT reflects the relatively radioresistant tissues imaged. In body CT, kVp does increase the conversion ratio up to 25% when adjusting from 80 to 140 kV. With increasing public awareness of radiation exposure and potential cancer risk, reporting of such values is likely to increase in the future.

Reference: Huda W, Ogden KM, Khorasani MR. Converting dose-length product to effective dose at CT. *Radiology* 2008;248(3):995–1003.

15 **Answer C.** In the current practice of CT imaging, parameters such as kV are still in the control of the operator, although automation in CT acquisition is increasing. Most current CT scanners employ mA dose modulation where mAs varies throughout the gantry rotation to account for the natural nonround configuration of the human body. Measures of image quality, such as the noise index, allows for mA modulation while still allowing for some operator control in the trade-off of radiation dose for image quality. Reduced dose chest CT generally employs this method, accepting increased image noise for relative decrease in radiation dose. A decrease in noise index would therefore increase radiation dose.

This question aims primarily at recognizing the relatively linear relationship between reducing the mAs and z-axis relative to radiation dose reduction versus the nonlinear relationship between kV and radiation dose. By decreasing the kV from 120 to 100 in the setting of coronary CTA, studies have shown a reduction in radiation dose between 47% and 53%. Additionally, in CT contrast studies, the decreased kV also enhances the image contrast from iodinated contrast relative to the surrounding soft tissues due to the k-edge of iodine.

Reference: Kanal KM, Stewart BK, Kolokythas O, et al. Impact of operator-selected image noise index and reconstruction slice thickness on patient radiation dose in 64-MDCT. *AJR Am J Roentgenol* 2007;189;219–225.

2 Normal Anatomy

QUESTIONS

1 Characterize the structure interposed between the aorta and carina.

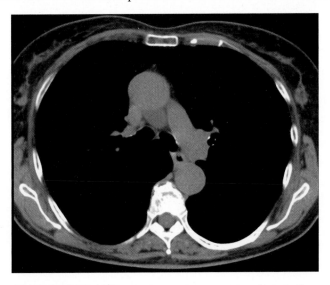

    A. Lymphadenopathy
    B. Normal anatomic variant
    C. Mediastinal cyst
    D. Vascular aneurysm

2 What is responsible for forming a juxtaphrenic peak?
    A. Superior pulmonary ligament
    B. Inferior pulmonary ligament
    C. Phrenic nerve
    D. Diaphragmatic eventration

3 Name the anatomic structure.

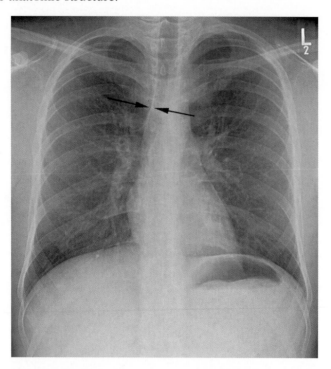

    A. Anterior junctional line
    B. Posterior junctional line
    C. Posterior wall of the bronchus intermedius
    D. Right paratracheal stripe

4 What forms the medial border of the right paratracheal stripe?

    A. Pleura
    B. Ascending aorta
    C. Trachea
    D. Superior vena cava

5 What muscle is identified on this CT?

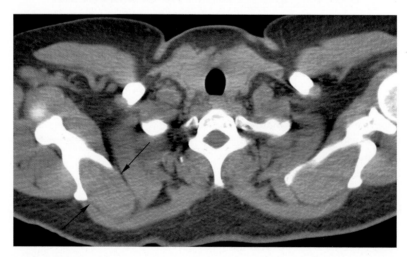

    A. Supraspinatus
    B. Infraspinatus
    C. Subscapularis
    D. Teres minor

6 Which segment of lung has been resected?

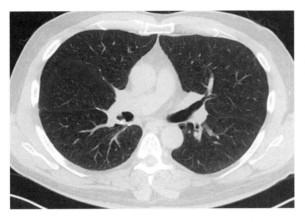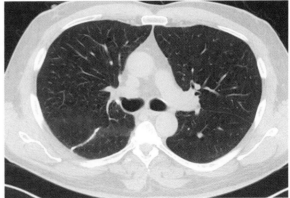

   A. Posterior right upper lobe
   B. Medial right middle lobe
   C. Superior right lower lobe
   D. Medial basilar right lower lobe

7 Name the structure identified.

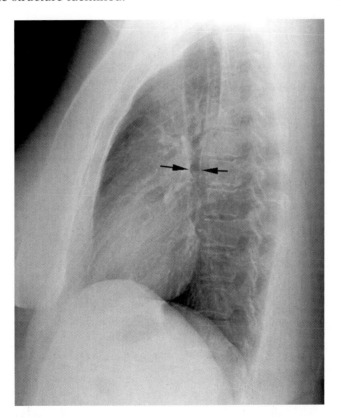

   A. Right upper lobe bronchus
   B. Left upper lobe bronchus
   C. Left mainstem bronchus
   D. Right middle lobe bronchus

8 Name the normal variant.

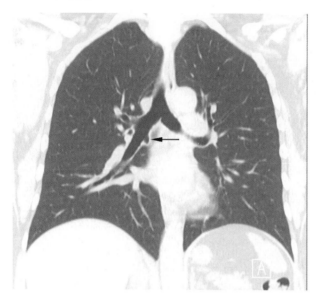

A. Tracheal bronchus
B. Bronchial atresia
C. Bronchus intermedius
D. Cardiac bronchus

9a Which window or clear space is demonstrated in this radiograph?

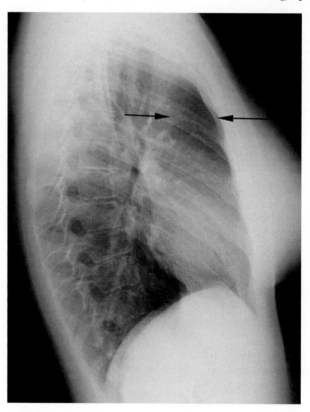

A. Retrotracheal
B. Retrocardiac
C. Retrosternal
D. Raider triangle

9b The retrosternal window on lateral view correlates with which structure on frontal view?

    A. Anterior junctional line
    B. Posterior superior junctional line
    C. Azygoesophageal recess
    D. Right paratracheal stripe

10 What anatomic structure is identified in the CT?

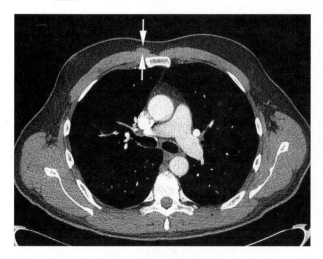 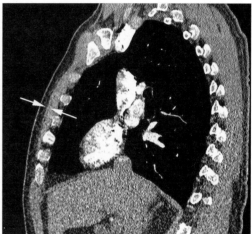

    A. Internal mammary lymph node
    B. Sternalis muscle
    C. Pectoralis minor muscle
    D. Internal mammary artery

11 What contrast enhancing structure is identified immediately to the left of the aortic arch on these images?

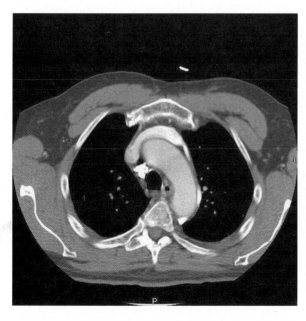 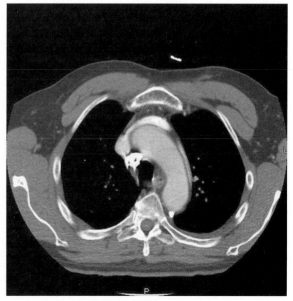

    A. Superior intercostal vein
    B. Bronchial artery
    C. Duplicated superior vena cava
    D. Left upper lobe anomalous pulmonary venous return

12a What is the name of the space denoted by the arrow?

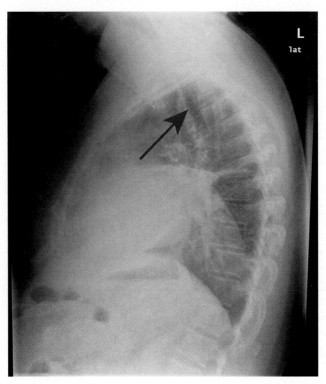

A. Anterior esophageal stripe
B. Tracheoesophageal stripe
C. Anterior junctional line
D. Posterior junctional line

12b What is the upper limit of normal for width of this anatomic space?

A. 2 mm
B. 5 mm
C. 10 mm
D. 15 mm

13 What is the name of the fissure that separates the medial basal bronchopulmonary segment from the other lower lobe segments?

A. Superior accessory fissure
B. Inferior accessory fissure
C. Medial accessory fissure
D. Minor accessory fissure

14 Which of the following would run in the periphery of the secondary pulmonary lobule?

A. Pulmonary vein
B. Pulmonary artery
C. Respiratory bronchiole
D. Terminal bronchiole

15 What vessel is most at risk of injury given the position of the percutaneous pleural catheter?

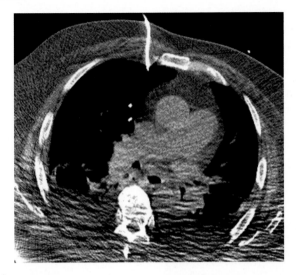

    A. Superior vena cava
    B. Ascending aorta
    C. Right brachiocephalic vein
    D. Right internal thoracic artery

16 What cardiac valve is identified on this lateral chest radiograph by its severe degree of calcification?

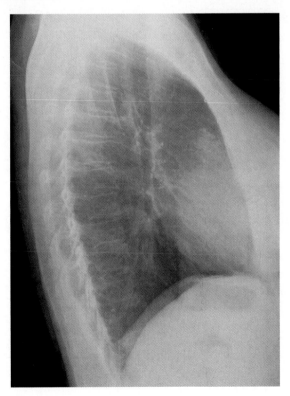

    A. Aortic
    B. Pulmonary
    C. Mitral
    D. Tricuspid

17a In the intercostal spaces, what is the cranial-to-caudal order of the neurovascular bundle?

    A. Vein → artery → nerve
    B. Nerve → artery → vein
    C. Artery → vein → nerve
    D. Nerve → vein → artery

17b What is the best descriptor for positioning of the neurovascular bundle in the intercostal space?

    A. Cranial (along the undersurface of the superior rib)
    B. Central (midway between the two ribs)
    C. Caudal (along the superior surface of the inferior rib)
    D. Variable (positioning depends on rib level)

18a What long tubular structure is identified by arrows on these two images?

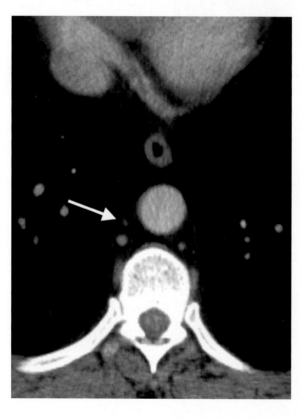
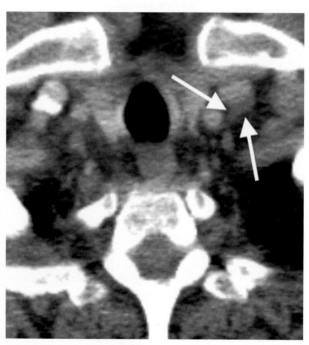

    A. Azygos vein
    B. Thoracic duct
    C. Hemiazygos vein
    D. Accessory hemiazygos vein

18b What structure does the thoracic duct typically drain into?

    A. Left subclavian vein and internal jugular vein confluence
    B. Right subclavian vein and internal jugular vein confluence
    C. Superior vena cava
    D. Inferior vena cava

18c Which of the following areas is not typically drained (directly or indirectly) via the thoracic duct?

    A. Right upper extremity
    B. Left upper extremity
    C. Right lower extremity
    D. Left lower extremity

19a What is responsible for the marbled fat appearance in the anterior mediastinum of this adult?

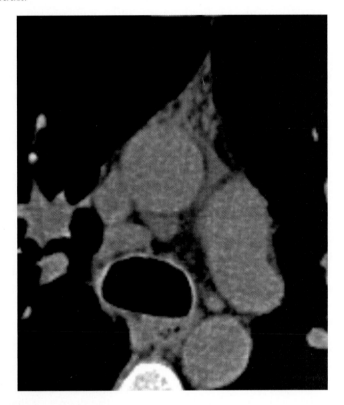

    A. Mediastinal hemorrhage
    B. Infectious mediastinitis
    C. Normal thymus
    D. Thymolipoma

19b In which decade of life should complete fatty replacement of the thymus be expected in all patients?

    A. Second
    B. Fourth
    C. Sixth
    D. Eighth

20 What forms the superior margin of the azygoesophageal recess?

    A. Azygos arch
    B. Aortic arch
    C. Accessory hemiazygos vein
    D. Innominate artery

ANSWERS AND EXPLANATIONS

1 **Answer B.** Occasionally misinterpreted as lymphadenopathy, mass, or mediastinal cyst, a prominent superior pericardial aortic recess is a normal anatomic variant and generally requires no further follow-up. Imaging findings that confirm the presence of the superior pericardial recess include (1) characteristic position of known pericardial recess, here along the posterior aorta, (2) crescentic shape, (3) fluid density and nonenhancing, and (4) benign appearance relative to adjacent structures. The superior aortic recess can even extend superiorly into the right paratracheal mediastinum. Some benign cystic lesions could overlap with these findings warranting follow-up, but multiplanar reformats in sagittal or coronal plane may better demonstrate extension from the pericardial region. Lymphadenopathy and vascular aneurysm would not have all of these findings.

Reference: Truong MT, et al. Pictorial essay: anatomy of pericardial recesses on multidetector CT: implications for oncologic imaging. *AJR Am J Roentgenol* 2003;181:1109–1113.

2 **Answer B.** The juxtaphrenic peak is associated with upper lung volume loss of any cause and resulting appearance of a small triangular opacity at the apex of the diaphragm on frontal chest x-ray. The peak is formed due to the inferior accessory fissure of an intrapulmonary septum related to the inferior pulmonary ligament. The superior pulmonary ligament would not touch the diaphragm. The phrenic nerve is generally not identifiable on imaging unless pathologic. Diaphragmatic eventration could account for a similar abnormality but is not associated with this term specifically and generally manifests as an additional smooth convexity of the diaphragm.

Reference: Hansell DM, Bankier AA, MacMahon H, et al. Fleischner Society: glossary of terms for thoracic imaging. *Radiology* 2008;246(3).

3 **Answer C.** On radiographs, the right paratracheal stripe is formed by the right tracheal wall (medially) and the medial pleura (laterally). It typically measures <4 mm although it can be affected by the degree of inspiration and predominance of mediastinal fat. Pathology that can cause widening of the stripe is frequently best evaluated by CT and includes lymphadenopathy (most common), mediastinal hemorrhage, mediastinal mass, or vessel enlargement.

Reference: Hansell DM, Bankier AA, MacMahon H, et al. Fleischner Society: glossary of terms for thoracic imaging. *Radiology* 2008;246(3).

4 **Answer D.** The ability to recognize expected lines and stripes on chest radiograph can assist in recognizing or explaining abnormal findings such as unilateral volume loss shifting a junctional line or widening of the right paratracheal stripe in lymphadenopathy. Alternatively, recognizing these lines or stripes as normal will alleviate the possibility of characterizing one as abnormal and assigning disease where none exists. In this case, the arrows highlight the right paratracheal stripe, a shadow outlined by tracheal air and the air-filled right upper lobe. Anatomic structures that reside in this region include tracheal wall including the epithelium and tracheal cartilage, mediastinal fat containing lymph nodes and minor vessels, and visceral and parietal pleural layers. A thickness of >4 mm suggests thickening such as adenopathy.

The other options provided are midline structures either on a normal frontal chest radiograph or a lateral radiograph finding. The anterior junctional line courses from right superior to left inferior over the superior midline mediastinum on frontal radiograph and represents the pleural layers of the right and left upper lobes meeting anterior to the great vessels. The posterior junctional line is similar in that it represents the meeting of pleural layers of the right and left upper lobes, but posterior to the trachea and esophagus, and appears overlying the trachea just left of midline and may extend superior to the clavicles. Finally, the posterior wall of the bronchus intermedius (PWBI) is found on lateral exam as a thin linear shadow and part of the intermediate stem line coursing through the left mainstem bronchus in the well-positioned lateral.

Reference: Gibbs JM, et al. Lines and stripes: where did they go? From conventional radiography to CT. *Radiographics* 2007;27:33–48.

5   Answer A.   Despite the focus of chest imaging on thoracic pathology, adjacent anatomic regions are included on chest images, to include the neck base, bilateral shoulders, and upper abdomen, and recognizing normal and abnormal CT appearances of these adjacent structures is part of every exam. Chest wall lesions or invasion can involve the musculature, which necessitates clearly defining each muscle on chest CT. The rotator cuff on axial chest CT is relatively straightforward. The scapula creates a "T" shape dividing the muscles into subscapularis deep (or anterior) to the scapula, infraspinatus lateral and inferior to the spine of the scapula, and supraspinatus medial and superior to the spine of the scapula. Teres minor courses along the lateral aspect of infraspinatus.

Reference: E-Anatomy. www.imaios.com/en/e-Anatomy. Last accessed December 29, 2014.

6   Answer C.   Outside of the occasional anatomic variant, the divisions of the tracheobronchial tree into 2 lungs, 5 lobes, and 18 segments are relatively constant as are their relationships on CT imaging. When a segment or lobe has been removed, knowing the expected relationships allows for successful characterizing of the prior resection. The upper and right middle lobar bronchi originate anterior to the lower, and lobectomy of one of these lobes results in surgical clips and bronchial stump anterior to the residual airway. Conversely, resection of a lower lobe results in clips or a stump posterior to the residual airway. A segmentectomy can be more difficult to accurately characterize and requires knowledge of the normal branching. In this case, the suture line courses along the superior right lower lobe and inferior posterior right upper lobe, in the region of the right lower lobe superior segment and posterior right upper lobe segment. The surgical clips and stump are demonstrated along the posterior bronchus intermedius at the expected origin of the right lower lobe superior segmental bronchus.

Reference: Webb WR, Higgins CB. *Thoracic imaging: Pulmonary and cardiovascular radiology*, 2nd ed. Philadelphia, PA: Lippincott Williams & Wilkins, 2011:165–174; Chapter 6: The Pulmonary Hila.

7   Answer C.   The asymmetry of the hila creates complicated shadows on lateral exam but also allows for lateralization of findings when these shadows are well understood. The origin of the left upper lobe bronchus is hyparterial, meaning it arises below the left pulmonary artery as it courses laterally into the lung. In contrast, the right upper lobe bronchus arises above the pulmonary artery with the right mainstem bronchus passing along the posterior aspect of the pulmonary artery. This asymmetry results in the left mainstem bronchus outlined along its anterior, superior, and posterior aspects, making it well defined relative to the other hilar bronchi. Above the left mainstem bronchus, the horizontal portion of the right upper lobe bronchus is about the level of the carina. As stated before, the posterior wall of the bronchus intermedius can be seen passing vertically through the left mainstem bronchus radiolucency on a well-positioned lateral chest radiograph. The left upper lobe bronchus and right middle lobe bronchus do not have well-defined portions on the lateral chest radiograph.

Reference: Feigin DS. Lateral chest radiograph: a systematic approach. *Acad Radiol* 2010;17:1560–1566.

8 **Answer D.**   Congenital variation in the branching of the tracheobronchial tree is not uncommon ranging from 1% to 12% of individuals. In this case, a short segment of bronchus branches from the medial aspect of the bronchus intermedius, opposite the right upper lobe bronchus, and is known as an accessory cardiac bronchus. The bronchus may be blind ending or have some associated aerated cystic or alveolar tissue. Reports of associated infection or hemoptysis have required resection, although the majority are discovered incidentally in asymptomatic individuals. As the name suggests, a tracheal bronchus arises from the trachea and almost invariably provides an accessory bronchus to the right upper lobe. Bronchial atresia refers to an interruption in a normal bronchial branch with noncommunicating peripheral bronchi and associated portions of lung. Finally, the bronchus intermedius is a normal anatomic branch beyond the right upper lobe takeoff, so named as it is the only bronchus beyond a lobar branch, but still peripherally bifurcating into two additional lobar branches.

Reference: Ghaye B, Szapiro D, Fanchamps JM, et al. Congenital bronchial abnormalities revisited. *Radiographics* 2001;21:105–119.

9a **Answer C.**

9b **Answer A.**   The retrosternal window or clear space, also known as the "anterior clear space," represents a narrowing of the mediastinum anterior to the heart and great vessels and posterior to the sternum where the pleurae of the anterior upper lobes come close together or meet. On the lateral chest radiograph, the retrosternal window provides improved visualization of the anterior mediastinum, a potential blind spot on frontal radiograph as the overlying sternum and mediastinal structures often obscure lesions in the anterior mediastinum. Normal anatomical structures that reside in the anterior mediastinum and retrosternal region include mediastinal fat, lymph nodes, thymic tissue, and internal mammary vessels.

When the pleurae of the anterior upper lobes of the lungs approximate close enough to each other, the anterior junctional line may be seen on frontal chest radiograph. In addition to understanding expected shadows and borders on the normal chest radiograph, recognizing the anterior junctional line can also support the impression of hyperinflation or emphysema, which can accentuate the anterior junctional line.

Reference: Feigin DS. Lateral chest radiograph: a systematic approach. *Acad Radiol* 2010;17:1560–1566.

10 **Answer B.**   Seen occasionally on mammography, the sternalis muscle, also known as the rectus sternalis muscle, is present in 2% to 11% of individuals with equal distribution between males and females. Recognizing this normal variant on chest imaging can avoid mischaracterizing it as a mass. Coursing vertically along the medial anterior aspect of the pectoralis major muscle, sternalis muscle may be unilateral or bilateral.

References: Bradley FM, Hoover HC Jr., Hulka CA, et al. The sternalis muscle: an unusual normal finding seen on mammography. *AJR Am J Roentgenol* 1996;166:33–36.

Katara P, Chauhan S, Arora R, et al. A unilateral rectus sternalis muscle: rare but normal anatomic variant of anterior chest wall musculature. *J Clin Diagn Res* 2013;7(12):2665–2667.

Nuthakki S, Gross M, Fessell D. Sonography and helical computed tomography of the sternalis muscle. *J Ultrasound Med* 2007;26:247–250.

11 **Answer A.** There is an enhancing structure coursing roughly parallel to the aortic arch. This is the normal left superior intercostal vein. This vein typically drains the second through fourth intercostal spaces, typically drains into the left brachiocephalic vein and frequently communicates with the accessory hemiazygos or hemiazygos vein. It can occasionally be seen "en face" on an AP or PA chest radiograph where it is referred to as the "aortic nipple." It may enlarge in the presence of a more central obstruction where it can serve as a collateral pathway. The bronchial arteries typically arise from the anterior descending thoracic aorta directly at the T3 to T8 level. Both a duplicated SVC and anomalous left upper lobe pulmonary vein would demonstrate a more vertical course than shown here.

Reference: Demos TC, Posniak HV, Pierce KL, et al. Venous anomalies of the thorax. *AJR Am J Roentgenol* 2004;182(5).

12a **Answer B.**

12b **Answer B.** The tracheoesophageal stripe is identified on lateral chest radiographs as between the air-filled wall of the trachea and the anterior wall of an air-filled esophagus. It typically measures up to 5 mm in size. If the posterior trachea does not abut the esophagus, it is generally smaller, up to 2.5 mm, and referred to as the posterior tracheal stripe. Thickening of this stripe (as in this example) generally warrants correlation with CT to evaluate for esophageal lesion, vascular lesion, or other mediastinal pathology.

Reference: Gibbs JM, Chandrasekhar CA, Ferguson EC, et al. Lines and stripes: where did they go?—from conventional radiography to CT. *Radiographics* 2007;27(1).

13 **Answer B.** The inferior accessory fissure separates the medial basal bronchopulmonary segment from the other basilar segments and is typically vertically oriented and frequently complete. It is more common on the right. The superior accessory fissure is in the same plane as the right minor fissure and separates the lower lobe superior segment from the basilar segments. There is no such thing as a medial accessory fissure or minor accessory fissure.

Reference: Godwin JD, Tarver RD. Accessory fissures of the lung. *AJR Am J Roentgenol* 1985;144(1): 39–47.

14 **Answer A.** The secondary pulmonary lobule serves as the functional unit of the lung and is critical to HRCT evaluation. They are polyhedral in shape measuring approximately 1.5 cm in size with fibrous septa walls (containing pulmonary veins and lymphatics). The center of the lobule is formed by the terminal bronchiole and pulmonary artery (as well as a central set of lymphatics).

Reference: Hansell DM, Lynch DA, McAdams HP, et al. *Imaging of diseases of the chest*, 5th ed. Mosby, 2009.

15 **Answer D.** The bilateral internal thoracic arteries (internal mammary arteries) serve as blood supply to the anterior chest wall extending from the clavicles to the umbilicus. They most frequently arise directly from the subclavian artery and pass posterior to the subclavian vein with a vertical course between the transversus thoracis muscle posteriorly and the costal cartilages anteriorly. The distal bifurcation results in the musculophrenic artery and superior epigastric artery. Placement of a chest tube via an anteromedial approach (close to the sternum as seen here) places this artery at risk. Injury can be catastrophic with severe chest wall, pleural and mediastinal hemorrhage. This patient required massive transfusion and artery coil embolization as a result of this placement.

The artery provides an important collateral to the inferior epigastric arteries if there is a coarctation or descending aortic occlusion.

Reference: Webb WR, Higgins CB. *Thoracic imaging: Pulmonary and cardiovascular radiology*, 2nd ed. Philadelphia, PA: Lippincott Williams & Wilkins, 2011.

16 **Answer B.** The lateral radiograph demonstrates severe dystrophic calcification projecting high and anterior relative to the cardiac shadow. The location is that of the pulmonary valve. The other valves would be more posterior and inferior than demonstrated. This patient had long-standing pulmonary stenosis.

Reference: Hansell DM, Lynch DA, McAdams HP, et al. *Imaging of diseases of the chest*, 5th ed. Mosby, 2009.

17a **Answer A.**

17b **Answer A.** The intercostal space neurovascular bundle is ordered vein, artery, and then nerve from superior to inferior (VAN is the acronym to remember). The location of the neurovascular bundle as immediately under the superior rib (cranial in the intercostal space) is critical for those performing interventional procedures to avoid vascular injury. Despite the classic distribution of the intercostal structures, three-dimensional CT angiographic images of the intercostal arteries can demonstrate the potential tortuous route of these arteries. Intercostal vessels can bleed profusely if injured, especially if they bleed into the pleural space.

Reference: Hansell DM, Lynch DA, McAdams HP, et al. *Imaging of diseases of the chest*, 5th ed. Mosby, 2009.

18a **Answer B.**

18b **Answer A.**

18c **Answer A.** The thoracic duct serves as the common trunk for a majority of the lymphatic vessels. The duct serves as a continuation of the cisterna chyli (typically located around L1). It courses through the aortic hiatus and ascends in the right posterior mediastinum between the aorta and azygos vein (shown). The hemiazygos and accessory hemiazygos are in the left posterior mediastinum. The thoracic duct is typically identifiable (although small) in patients with a moderate degree of mediastinal fat, but not identifiable on thinner patients. It crosses midline around T5 and continues to the thoracic inlet, anterior to the subclavian artery and anterior scalene before draining into the angle of the left subclavian and internal jugular veins. Variant drainage includes drainage directly into one of the other neck vessels (internal jugular, external jugular, brachiocephalic of subclavian). Understanding this anatomy is important for cases of chylothorax to guide potential surgical or interventional therapy. The duct drains the lower extremities, abdomen, left chest, left upper extremity, and left neck.

Reference: Liu ME, Branstetter BF, Whetstone J, et al. Normal appearance of the distal thoracic duct. *AJR Am J Roentgenol* 2006;187:1615–1620.

19a **Answer C.**

19b **Answer D.** The appearance is that of normal thymus. Mediastinal hemorrhage would be expected to demonstrate more areas of mixed high and low attenuation from either direct vessel injury or, more commonly, rupture of the vasa vasorum surrounding the mediastinal vessels. Thymolipoma would demonstrate a combination of fat density and soft tissue; however, there is no actual mass in this case. Similarly, infectious mediastinitis would be much more likely to produce an indurated space-occupying appearance than is demonstrated.

The thymus involutes with age resulting in continual decrease in thymic mass relative to body size. The thymus actually continues to grow in absolute terms until puberty but will start occupying a significantly smaller portion of relative size from infancy. In a study of 309 individuals ranging in age from 6 weeks to 81 years, some remnant thymic tissue was visualized on CT up to the age of 70 years with those in the eighth decade (older than 70) all demonstrating complete fatty replacement of the thymus on CT. The stranded mixed soft tissue and fat appearance shown is typical. Configuration is normally bilobed or triangular. Presence of a significant solid component should raise the possibility of developing thymic neoplasm.

References: Francis IR, Glazer GM, Bookstein FL, et al. The thymus: reexamination of age-related changes in size and shape. *AJR Am J Roentgenol* 1985;145:249–254.

Nishino M, Ashiku SK, Kocher ON, et al. The thymus: a comprehensive review. *Radiographics* 2006;26(2):335–348.

20 **Answer A.**   The azygoesophageal recess is a posterior mediastinal recess located in the right chest. The azygos arch forms the cranial margin. The azygos vein and pleura form the posterior margin. The esophagus generally forms the medial margin.

Reference: Hansell DM, Bankier AA, MacMahon H, et al. Fleischner Society: glossary of terms for thoracic imaging. *Radiology* 2008;246(3).

3 Terms and Signs

QUESTIONS

1a CT of the chest was performed for evaluation of chronic cough. Which of the following terms best describes the salient abnormality?

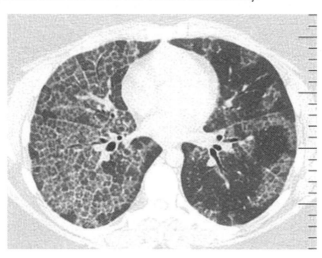

    A. Consolidation
    B. Crazy-paving pattern
    C. Interlobular septal thickening
    D. Centrilobular nodules

1b Given the history of chronic cough and significant occupational inhalational exposure to silica, which of the following causes of crazy-paving pattern is most likely?

    A. Lipoid pneumonia
    B. Pulmonary alveolar proteinosis
    C. *Pneumocystis jirovecii* pneumonia
    D. Pulmonary hemorrhage

2   A 35-year-old male presents with uveitis and mild shortness of breath. Chest radiograph is obtained. What sign best describes the radiograph image provided?

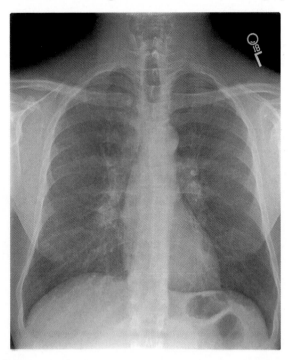

A. Galaxy sign
B. Fleischner sign
C. 1-2-3 sign
D. Golden S sign

3a A 32-year-old female presents with refractory asthma and chronic sinusitis. Prior bronchoscopy had revealed eosinophilia on bronchoscopic alveolar lavage (BAL). What sign is present on this patient's radiograph?

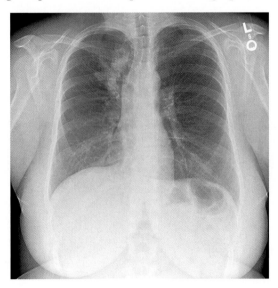

A. Tree-in-bud
B. Hilum overlay
C. Air crescent
D. Finger-in-glove

3b Based on the imaging findings and clinical history, what is the most likely diagnosis?

    A. Allergic bronchopulmonary aspergillosis
    B. Aspergilloma
    C. Semi-invasive aspergillosis
    D. Angioinvasive aspergillosis

3c A follow-up CT of the chest was obtained on the patient and provided below. Do the imaging findings support your prior diagnosis?

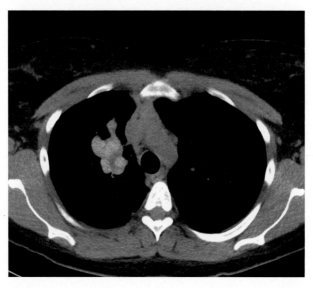

    A. Yes, contrast enhancement of bronchial impaction is common in ABPA.
    B. Yes, high density of bronchial impaction is common in ABPA.
    C. No, a vasculitis such as Churg-Strauss disease should be considered.
    D. No, high density of bronchial impaction suggests a diagnosis other than ABPA.

4a On these inspiratory images, what is the primary radiologic finding?

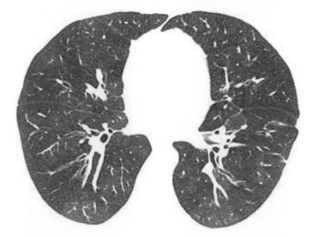

    A. Mosaic attenuation
    B. Consolidation
    C. Bronchiectasis
    D. Architectural distortion

4b Expiratory images of the same patient demonstrate that the previously noted mosaic attenuation is due to which of the following?

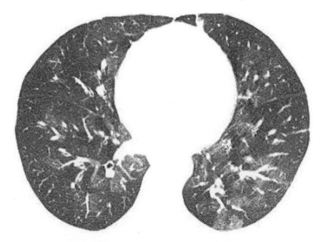

    A. Air trapping
    B. Pulmonary vascular disease
    C. Ground-glass opacity
    D. Photon starvation artifact

4c If this patient had a history of prior toxic fume inhalation injury, which of the following etiologies is most likely?

    A. Hypersensitivity pneumonitis
    B. Asthma
    C. Obliterative bronchiolitis
    D. Follicular bronchiolitis

4d Which of the following connective tissue diseases is most highly associated with obliterative bronchiolitis?

    A. Scleroderma
    B. Rheumatoid arthritis
    C. Lupus
    D. Sjogren syndrome

5a What sign is demonstrated in the CT image provided?

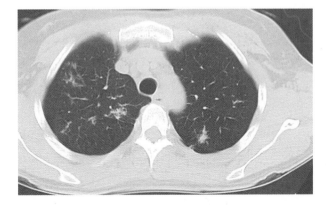

    A. Crescent sign
    B. Headcheese sign
    C. Halo sign
    D. Galaxy sign

5b   Which diagnosis best correlates with the galaxy sign?

    A. Sarcoidosis
    B. Bronchogenic carcinoma
    C. Lymphangitic carcinomatosis
    D. Organizing pneumonia

6   What radiographic sign best describes the image finding below?

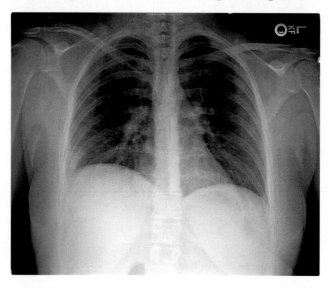

    A. S Sign of Golden
    B. Westermark sign
    C. Hampton hump
    D. Fleischner sign

7   What structure forms the superior border of the aortopulmonary window?

    A. Left pulmonary artery
    B. Aortic arch
    C. Ligamentum arteriosum
    D. Parietal pleura

8   Which of the following is the most unlikely cause of a "beaded septum" sign?

    A. Sarcoidosis
    B. Lymphangitic carcinomatosis
    C. Neurogenic pulmonary edema
    D. Coal worker's pneumoconiosis

9   Pulmonary infarction most commonly involves which of the following vessels?

    A. Bronchial arteries
    B. Pulmonary arteries
    C. Pulmonary veins
    D. Intercostal arteries

10a What term best describes the pattern in the CT image provided?

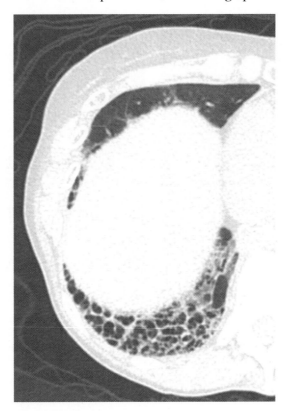

    A. Emphysema
    B. Honeycombing
    C. Mosaic attenuation
    D. Air trapping

10b An additional CT image from the same study is provided below. What is the most likely diagnosis?

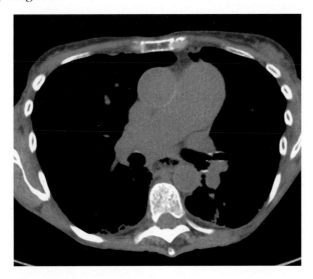

    A. Idiopathic pulmonary fibrosis
    B. Hypersensitivity pneumonitis
    C. Scleroderma
    D. Asbestosis

11a What is the best descriptor of the pattern of nodule distribution shown?

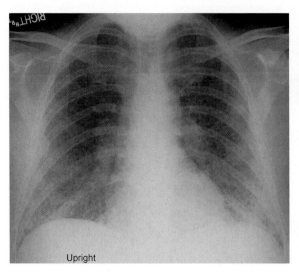
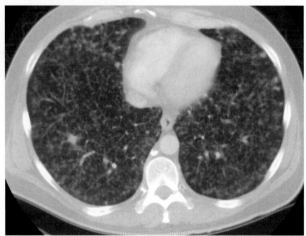

A. Centrilobular
B. Peribronchovascular
C. Miliary
D. Perilymphatic

11b What is the most unlikely diagnosis for a miliary distribution of nodules?

A. Sarcoidosis
B. Disseminated fungal infection
C. Disseminated mycobacterial infection
D. Metastasis

12 Tree-in-bud nodules is a combination of branching opacities and what nodule type?

A. Centrilobular
B. Perilymphatic
C. Random
D. Subpleural

13 The Monod sign indicates what underlying pathology?

A. Mycetoma
B. Angioinvasive fungal infection
C. Cavitary neoplasm
D. Granulomatosis with polyangiitis

14 What is the maximum size limit of a pulmonary bleb?

A. 0.5 cm
B. 1.0 cm
C. 2.0 cm
D. 3.0 cm

15 Which of these radiologic signs is demonstrated?

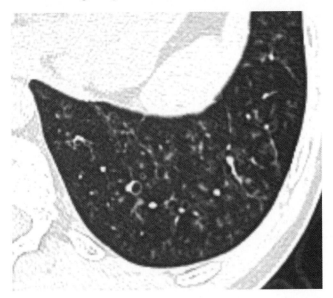

A. Silhouette sign
B. Signet ring sign
C. Reversed halo sign
D. Halo sign

ANSWERS AND EXPLANATIONS

1a   **Answer B.**

1b   **Answer B.**   The CT demonstrates geographic and lobular areas of ground-glass attention AND interlobular septal thickening. These findings in combination are referred to as crazy-paving pattern. There are numerous causes of this pattern in both acute and chronic lung disease ranging from infectious, neoplastic, idiopathic, inhalational, and sanguineous disorders. Although rare, pulmonary alveolar proteinosis is specifically associated with this pattern and alveolar proteinosis is associated with prior silica exposure (in additional to idiopathic causes).

Reference: Marshall GB, Farnquist BA, MacGregor JH, et al. Signs in thoracic imaging. *J Thorac Imaging* 2006;21:76–90.

2   **Answer C.**   In the radiograph provided, the bilateral hila demonstrate symmetric fullness with thickening of the right paratracheal stripe, accounting for the 1 (right hilum), 2 (left hilum), 3 (right paratracheal stripe) sign of lymphadenopathy in the setting of sarcoidosis. While this sign is highly suggestive of sarcoidosis, the differential would include other granulomatous diseases such as silicosis, coal worker's pneumoconiosis, or granulomatous infection. Less likely, but not excluded, would be a neoplastic process such as lymphoma or small cell carcinoma.

Reference: Webb WR, Higgins CB. *Thoracic imaging: Pulmonary and cardiovascular radiology*, 2nd ed. Philadelphia, PA: Lippincott Williams & Wilkins, 2011:466; Chapter 15: The Pulmonary Hila.

3a   **Answer D.**

3b   **Answer A.**

3c   **Answer B.**   Finger-in-glove is a characteristic finding in allergic bronchopulmonary aspergillosis (ABPA), which often presents as refractory asthma. Bronchial atresia or other chronic bronchial obstruction would be alternative considerations although the clinical history to include bronchial eosinophilia correlates better with ABPA. High density of the bronchial impaction is also characteristic of ABPA caused by the dense collection of aspergillus in the secretions. In a recent study of 155 patients with diagnosed ABPA, hyperattenuation of the mucoid impaction on CT correlated with greater serologic severity and increased frequency of relapses. Additional imaging findings seen on CT for ABPA would include upper lobe predominant bronchiectasis, bronchial wall thickening, and tree-in-bud opacities.

References: Agarwal R, Gupta D, Aggarwal AN, et al. Clinical significance of hyperattenuating mucoid impaction in allergic bronchopulmonary aspergillosis: an analysis of 155 patients. *Chest* 2007;132:1183–1190.

Marshall GB, Farnquist BA, MacGregor JH, et al. Signs in thoracic imaging. *J Thorac Imaging* 2006;21:76–90.

4a   **Answer A.**

4b   **Answer A.**

4c   **Answer C.**

4d Answer B.   The inspiratory CT demonstrates geographic areas of mosaic attenuation, defined as patchwork regions of differing attenuation by the Fleischner Society Glossary. Differential considerations include (1) interstitial lung disease, (2) air trapping, and (3) occlusive pulmonary vascular disease. Of these causes, air trapping is accentuated by expiration (as demonstrated on the expiratory images of this patient). This air trapping is characteristic of small airways disease such as hypersensitivity pneumonitis, obliterative (constrictive) bronchiolitis, or asthma. Causes of obliterative bronchiolitis include prior infection (especially adenovirus or respiratory syncytial virus), collagen vascular disease (especially rheumatoid arthritis), drug toxicity, industrial toxic inhalation injury, and chronic transplant rejection (both heart/lung and graft versus host disease in bone marrow transplant).

Reference: Hansell DM, Bankier AA, MacMahon H, et al. Fleischner Society: glossary of terms for thoracic imaging. *Radiology* 2008;246(3):697–722.

5a Answer D.

5b Answer A.   Multifocal pulmonary nodules on CT have a broad potential differential, and various signs assist in narrowing the differential. The "galaxy sign" represents a conglomeration of smaller nodules with the fine nodularity seen on the margins of the lesion. Granulomatous diseases are most likely to produce this conglomerate nodularity, and while sarcoidosis is characteristic in producing the galaxy sign, it has been described in pulmonary tuberculosis. The provided image also demonstrates perilymphatic nodularity with septal studding further supporting the diagnosis of sarcoidosis. Focal pulmonary nodules and perilymphatic thickening/nodularity raise concern for bronchogenic carcinoma and lymphangitic carcinomatosis, but the satellite nodules associated with the galaxy sign decrease the likelihood of malignancy. While organizing pneumonia causes several classic signs, the galaxy sign and perilymphatic nodularity would be atypical.

References: Heo J, Choi YW, Jeon SC, et al. Pulmonary tuberculosis: another disease showing clusters of small nodules. *AJR Am J Roentgenol* 2005;184:639–642.

Nakatsu M, Hatabu H, Morikawa K, et al. Large coalescent parenchymal nodules in pulmonary sarcoidosis: "Sarcoid Galaxy" sign. *AJR Am J Roentgenol* 2002;178:1389–1393.

6 Answer C.   The image provided demonstrates a focal round consolidation in the lateral right lung base. While not specific, the basilar and peripheral locations in the appropriate clinical setting are characteristic of focal pulmonary infarct associated with pulmonary thromboembolism. Generally, the dual blood supply to the lung from the pulmonary and bronchial arteries requires a relatively large pulmonary embolus to cause pulmonary infarct. Westermark and Fleischner signs are both associated with pulmonary embolism; the former indicating relative oligemia and radiographic decrease in lung attenuation and the latter indicating vascular distention on radiograph by a large central pulmonary embolism.

Reference: Marshall GB, Farnquist BA, MacGregor JH, et al. Signs in thoracic imaging. *J Thorac Imaging* 2006;21:76–90.

7 Answer B.   The aortic arch forms the superior border. The other choices form the inferior (left pulmonary artery), medial (ligamentum arteriosum), and lateral borders (parietal pleura of the left lung). The anterior border is formed by the ascending aorta, and the posterior border is formed by the descending aorta.

Reference: Hansell DM, Bankier AA, MacMahon H, et al. Fleischner Society: glossary of terms for thoracic imaging. *Radiology* 2008;246(3):697–722.

8 **Answer C.** The beaded septum sign denotes nodular interlobular septal thickening. The most common cause is lymphangitic carcinomatosis with other causes of diffuse perilymphatic nodules such as sarcoidosis and pneumoconiosis being less common. Although pulmonary edema is associated with interlobular septal thickening, the nodular thickening of the "beaded septum" sign would be very unusual without additional underlying pathology.

Reference: Hansell DM, Bankier AA, MacMahon H, et al. Fleischner Society: glossary of terms for thoracic imaging. *Radiology* 2008;246(3):697–722.

9 **Answer B.** Infarction is the result of pulmonary artery occlusion in almost all cases. Pulmonary vein–related infarction is recognized but extremely uncommon. Ischemic necrosis may or may not be present due to the bronchial arteries remaining patent and serving as a secondary vascular supply. Pulmonary embolism and pulmonary involvement of vasculitis are the most frequent causes.

Reference: Hansell DM, Bankier AA, MacMahon H, et al. Fleischner Society: glossary of terms for thoracic imaging. *Radiology* 2008;246(3):697–722.

10a **Answer B.**

10b **Answer C.** According to the Fleischner Society "Glossary of Terms for Thoracic Imaging," pulmonary fibrotic cystic airspaces with thick walls define honeycombing and therefore honeycombing represents fibrotic changes of the lung. Generally peripheral in distribution, honeycombing is a useful finding for consideration of fibrosing interstitial pneumonias. Emphysema can have some overlap in appearance, particularly in the setting of combined pulmonary fibrosis and emphysema (CPFE), although the thicker walls and basilar peripheral distribution are not characteristic of emphysema. Mosaic attenuation and air trapping do not produce well-defined walls but rather distinct areas of variable lung density on inspiratory and expiratory CT imaging, respectively.

While any of the diagnoses provided could cause honeycombing at the lung bases, the significant enlargement of the pulmonary artery and the dilated debris-filled esophagus best correlate with scleroderma, also called systemic sclerosis.

References: Bhalla M, Silver RM, Shepard JO, et al. Chest CT in patients with scleroderma: prevalence of asymptomatic esophageal dilatation and mediastinal lymphadenopathy. *AJR Am J Roentgenol* 1993;161:269–272.

Hansell DM, Bankier AA, MacMahon H, et al. Fleischner Society: glossary of terms for thoracic imaging. *Radiology* 2008;246(3):697–722.

Solomon JJ, Olson AL, Fischer A, et al. Scleroderma lung disease. *Eur Respir Rev* 2013;22(127):6–19.

11a **Answer C.**

11b **Answer A.** The nodule distribution is miliary. The miliary pattern is characterized by innumerable tiny nodules <3 mm in size diffusely throughout the lungs. It is technically a subclass of randomly distributed nodules, but the random descriptor is generally reserved for larger and less profuse nodules. This distribution implies hematogenous spread of infection or malignancy with common pathogens being tuberculosis, fungal infection (such as histoplasmosis), and thyroid cancer. Sarcoid can present with miliary pattern but is quite unusual by comparison. Centrilobular nodules are generally airway-centered processes such as endobronchial infection, respiratory bronchiolitis, or subacute hypersensitivity pneumonitis. Perilymphatic nodules are a more common presentation for sarcoidosis or pneumoconiosis. This was a case of disseminated histoplasmosis.

Reference: Hansell DM, Bankier AA, MacMahon H, et al. Fleischner Society: glossary of terms for thoracic imaging. *Radiology* 2008;246(3):697–722.

12 Answer A.   The tree-in-bud pattern reflects endobronchial filling of the branching distal airways and as such is a type of centrilobular nodule pattern. The differential diagnosis includes a variety of infectious and inflammatory bronchiolar conditions, but most common causes include endobronchial spread of infection and aspiration. In the past, the term tree-in-bud was synonymous with endobronchial spread of tuberculosis, but this is now recognized as a finding present in multiple other diseases.

Reference: Nupur V, Jonathan HC, Tan-Lucien HM. Tree-in-bud sign. *J Thorac Imaging* 2012;27(2):W27.

13 Answer A.   The Monod sign reflects a mycetoma mass within a preexisting cavity. Frequently, the mass is gravity dependent and can move with prone or decubitus imaging. The mycetoma itself forms from conglomerate hyphae, mucin, fibrin, and debris. Overlapping appearance with cavitary masses and nodules can sometimes occur, and some use the "air crescent sign" (originally reserved for angioinvasive fungal disease with immune reconstitution) to also refer to a mycetoma. Intracavitary hematoma can present similarly as well.

Reference: Ashley N, Peter S, Thomas SL. et al. Monod sign. *J Thorac Imaging* 2013;28(6):W120.

14 Answer B.   A bleb is an air-containing cystic space in the subpleural lung with a maximum diameter of 10 mm. Bullae are similar airspaces measuring larger than 1 cm. Both usually demonstrate a wall no thicker than 1 mm and are seen in associate with emphysema. The term "giant" bulla is generally reserved for a bulla occupying more than 30% of a hemithorax although some simply use the term more generally to mean any dominantly large bulla.

References: Hansell DM, Bankier AA, MacMahon H, et al. Fleischner Society: glossary of terms for thoracic imaging. *Radiology* 2008;246(3):697–722.

Palla A, Desideri M, Rossi G, et al. Elective surgery for giant bullous emphysema: a 5-year clinical and functional follow-up. *Chest* 2005;128:2043.

15 Answer B.   The signet ring sign represents a dilated bronchus (the ring) with a smaller adjacent pulmonary artery (the signet). The bronchus should be similar in size to the adjacent artery and when dilated represents bronchiectasis. By definition, bronchiectasis is irreversible, and it should be noted that occasionally bronchial dilatation can resolve. More rarely, some causes of pulmonary arterial vasoconstriction can result in a similar appearance such as chronic thromboembolic disease.

   Note that this signet ring sign has no relation to the musculoskeletal sign reflecting scapholunate dissociation or the presence of renal papillary necrosis in genitourinary imaging.

References: Hansell DM, Bankier AA, MacMahon H, et al. Fleischner Society: glossary of terms for thoracic imaging. *Radiology* 2008;246(3):697–722.

Ouellette H. The signet ring sign. *Radiology* 1999;212(1).

QUESTIONS

1a A 56-year-old man with acute respiratory distress syndrome has been in the ICU for 10 days and presents with the chest radiograph shown. What is the most acute finding?

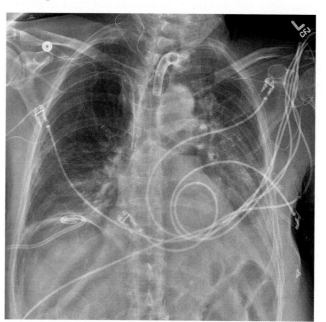

A. Pleural effusion
B. Esophageal intubation
C. Pneumoperitoneum
D. Pneumonia

1b What accounts for the well-demarcated bowel loops?

A. Oral contrast
B. Air on both sides of the bowel wall
C. Ascites surrounding bowel loops
D. Bowel wall thickening

2a What is the optimum position of an endotracheal tube in an adult patient?

   A. Midthoracic trachea

   B. At the level of the clavicles

   C. Right mainstem bronchus

   D. Greater than 6 cm above the carina

2b How does an endotracheal tube (ETT) tip move relative to head positioning?

   A. ETT moves down when head is elevated.

   B. ETT moves down when head is lowered.

   C. ETT moves up when head is lowered.

   D. ETT doesn't move with head positioning.

3a What is the cause of the radiodensity indicated by the arrow?

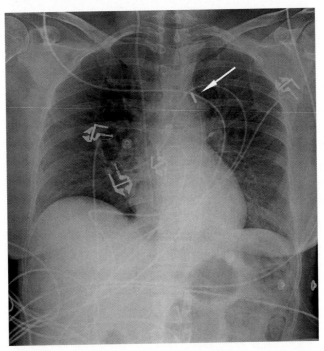

   A. Patent ductus arteriosus occlusion clip

   B. Lower extremity central venous catheter

   C. Intra-aortic balloon pump

   D. Swan-Ganz catheter

3b What complication is the primary concern for the malpositioned intra-aortic balloon pump (IABP) as shown?

   A. Stroke

   B. Aortic dissection

   C. Aortic rupture

   D. Limb paralysis

4 On a chest radiograph, what is the approximate location of the superior vena cava and the right atrial junction (superior cavoatrial junction)?

   A. Midthoracic trachea

   B. Carina

   C. T9/T10 disc space

   D. Two vertebral body heights below the carina

5a This is a chest radiograph for left central line placement. If no prior imaging is available, what is the next best step in the management of the patient?

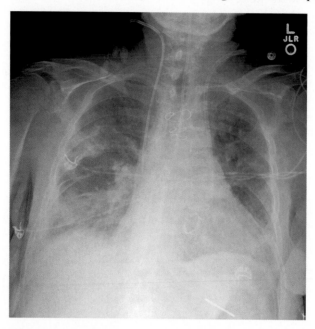

A. Follow-up chest radiograph in 6 hours.
B. Evaluate flow return and obtain blood gas.
C. Pull and replace the left central line.
D. Place a left thoracostomy tube.

5b A prior CT scan was reviewed on the same patient. What is the most likely explanation for the course of the left central line?

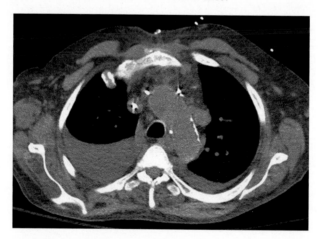

A. Placement in the left subclavian artery
B. Placement in the left common carotid artery
C. Extravascular placement
D. Placement in a left superior vena cava

6 An intubated patient in the ICU had morning chest radiographs taken 6 hours apart. What is the most likely cause for the left lung findings?

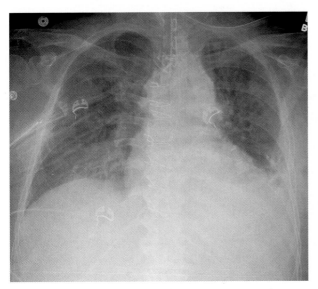 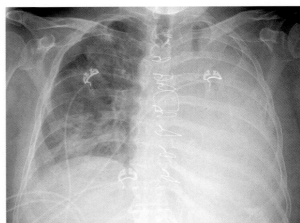

A. Pneumonia
B. Hematoma
C. Malignancy
D. Mucous plug

7a A left ventricular assist device (LVAD) is shown. What part of the device is indicated by the arrow?

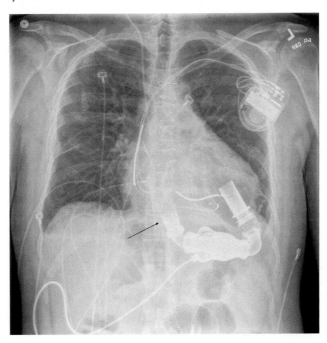

A. Reservoir
B. Outflow cannula
C. Drive line
D. Pump

7b Where is blood flow directed after leaving the outflow cannula?

    A. Aorta

    B. Left ventricle

    C. Left atrium

    D. Pulmonary artery

8a Where is the indicated lead positioned?

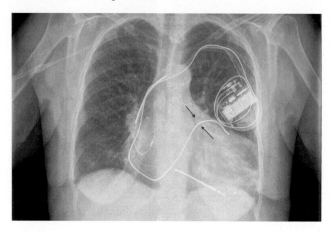

    A. Pulmonary artery

    B. Left atrium

    C. Coronary sinus

    D. Right ventricle

8b What is the primary indication for placement of biventricular pacemaker?

    A. Bradycardia

    B. Heart failure

    C. History of ventricular fibrillation

    D. Supraventricular tachycardia

9 What is the best way to differentiate extrapleural hematoma from hemothorax?

    A. Free layering configuration

    B. Increased density

    C. Blood return in chest tube

    D. Displacement of extrapleural fat

10 How can esophageal intubation be most reliably diagnosed?

    A. pH probe

    B. Expiratory radiograph

    C. Posterior oblique radiograph

    D. New atelectasis on radiograph

11 What is the ideal position for a pulmonary artery (Swan-Ganz) catheter?

    A. Central pulmonary arteries

    B. Superior cavoatrial junction

    C. Fifth-generation pulmonary artery

    D. Level of the pulmonary valve

12a What is the primary abnormality?

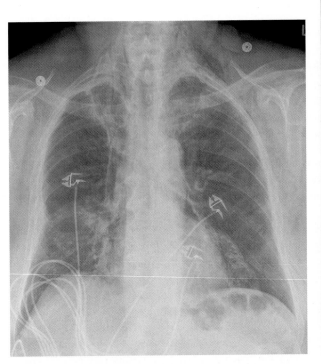 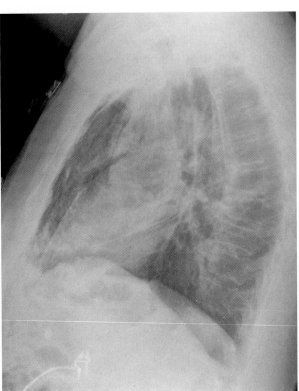

A. Pneumothorax
B. Pneumopericardium
C. Pneumoperitoneum
D. Pneumomediastinum

12b In a different patient, what accounts for the lucency inferior to the heart?

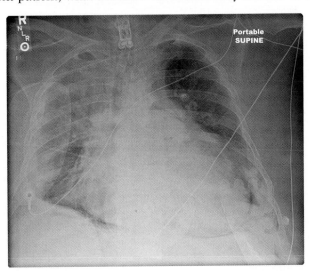

A. Pneumothorax
B. Pneumopericardium
C. Pneumoperitoneum
D. Pneumomediastinum

13 What secondary sign may indicate myocardial perforation by a pacemaker electrode?

   A. Pericardial effusion
   B. Hemothorax
   C. Pneumomediastinum
   D. Pneumothorax

14 What is the role of a Sengstaken-Blakemore tube?

   A. Direct drainage of bleeding gastric ulcer
   B. Enteric feeding following gastrectomy
   C. Balloon tamponade of bleeding esophageal varices
   D. Temporary plombage treatment of mycobacterial pneumonia

15a Evaluate these two sequential radiographs taken 3 hours apart (initial on the left and follow-up on the right). What intervention between the two images accounts for the right thorax changes?

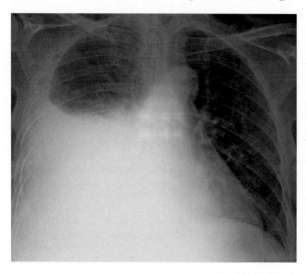 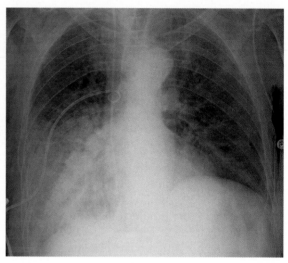

   A. Central venous catheter placement
   B. Pleural drain placement
   C. Endotracheal tube placement
   D. Change in patient position

15b What accounts for the new right lower lung consolidation?

   A. Pneumothorax
   B. Aspiration pneumonia
   C. Reexpansion pulmonary edema
   D. Pulmonary hemorrhage

16a What is the most common location for lead fracture of a transvenous pacer?

   A. At the pacemaker attachment
   B. Terminal lead tip
   C. Venous access site
   D. Cavoatrial junction

16b What is a common cause of pacemaker lead fracture?

   A. Metal fatigue
   B. Friction motion between leads
   C. Electrical short circuit
   D. Compression between the clavicle and first rib

17 What is generally the most appropriate initial management of vascular catheter fracture and dislodgement?

A. No treatment
B. Snare
C. Vascular surgery
D. Suction aspiration

18 A patient develops hemoptysis 6 weeks following a prolonged ICU stay, which included long-term pulmonary artery catheter use for fluid management. What is the most likely etiology?

A. Pulmonary artery pseudoaneurysm
B. Bleeding gastric ulcer
C. Bronchopleural fistula
D. Bronchial artery fistula

19a What is this imaging sign commonly called?

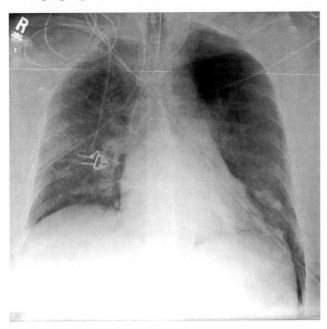

A. Deep sulcus sign
B. Silhouette sign
C. Air crescent sign
D. Scimitar sign

19b Where is the air located associated with the deep sulcus sign?

A. Posterior lateral pleural space
B. Anterior lateral pleural space
C. Left upper quadrant
D. Lateral chest wall

20 A chest x-ray was obtained for evaluation of feeding tube placement. What best describes the location of the feeding tube tip?

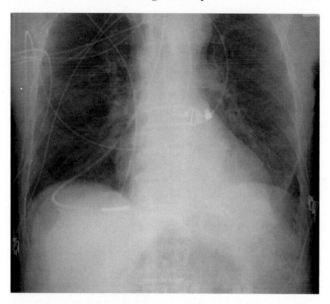

A. In the right lower lobe bronchus
B. In the right middle lobe bronchus
C. In the right pleural space
D. In a large hiatal hernia

ANSWERS AND EXPLANATIONS

1a **Answer C.**

1b **Answer B.**   Pneumoperitoneum can result from a variety of benign and emergent conditions and can be a harbinger of a serious underlying condition. Commons causes include surgery, peritoneal dialysis, or recent instrumentation. Toxic causes include bowel ischemia, infectious or inflammatory gastrointestinal conditions, or penetrating trauma. Steroids and NSAIDs can cause asymptomatic, benign pneumoperitoneum. "Free air" rises to a nondependent location in a body cavity. In the upright position, pneumoperitoneum will be seen as curvilinear lucencies outlining the abdominal surface of the diaphragm. In the ICU, supine radiography is employed in intubated nonambulatory patients. Right upper quadrant air can be seen in the subdiaphragmatic space distinct from the liver. Normal bowel gas only outlines the intraluminal surface. The serosal surfaces have similar radiographic soft tissue attenuation as the surrounding mesenteric fat and are not as well delineated. When gas is on the extraluminal surface of the bowel wall, this creates a radiodense line known as the Rigler sign.

Reference: Ly JQ. The Rigler sign. *Radiology* 2003;228(3):706–707.

2a **Answer A.**

2b **Answer B.**   Endotracheal tubes provide ventilatory support to critically ill patients to aid with oxygenation. Malposition can occur in up to 15% of patients. Postplacement chest radiography of intubated patients can detect malposition prior to complications. Optimal position is in the midthoracic trachea approximately 5 cm above the carina with the head in the neutral position where the mandible overlies the lower cervical spine on frontal view. Head flexion causes the tube to move caudally while head extension causes it to move cranially ("the hose follows the nose"). High placement of an ETT can lead to extubation, hypopharyngeal intubation, gastric distension, and poor ventilation as well as lead to vocal cord injury. Low placement can result in mainstem bronchus intubation, ipsilateral lung overinflation, and increased risk of pneumothorax and atelectasis of the opposite lung. Bronchial intubation usually occurs on the right due to the more vertical course of the right mainstem bronchus. Esophageal intubation can be fatal and may present as an ETT lateral to the trachea, an esophageal air column parallel to the trachea, or gastric distension. Obtaining a right posterior oblique radiograph can aid in diagnosis by separating the trachea and the inadvertently intubated esophagus.

Reference: Godoy MCB, Leitman BS, de Groot PM, et al. Chest radiography in the ICU: part I, evaluation of airway, enteric, and pleural tubes. *AJR Am J Roentgenol* 2012;198:563–571.

3a **Answer C.**

3b **Answer A.**   The intra-aortic balloon pump (IABP) is used to augment coronary artery perfusion in patients in cardiogenic shock. It contains an inflatable balloon around a catheter with a short radiopaque tip. It is inserted via a femoral artery approach until the tip is in the upper descending aorta and the radiopaque tip is positioned 2 cm caudal to the aortic arch and distal to the left subclavian artery. Inflation during diastole increases coronary artery and carotid flow, and deflation during systole reduces left ventricular afterload. The gas-filled balloon should not be confused with an abnormal air collection.

Complications of malposition include occlusion of aortic branches, which can lead to cerebral ischemia or left limb ischemia. Caudal aortic placement can lead to renal or mesenteric ischemia. Aortic dissection has also been reported in 1% to 4% of insertions.

Reference: Godoy M, Leitman B, Groot P, et al. Chest radiography in the ICU: part 2, evaluation of cardiovascular lines and other devices. *AJR Am J Roentgenol* 2012;198:572–581.

4 **Answer D.** The superior cavoatrial junction (CAJ) is the point between the superior vena cava (SVC) and the true right atrium. The CAJ is the midpoint on an oblique line between the crista terminalis anteriorly and the crista dividens posteriorly. Because the SVC has a most posterior insertion on the right atrium, the CAJ is located more inferior than usually anticipated on chest radiography. Various techniques have been described to confirm adequate positioning of central venous catheters, to include two vertebral body heights below the carina, within 4 cm of the carina, and alignment with the inferior bronchus intermedius.

References: Baskin KM, Jimenez RM, Cahill AM, et al. Cavoatrial junction and central venous anatomy: implications for central venous access tip position. *J Vasc Interv Radiol* 2008;19(3):359–365.

Ridge CA, Litmanovich D, Molinari F, et al. Radiographic evaluation of central venous catheter position: anatomic correlation using gated coronary computed tomographic angiography. *J Thorac Imaging* 2013;28(2):129–133.

Webb WR, Higgins CB. *Thoracic imaging: pulmonary and cardiovascular radiology*, 2nd ed. Philadelphia, PA: Lippincott Williams & Wilkins, 2011. Chapter 11: Pulmonary Edema, ARDS and Radiology in the ICU:p. 368.

5a **Answer B.**

5b **Answer D.** Central venous lines provide venous access to administer fluids, medications, and pressure monitoring. Common types of central lines include internal jugular and subclavian lines and peripherally inserted central catheters (PICC). Optimal position of a central line tip is in the downstream superior vena cava at the cavoatrial junction. Intracardiac placement risks cardiac injury or rhythm disturbances while high positioning could lead to thrombus formation or intravenous introduction of potentially toxic drugs that are meant to be diluted. Malpositioned catheters may lie in the internal jugular, contralateral subclavian, or azygos veins. Inadvertent arterial positioning can lead to thromboembolic events and stroke.

Variant anatomy can cause unexpected positioning on radiography and can be confirmed by review of cross-sectional imaging. A persistent left SVC is not an infrequent anomaly, which can cause an aberrant course of a left central line projecting along the left upper mediastinum. A diligent search for a vascular anomaly should be undertaken with available images. If no cause is found, communication with the care team should raise the possibility of arterial catheterization. Intravenous fluids should be maintained to prevent thrombus formation. Confirmation of arterial catheterization includes evaluation of blood color, arterial blood gas measurements, catheter transduction, and assessment of pulsatile waveform. A CT scan or contrast injection under fluoroscopy can confirm the diagnosis. The line should remain in place and consultation obtained for endovascular or surgical management.

References: Godoy MC, Leitman BS, de Groot PM, et al. Chest radiography in the ICU: part 2, evaluation of cardiovascular lines and other devices. *AJR Am J Roentgenol* 2012;198(3):572–581.

Pikwer A, Acosta S, Kölbel T, et al. Management of inadvertent arterial catheterisation associated with central venous access procedures. *Eur J Vasc Endovas Surg* 2009;38(6):707–714.

6 **Answer D.** Central endobronchial obstruction can cause obstructive atelectasis following reabsorption of gas from the alveoli. A central mucous plug can cause relatively rapid and impressive whole lung atelectasis. By knowing the intubation status of the patient and recognizing the ipsilateral volume loss, one can make a confident diagnosis of a mucous plug and not mistake the "white out" appearance for a large pleural effusion. Bronchoscopy can confirm the diagnosis and clear the mucoid impaction.

Reference: Collins J, Stern EJ, eds. *Chest radiology: the essentials.* Philadelphia, PA: Lippincott Williams & Wilkins, 2008.

7a **Answer B.**

7b **Answer A.** Left ventricular assist devices (LVADs) are implantable devices used for patients in end-stage heart failure prior to heart transplantation, during cardiac recovery, or for those patients ineligible for transplant. Several different types of LVADs are in use (HeartMate II shown, Thoratec, Inc.). Basic design features usually include an inflow cannula attached to the left ventricle, a pump, and an outflow cannula attached to the aorta. The connection between the outflow cannula and the ascending aorta is normally radiolucent, and the position must be inferred by radiography. Potential complications include postoperative hemorrhage, pericardial tamponade, thrombus formation, aortic valve stenosis, aortic valve insufficiency, right-sided heart failure, and infection. These complications are generally best evaluated by chest CT.

Reference: Carr CM, Jacob J, Park SJ, et al. CT of left ventricular assist devices 1. *RadioGraphics* 2010;30(2):429–444.

8a **Answer C.**

8b **Answer B.** On a frontal chest radiograph, the approximate position of the coronary sinus runs at an oblique angle from the inferior right heart border to the superior left heart border. A pacer lead in the coronary sinus allows for pacing of the left ventricle and in this patient indicates placement of a dual-chamber biventricular pacer. Heart failure is the primary indication for biventricular pacing, as they have shown improved cardiac function in refractory heart failure patients.

References: Costelloe CM, et al. Radiography of pacemakers and implantable cardioverter defibrillators. *AJR Am J Roentgenol* 2012;199(6):1252–1258.

Singh JP, Gras D. Biventricular pacing: current trends and future strategies. *Eur Heart J* 2012;33(3):305–313.

9 **Answer D.** The pleura is surrounded by a thin layer of fat external to the parietal layer of the pleura. An extrapleural hematoma occurs outside the fat layer causing inward medial displacement of the extrapleural fat. Other indications of an extrapleural hematoma, as may be seen due to thoracentesis, include a focal lobular contour and fixed position despite repositioning of the patient.

Reference: Godoy MCB, Leitman BS, de Groot PM, et al. Chest radiography in the ICU: part I, evaluation of airway, enteric, and pleural tubes. *AJR Am J Roentgenol* 2012;198:563–571.

10 **Answer C.** Esophageal intubation can be fatal and as mentioned before may present as an ETT lateral to the trachea, an esophageal air column parallel to the trachea, or gastric distension. Obtaining a right posterior oblique radiograph can aid in diagnosis by separating the trachea and the intubated esophagus.

Reference: Godoy MCB, Leitman BS, de Groot PM, et al. Chest radiography in the ICU: part I, evaluation of airway, enteric, and pleural tubes. *AJR Am J Roentgenol* 2012;198:563–571.

11 **Answer A.** The Swan-Ganz catheter is a pulmonary artery catheter for hemodynamic monitoring of critically ill patients. The pulmonary capillary wedge pressure (PCWP) can be measured as an estimate for left atrial pressure. This can help differentiate cardiogenic from noncardiogenic pulmonary edema as left heart pressures will be elevated in cardiogenic causes. The catheter is usually inserted through the internal jugular or subclavian veins. Ideal position is in the proximal right or left pulmonary arteries within 2 cm of the hilum. Distal location can result in pulmonary artery injury, rupture, occlusion, dissection, infarction, pseudoaneurysm, or fistula.

Reference: Godoy M, Leitman B, Groot P, et al. Chest radiography in the ICU: part 2, evaluation of cardiovascular lines and other devices. *AJR Am J Roentgenol* 2012;198:572–581.

12a **Answer D.**

12b **Answer D.** Pneumomediastinum can result from a variety of causes including alveolar rupture, tracheobronchial tree laceration, gastrointestinal tract injury (especially the esophagus), or extraluminal gas tracking into the thorax from other sites. Mechanically ventilated patients are at increased risk for pneumomediastinum. The first case shown was related to recent bronchoscopy. The streaky lucencies overlying the mediastinum on the frontal and lateral projections are typical.

Mediastinal gas collecting along the inferior margin of the heart can sometimes outline the superior diaphragmatic surface. Usually, the anterior medial left hemidiaphragm is not distinguishable due to the isodense soft tissue interface between the diaphragm and the heart. A pneumomediastinum air gap separates these two surfaces allowing visibility of the left side of the diaphragm which creates a continuous diaphragm sign as seen in the second case shown.

References: Bejvan SM, Godwin JD. Pneumomediastinum: old signs and new signs. *AJR Am J Roentgenol* 1996;166(5):1041–1048.

Schmitt ER, Burg MD. Continuous diaphragm sign. *West J Emerg Med* 2011;12(4):526–527.

13 **Answer A.** Myocardial injury following cardiac device placement is uncommon. It most commonly occurs in the right ventricle. Myocardial perforation may be identified if the lead tip projects outside the borders of the heart or if there is pericardial effusion or tamponade. Pneumothorax can be seen as a complication of pacer lead placement although pneumothorax, pneumomediastinum, and hemothorax would be rare in myocardial perforation from a pacemaker lead.

Reference: Godoy M, Leitman B, Groot P, et al. Chest radiography in the ICU: part 2, evaluation of cardiovascular lines and other devices. *AJR Am J Roentgenol* 2012;198:572–581.

14 **Answer C.** Bleeding esophageal varices can be a life-threatening condition, and prompt treatment is necessary for patient stabilization. Volume repletion, with pharmacologic and surgical interventions, is a mainstay of treatment. Mechanical balloon tamponade can be accomplished with a Sengstaken-Blakemore tube. It is inserted through the mouth or nose and the balloon tip inflated for compression of bleeding varices. Tubes that have an opening near the top are called Minnesota tubes. Complications include esophageal perforation, rupture, ulceration, and necrosis. Due to modern endoscopic advances, Sengstaken-Blakemore tubes are much less frequently employed than in the past.

Reference: Shen TC, Tu CY. Common procedure-related complications in the ICU: a pictorial review. *J Intern Med Taiwan* 2013;24(6):453–460.

15a Answer B.

15b Answer C.   There is a large right pleural effusion on initial x-ray. On subsequent radiograph, there is a small-bore pleural catheter with near-total resolution of the right effusion. However, there has been interval development of significant right mid and lower lung airspace disease. The process is quite unilateral. No pleural line or evidence of pneumothorax is seen. Aspiration pneumonia is possible, but this large of an aspiration even would be expected to be bilateral. Reexpansion pulmonary edema is the correct diagnosis. Clinical symptoms can be severe and usually appear within the first 2 hours but can take up to 2 days, lasting 1 to 2 days or more. Unilateral airspace opacity is the most usual finding.

The underlying mechanism is not well understood but presumed to be capillary leak edema related to more long-standing lung collapse and atelectasis. Risk factors for developing reexpansion edema include rapid lung expansion from draining either large pneumothoraces or effusions that have been present for more than 7 days. The clinical setting is critical to making this diagnosis.

Some guidelines suggest draining no more than 1 to 1.5 L of pleural fluid per day to prevent this from occurring.

References: Echevarria C, Twomey D, Dunning J, et al. Does re-expansion pulmonary oedema exist? *Interact Cardiovasc Thorac Surg* 2008;7(3):485–489.

Godoy MCB, Leitman BS, de Groot PM, et al. Chest radiography in the ICU: part I, evaluation of airway, enteric, and pleural tubes. *AJR Am J Roentgenol* 2012;198:563–571.

16a Answer C.

16b Answer D.   Pacemakers are used to treat a variety of cardiac conduction disturbance and can be either temporary or permanent. Permanent pacers have a pulse generator with a battery pack and control unit that is implanted into the anterior chest wall. One or more leads are positioned endovascularly as needed. Biventricular pacing can treat congestive heart failure, and an automatic implantable cardioverter–defibrillator (AICD) may be added to reduce the risk of ventricular tachyarrhythmias. Complications can include pneumothorax, vascular injury, myocardial perforation, and lead fracture. Lead fractures can occur at the venous access site, from compression between the clavicle and first rib; at the battery pack; or at the lead tip. Patients who rotate the generator in the subcutaneous skin pocket ("twiddler's syndrome") can cause lead traction and dislodgement.

Reference: Godoy MC, Leitman BS, de Groot PM, et al. Chest radiography in the ICU: part 2, evaluation of cardiovascular lines and other devices. *AJR Am J Roentgenol* 2012;198(3):572–581.

17 Answer B.   When an intravascular foreign body is discovered, careful evaluation can determine the necessity of removing the object, best approach, safety concerns, and technique. A snare loop is the simplest and most commonly found device that can retrieve a variety of foreign bodies. A snare consists of an adjustable loop that works similar to a "lasso" to tighten around intravascular catheters for extraction.

Reference: Kaufman JA, Lee MJ. *Vascular and interventional radiology*. Philadelphia, PA: Elsevier Health Sciences, 2013.

18 Answer A.   Swan-Ganz pulmonary artery catheters are commonly used in ICU patients for hemodynamic monitoring. Complications include malposition, looping, coiling, knotting, and pneumothorax. Rarer complications include pulmonary artery rupture, dissection, pseudoaneurysm formation, and fistula formation with the bronchial tree. Iatrogenic pseudoaneurysm can sometimes progress and rupture, resulting in hemoptysis.

Reference: Godoy MC, Leitman BS, de Groot PM, et al. Chest radiography in the ICU: part 2, evaluation of cardiovascular lines and other devices. *AJR Am J Roentgenol* 2012;198(3):572–581.

19a **Answer A.**

19b **Answer B.** Pneumothorax in a supine patient collects anteriorly and basally in the nondependent portion of the chest. When it accumulates laterally, the lateral costophrenic angle is accentuated producing the deep sulcus sign. Other signs of pneumothorax include diaphragmatic depression, increased sharpness of the cardiac borders and pericardial fat pads, inferior pleural line, or double diaphragmatic contour. Lateral decubitus views may be helpful for future evaluation.

Reference: Kong A. The deep sulcus sign. *Radiology* 2003;228(2):415–416.

20 **Answer C.** A feeding tube is identified overlying the right lung. The course of the tube extends into the right bronchial tree but makes an L-shaped curve that is not compatible with being inside the lung parenchyma. This tube has pierced the visceral pleura and resides within the pleural space. This should be considered an emergent finding, and the caregivers should be prepared for a high likelihood that this patient will require a chest tube after removal of the feeding tube. There is no identifiable hiatal hernia although feeding tubes can loop inside hernias on occasion.

Reference: Godoy MCB, Leitman BS, de Groot PM, et al. Chest radiography in the ICU: part I, evaluation of airway, enteric, and pleural tubes. *AJR Am J Roentgenol* 2012;198:563–571.

5 Pulmonary Pathology

QUESTIONS

Section 1: Infectious Pneumonia

1a In the CT image, a distinguishing feature that differentiates between Cytomegalovirus pneumonia and *Pneumocystis jiroveci* pneumonia is:

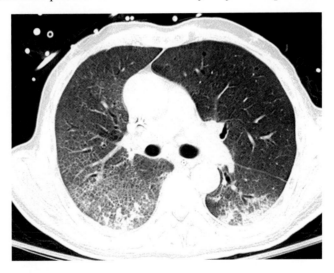

A. "Crazy paving"
B. Consolidation
C. The presence of cysts
D. Not present

1b At what CD4+ cell count does PJP infection generally begin to arise?

A. 400 cells/mm^3
B. 200 cells/mm^3
C. 100 cells/mm^3
D. 50 cells/mm^3

2   This 66-year-old nursing home patient with pneumonia has a past medical history of diabetes, chronic respiratory insufficiency requiring tracheostomy, and chronic renal insufficiency. Considering the CT appearance, the most likely etiologic agent of pneumonia is:

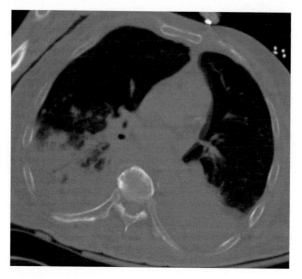

A. *Pseudomonas aeruginosa*
B. Cytomegalovirus
C. *Pneumocystis jiroveci*
D. Histoplasmosis

3a   Two weeks after significant head injury, this 74 year old patient developed overnight respiratory decline in the ICU. CT pulmonary angiogram obtained and shown below. After obtaining a protected bronchial washing for culture, the best intervention is to commence therapy with:

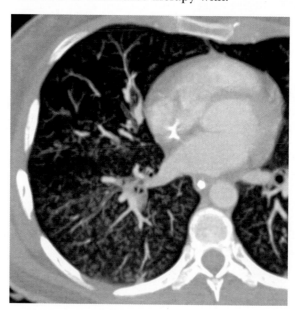

A. Sulfamethoxazole and trimethoprim
B. Isoniazid and rifampin
C. Levofloxacin
D. Ceftazidime and vancomycin

3b Which of the following is a risk factor for community-acquired methicillin-resistant *Staphylococcus aureus* (MRSA) infection?

A. Female gender
B. Incarceration
C. High socioeconomic status
D. Silica exposure

4 This 37-year-old was referred to the outpatient imaging center with complaints of a nonproductive cough for 5 months. The most appropriate subsequent intervention is:

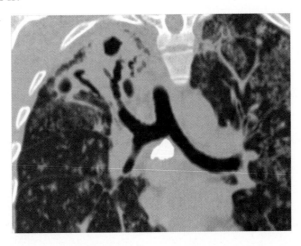

A. A left bronchial intubation
B. Bronchoscopy with bronchoalveolar lavage
C. Initiation of antimicrobial therapy
D. A video barium swallowing study

5 A 26-year-old patient with known HIV presents with respiratory distress. The most likely etiologic agent responsible for the findings present on the image provided is:

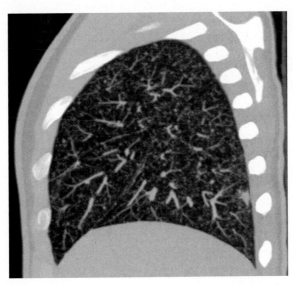

A. *Coccidioides immitis*
B. Cytomegalovirus
C. *Pneumocystis jiroveci*
D. *Nocardia asteroides*

6a   In the setting of septic emboli, what is the most common cardiac source of infection?

    A. Tricuspid valve
    B. Mitral valve
    C. Pulmonary valve
    D. Aortic valve

6b   What is the most common infectious agent to cause septic emboli?

    A. *Streptococcus pneumoniae*
    B. *Enterobacter aerogenes*
    C. *Haemophilus influenzae*
    D. *Staphylococcus aureus*

7a   A 79-year-old woman with COPD and newly diagnosed pancytopenia presents with rapid onset of respiratory distress. Of the pathogens listed, the most likely etiologic agent responsible for the findings present on the image provided is:

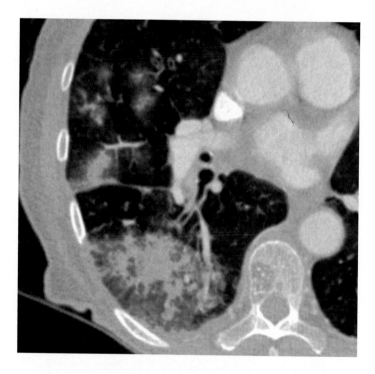

    A. *Streptococcus pneumoniae*
    B. *Cryptococcus neoformans*
    C. *Staphylococcus aureus*
    D. *Legionella pneumophila*

7b   Which CT finding not present on this exam would be common in *Legionella* pneumonia?

    A. Cavitation
    B. Pleural effusion
    C. Pneumothorax
    D. Chest wall invasion

8a Of the choices below, which imaging finding on the CT provided is the most common for pulmonary *Mycobacterium abscessus*?

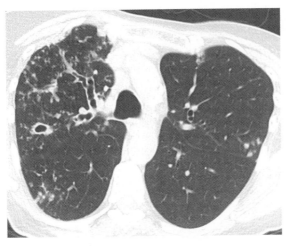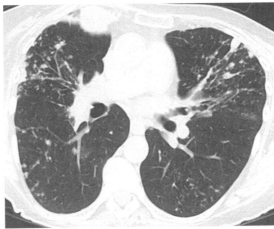

    A. Cavitation
    B. Bronchiectasis
    C. Consolidation
    D. Nodules

8b Which CT finding would be more characteristic in *Mycobacterium avium* complex (MAC) compared to *Mycobacterium abscessus*?

    A. Cavitation
    B. Bronchiectasis
    C. Consolidation
    D. Tree-in-bud pattern

8c In cancer patients who develop *M. abscessus* pulmonary infection, which is the most common associated risk factor?

    A. Underlying lung disease
    B. Hematopoietic stem cell transplant
    C. Male gender
    D. Hematologic neoplasm

9 This patient has undergone heart transplant. Of these choices, what is the most likely cause of the nodule?

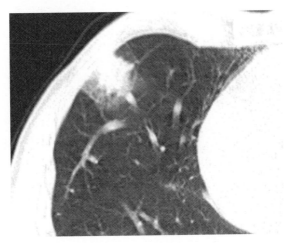

    A. *Aspergillus*
    B. Cytomegalovirus
    C. Posttransplant lymphoproliferative disease
    D. Round atelectasis

10   A 61-year-old male presents with declining pulmonary function tests. The etiology of the process evident on the image provided is most likely to be:

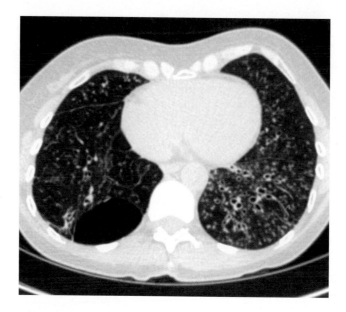

A. Allergic bronchopulmonary aspergillosis
B. Adult cystic fibrosis
C. Sarcoidosis
D. Recurrent infection

11   Chest radiographs obtained 6 days apart in this 19-year-old male with positive H1N1 viral culture. What is the most likely cause of progression in the second chest radiograph?

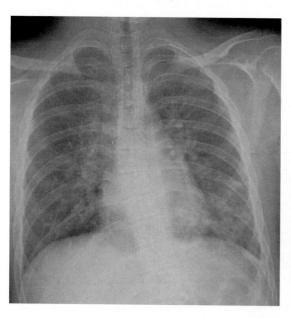 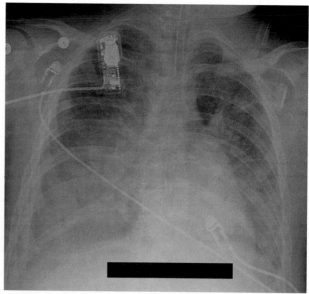

A. Pulmonary hemorrhage
B. Cardiogenic pulmonary edema
C. Alveolar proteinosis
D. Diffuse alveolar damage

12 A 42-year-old female with prior end-stage pulmonary sarcoidosis presents to the clinic with worsening respiratory distress 3 months after lung transplant. A CT of the chest shows new consolidation in the transplanted lung. The process most likely to be responsible for the consolidation is:

    A. Acute rejection pneumonitis

    B. Infectious process

    C. Organizing pneumonia

    D. Recurrence of sarcoid

13a What lung segment is largely spared by the pathologic process demonstrated in the right upper lobe?

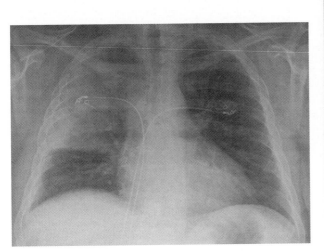 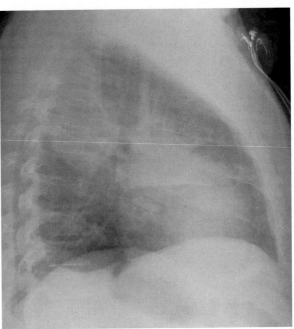

    A. Apical segment

    B. Posterior segment

    C. Anterior segment

    D. Apicoposterior segment

13b What is the most likely pathogen in the setting of a community-acquired pneumonia in an immunocompetent patient?

    A. *Streptococcus pneumonia*

    B. *Nocardia asteroides*

    C. Cytomegalovirus

    D. *Mycoplasma pneumoniae*

14 Which of the following pulmonary infections is characterized by hemorrhagic mediastinal adenopathy?

    A. *Mycobacterium tuberculosis*

    B. Inhalational anthrax

    C. Tularemia

    D. *Staphylococcus aureus*

15a What complication of airspace disease is identified in the right upper lobe?

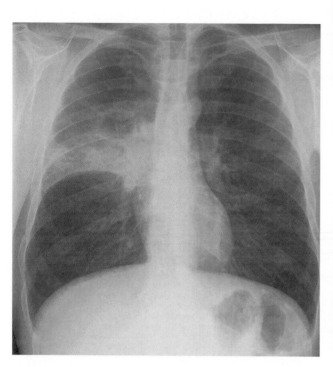
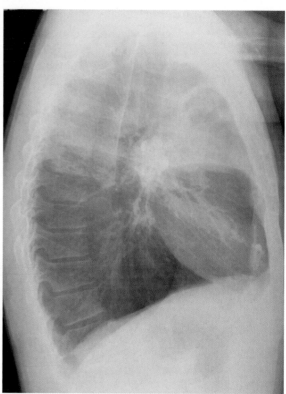

A. Pleural effusion
B. Pneumothorax
C. Cavitation
D. Pulmonary hemorrhage

15b What is the likely pathogen given that complication, presuming this is an infectious process?

A. Mixed anaerobic infection
B. *Staphylococcus aureus*
C. *Pseudomonas aeruginosa*
D. *Mycobacterium tuberculosis*

16 What is the most common radiologic presentation of Epstein-Barr virus infection?

A. Lobar consolidation
B. Bronchopneumonia
C. Interstitial pneumonia
D. Lymphadenopathy

17 What is the most common cause of lobar consolidation in an HIV patient?

A. Bacterial pneumonia
B. Viral pneumonia
C. Fungal pneumonia
D. Tuberculosis

18 Given a history of HIV infection and slow progressive worsening in constitutional symptoms, what is the likely diagnosis?

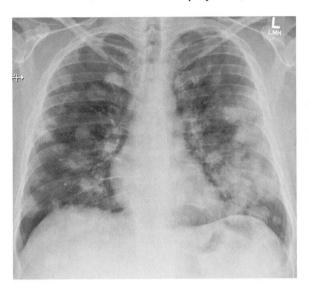 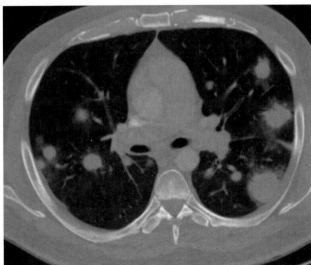

A. Septic emboli
B. Angioinvasive fungal infection
C. Lymphoma
D. Organizing pneumonia

19a A patient presents with the following imaging with a concurrent diffuse rash progressing from macules to blisters and finally scabbing. What is the likely cause of the pulmonary parenchymal abnormality?

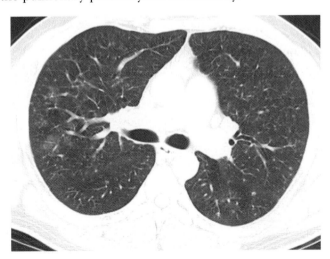

A. Varicella pneumonia
B. Respiratory bronchiolitis
C. Pulmonary hemorrhage
D. Hypersensitivity pneumonitis

19b What is the most common residual appearance of healed varicella pneumonia?
A. Linear scar formation
B. Round atelectasis
C. Diffuse calcified tiny pulmonary nodules
D. Pulmonary cysts

Section 2: Diffuse Lung Disease

20a Chest radiographs obtained in a 28-year-old black female with chronic dry cough, night sweats, elevated ACE level, and tender red nodules on shins most likely correspond to:

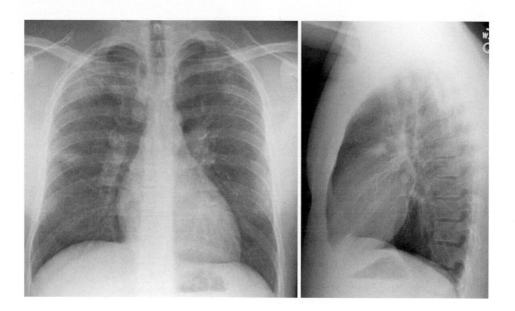

    A. Tuberculosis
    B. Sarcoidosis
    C. Hodgkin lymphoma
    D. Pulmonary lymphoproliferative disease

20b Staging of pulmonary sarcoidosis is based on correlation of functional impairment and what radiographic examination?

    A. CT chest with contrast
    B. CT chest without contrast
    C. Chest radiograph
    D. PET/CT

20c Typical perilymphatic nodularity in sarcoidosis is characterized by:

    A. Diffuse distribution without zonal predilection
    B. Significant characteristic FDG uptake on PET/CT
    C. Patchy distribution with upper and midlung predominance
    D. Direct correlation with worsened functional status in lung allograft

21a Frontal chest radiograph obtained in a 40-year-old female shows:

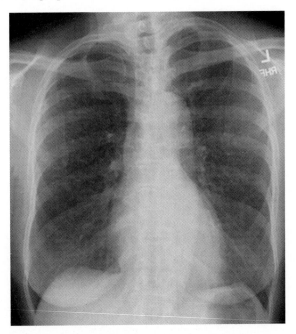

    A. Ground-glass opacities with central predilection
    B. Bilateral perihilar honeycombing
    C. Evidence of prior radiation treatment
    D. Bilateral reticular opacities with scattered cystic lesions

21b Axial and coronal CT images of the same patient are shown. The most important clinical information to correlate with imaging findings would be:

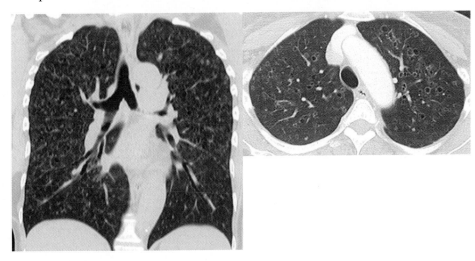

    A. Smoking history
    B. Presence of vegetations on cardiac valves
    C. Recent viral upper respiratory infection
    D. Exposure to environmental inhaled antigens

21c Regarding pulmonary Langerhans cell histiocytosis (PLCH), the correct statement is:

A. End-stage PLCH is characterized by cellular interstitial infiltrates composed of Langerhans cells, lymphocytes, macrophages, eosinophils, plasma cells, and fibroblasts.

B. Mere presence of Langerhans cells in the lesions is enough for diagnosis.

C. TGF-beta is an essential factor in the development of Langerhans cells and airway-centered fibrosis.

D. Pneumothorax is frequent complication but is significantly reduced by steroid use.

22a What is the best next step based on radiographic assessment of a 36-year-old female with acute exacerbation of chronic shortness of breath?

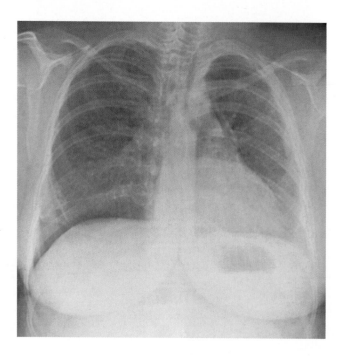

A. Repeat chest x-ray with an additional lateral view.

B. Perform CT chest with contrast.

C. Consider diuretics.

D. An emergent phone call to the referring clinician.

22b Isolated lymphangioleiomyomatosis is most frequently seen in which patient population?

A. Young females

B. Males and females equally

C. Young males

D. Elderly males

22c Based on coronal and axial images from the same patient, the most likely underlying diagnosis is:

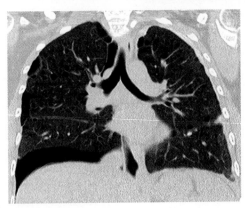

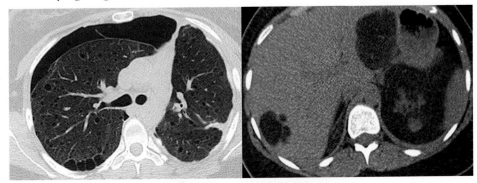

    A. Lymphangioleiomyomatosis (LAM)
    B. Pulmonary Langerhans cell histiocytosis (PLCH)
    C. Lymphocytic interstitial pneumonia (LIP)
    D. Chronic pneumocystis pneumonia

22d Which of the following would be most atypical for lymphangioleiomyomatosis?
    A. Progressive enlargement of thin-walled cysts over time
    B. Decreased lung volumes
    C. Reticular pattern on chest x-ray
    D. Hilar and abdominal lymphadenopathy

23a Frontal and lateral chest radiographs obtained from a 33-year-old male with history of voice hoarseness and recurrent pneumonia demonstrate:

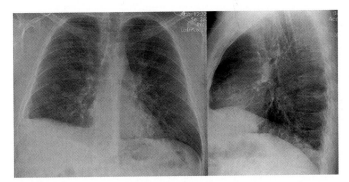

    A. Evidence of hydrostatic edema with associated right-sided pleural effusion
    B. Bilateral hilar lymphadenopathy with right lung base consolidation
    C. Partially cavitating lung nodules, bronchiectases, and elevated right hemidiaphragm
    D. Radiographic features suggestive of honeycombing, right more than left

23b Taken into consideration provided history and CT imaging findings, the leading diagnostic consideration would be:

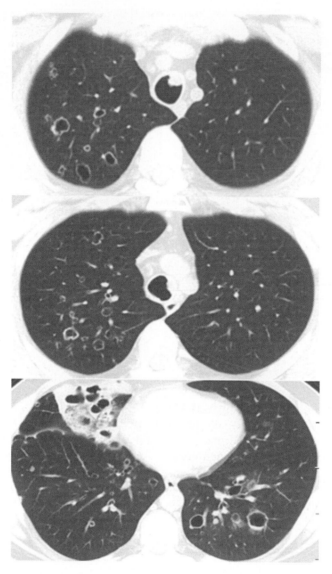

    A. *Mycobacterium avium* infection
    B. Relapsing polychondritis
    C. Wegener granulomatosis
    D. Respiratory papillomatosis

23c Regarding imaging assessment of the large airways for masses:

    A. Chest radiography is the modality of choice.
    B. Chest CT is the modality of choice.
    C. PET/CT is the modality of choice.
    D. Chest MRI is the modality of choice.

23d The difference between recurrent laryngeal papillomatosis in children and adults is:

    A. Not significant for incidence and severity
    B. Does not exist for the most common site of anatomic involvement
    C. Higher rate of extralaryngeal spread of respiratory papillomata in adults
    D. Higher rate of pulmonary nodule calcification in kids

24a What is the best next step based on radiographic assessment of a middle age female with xerostomia and dry eyes?

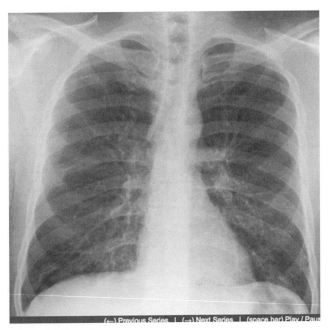

A. Chest CT
B. PET/CT
C. Biopsy
D. Repeat chest x-ray

24b Given the patient's CT findings, the most likely diagnosis is:

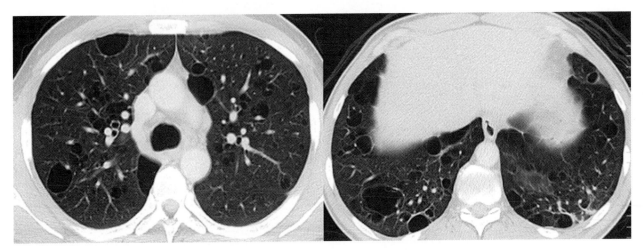

A. Pulmonary Langerhans cell histiocytosis
B. Lymphocytic interstitial pneumonia
C. Lymphangiomyomatosis
D. Idiopathic pulmonary fibrosis

24c The correct statement regarding lymphocytic interstitial pneumonia (LIP) is:

A. At least 25% of patients with Sjögren syndrome have LIP.
B. A majority of the patients with AIDS who have LIP are asymptomatic adults.
C. The course of the disease is unpredictable.
D. Half of patients with LIP progress into lymphoma.

25a A 43-year-old man with history of AIDS presents with chronic cough. What is the best description of the CT imaging abnormalities?

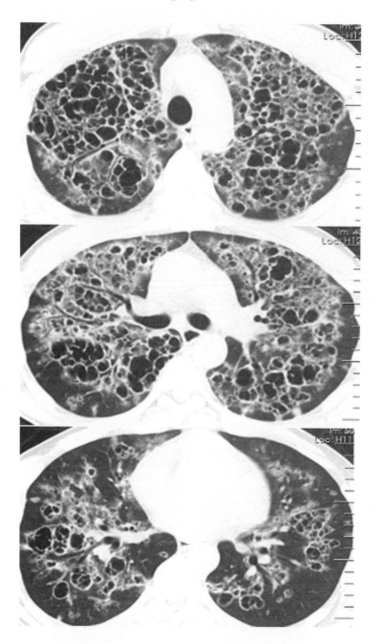

A. Extensive perivascular cysts superimposed on areas of consolidation
B. Upper and midlung predominant partially septated cystic lesions with variable wall thickness in a background of parenchymal opacities
C. Centrilobular emphysema superimposed on incompletely resolved alveolar pulmonary edema
D. Peripheral reticulation and cicatricial emphysema

25b The most likely diagnosis is:

A. *Pneumocystis jiroveci* infection
B. Pulmonary Langerhans cell histiocytosis (PLCH)
C. Septic emboli
D. Lymphangiomyomatosis (LAM)

26a A 60-year-old male who has previously worked in a foundry. What are the main radiographic abnormalities?

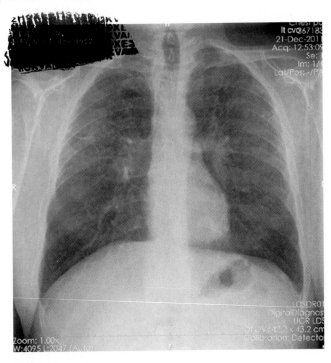

A. Kerley B lines and left hazy consolidative ground-glass opacities
B. Bibasilar peripheral reticulation and volume loss
C. Bilateral small nodules and hilar retraction
D. Patchy ill-defined consolidations

26b Given the CT findings and patient history, the most likely diagnosis is:

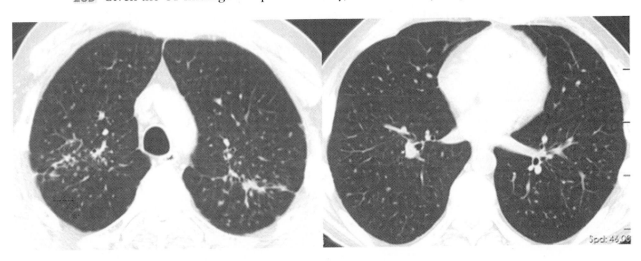

A. Pneumoconiosis
B. Granulomatosis with polyangiitis
C. Healed varicella
D. Miliary tuberculosis

26c The imaging feature most associated with simple classic silicosis is:

    A. Geographic ground-glass opacities with interlobular septal thickening

    B. Calcified pleural plaques

    C. Perilymphatic nodules

    D. Upper lobe confluent opacities with hilar retraction

27a Most likely diagnosis is:

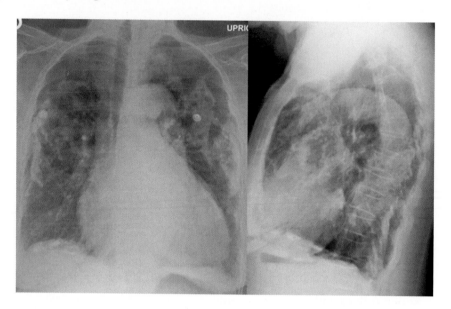

    A. Asbestos exposure

    B. Bilateral mesothelioma

    C. Multifocal round atelectasis

    D. Multifocal squamous cell carcinoma

27b CT images from a different patient with dyspnea. On the soft tissue window (not provided), bilateral diaphragmatic and lower lung parietal pleural calcifications are noted. The most likely explanation for CT findings is:

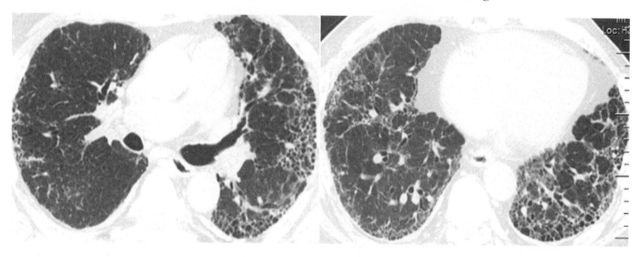

    A. Asbestosis

    B. Drug toxicity/reaction

    C. Idiopathic pulmonary fibrosis

    D. Post–ARDS-related fibrosis

27c The earliest sign of asbestosis on HRCT is:

  A. Bronchiectasis
  B. Parenchymal bands
  C. Curvilinear subpleural lines
  D. Honeycombing

27d The correct statement regarding utilization of HRCT in asbestosis is:

  A. Prone images should be obtained in early disease.
  B. HRCT should be avoided when radiograph is normal.
  C. HRCT should be used invariably for confirmation when diaphragmatic
     pleural calcifications are present.
  D. HRCT should be used as a problem-solving tool to distinguish advanced
     asbestos-related fibrosis from UIP and NSIP fibrosis.

27e The incidence of bronchogenic lung cancer in asbestos exposure is:

  A. The same to those without exposure
  B. Decreased in comparison to those without exposure
  C. Increased in comparison to those without exposure
  D. Controversial

28a Compare initial (left) and 1-month follow-up (right) CT images from the same
patient with remote history of scalp angiosarcoma. What is the most likely
cause of recurrent pneumothorax?

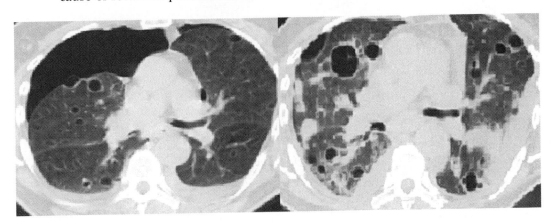

  A. Rupture of a subpleural bleb in emphysema
  B. Pulmonary Langerhans cell histiocytosis
  C. Metastatic disease
  D. Birt-Hogg-Dube syndrome

28b Typical imaging features of lung parenchymal metastases are:

  A. Variable-sized round nodules
  B. Air-space consolidation
  C. Solitary mass
  D. Pneumothorax

28c Cavitation is least common in which of the following types of metastasis?

  A. Adenocarcinoma
  B. Squamous cell carcinoma
  C. Transitional cell carcinoma
  D. Sarcoma

29a In a patient with a known occupational lung exposure in the aerospace industry, the related CT findings would be most likely due to:

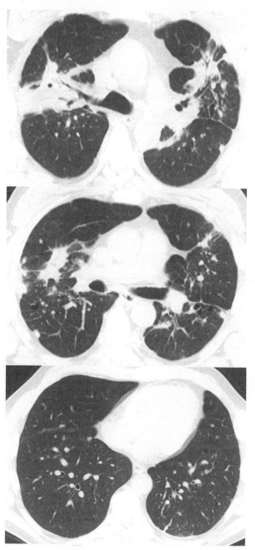

A. Sarcoidosis
B. Chronic beryllium disease
C. Usual interstitial pneumonia
D. Silicosis

29b The pathologic hallmark of chronic beryllium disease is:

A. Caseating granulomas indistinguishable from those in tuberculosis
B. Noncaseating granulomas indistinguishable from those in sarcoidosis
C. Caseating granulomas indistinguishable from those in granulomatosis with polyangiitis
D. Noncaseating granulomas indistinguishable from those in Langerhans cell histiocytosis

29c To diagnose chronic beryllium disease in a patient with beryllium exposure:

A. Characteristic CT findings are sufficient.
B. Positive beryllium-specific lymphocyte proliferation test is the test of choice.
C. Presence of noncaseating granulomas on transbronchial biopsy is diagnostic.
D. Open lung biopsy is invariably required.

30a In these radiographs from a 48-year-old female with history of heartburn and fingertip ulcerations, the main radiographic abnormality is:

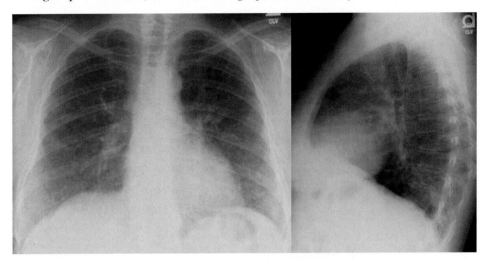

    A. Cardiomegaly
    B. Mediastinal lymphadenopathy
    C. Reticular pattern
    D. Pleural effusions

30b CT axial images taken 3 years apart from a 37-year-old female with mixed connective tissue disease. The imaging pattern is that of what interstitial pneumonia?

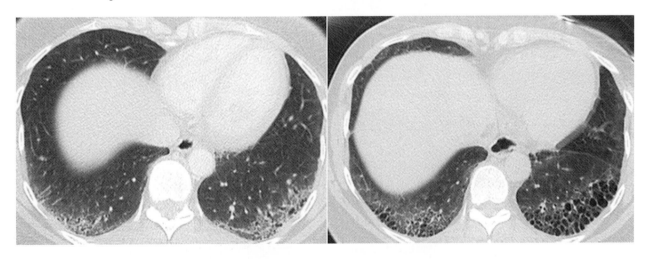

    A. Nonspecific interstitial pneumonia (NSIP)
    B. Usual interstitial pneumonia (UIP)
    C. Lymphocytic interstitial pneumonia (LIP)
    D. Organizing pneumonia (OP)

30c The classic imaging findings on HRCT in early-phase UIP-pattern lung fibrosis are:

    A. Honeycombing and reticulations with upper lung predominance
    B. Ground-glass opacities and traction bronchiectases without zonal predilection
    C. Subpleural reticulation with lower lung predominance
    D. Mediastinal lymphadenopathy

30d Which of the following is correct regarding idiopathic pulmonary fibrosis?
   A. Nonspecific interstitial pneumonia (NSIP) is the CT imaging pattern seen.
   B. Ground-glass opacities are better predictors of outcome than extent of reticulation.
   C. It could be seen in association with connective tissue disease.
   D. Characteristic CT features are present in 50% to 70% of patients.

31a CT axial images obtained from 58-year-old female with scleroderma. The pattern of lung fibrosis corresponds to:

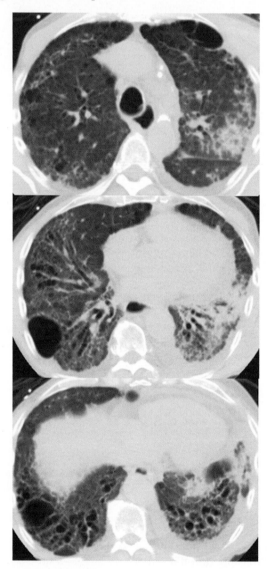

   A. Nonspecific interstitial pneumonia
   B. Usual interstitial pneumonia
   C. Idiopathic pulmonary fibrosis
   D. Cystic fibrosis

31b The most characteristic thin section CT findings of cellular NSIP are:
   A. Symmetric bilateral lower lung ground-glass opacities
   B. Mediastinal lymphadenopathy
   C. Bronchiolectasis
   D. Lower lung honeycombing

31c Which of the following is a well-recognized etiology of NSIP?

    A. Bacterial pneumonia
    B. Connective tissue disease
    C. Emphysema
    D. Tuberculosis

31d The correct statement regarding nonspecific interstitial pneumonia is:

    A. Five-year survival in fibrotic NSIP is similar to that in IPF.
    B. If honeycombing is a predominant feature, biopsy should be performed.
    C. Histologic evidence of NSIP is enough for final diagnosis of idiopathic form.
    D. Response to corticosteroids is variable depending on NSIP type.

32a Review these CT axial images obtained from a 48-year-old man with dyspnea on exertion and a strong smoking history. The most likely diagnosis is:

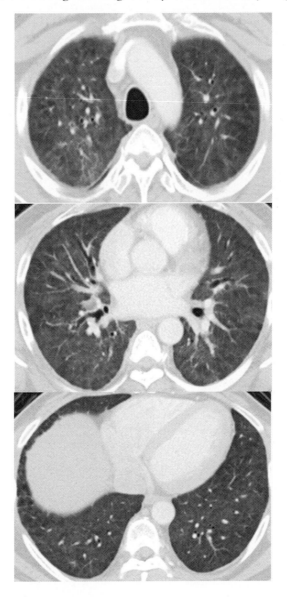

    A. Usual interstitial pneumonia
    B. Desquamative interstitial pneumonia
    C. Pulmonary edema
    D. Hypersensitivity pneumonitis

32b Desquamative interstitial pneumonia:

    A. Is highly associated with smoking
    B. Has similar distribution of findings to respiratory bronchiolitis
    C. Most frequently presents with a severe obstructive pattern on spirometry
    D. Is almost always associated with subpleural cysts

33a Please review frontal chest radiograph obtained in a 26-year-old female with severe respiratory failure. Imaging findings would be most typical of:

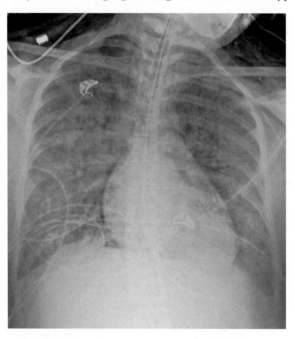

    A. Cardiogenic pulmonary edema
    B. Noncardiogenic pulmonary edema
    C. Lobar pneumonia
    D. Aspiration

33b CT axial images obtained from an otherwise healthy young patient with acute onset of respiratory failure leading to an emergent intubation. The best explanation for the underlying mechanism responsible for these imaging abnormalities is:

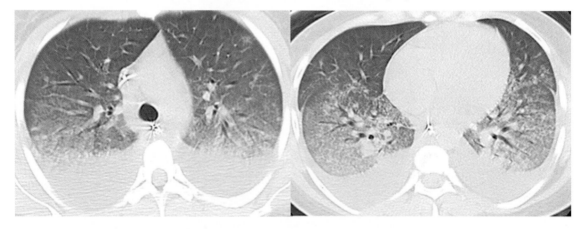

    A. Accumulation of lipoproteinaceous material in the alveoli
    B. Replacement of alveoli and interstitium by fibroblasts
    C. Diffuse alveolar damage
    D. Increased oncotic pressure

33c CT axial images from the same patient several months later. The pattern of fibrosis is likely caused by:

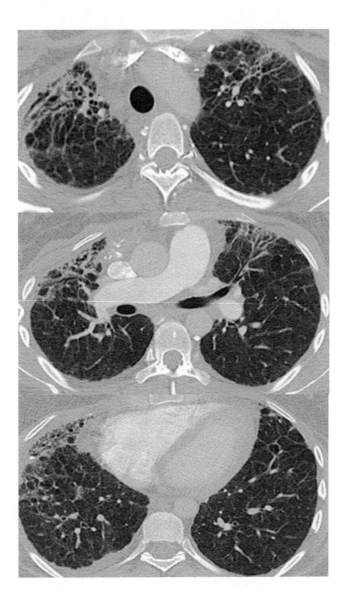

A. Nonspecific interstitial pneumonia
B. Fibroproliferative ARDS
C. Sarcoid
D. Idiopathic pulmonary fibrosis

33d In diffuse alveolar damage (DAD):

A. The survival in acute and organizing phase of DAD is similar.
B. DAD is unlikely to be present in accelerated idiopathic pulmonary fibrosis.
C. There is clear demarcation between acute and chronic lung parenchymal changes in DAD.
D. Recovery correlates with degree of basement membrane damage and reparative processes.

34a A 72-year-old female with fatigue. Differential diagnosis favors:

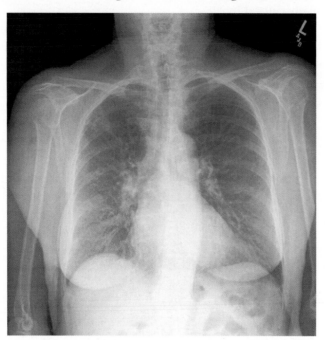

    A. Emphysema
    B. Pulmonary edema
    C. Lymphangitic carcinomatosis
    D. Silicosis

34b Please review CT images. Imaging findings include:

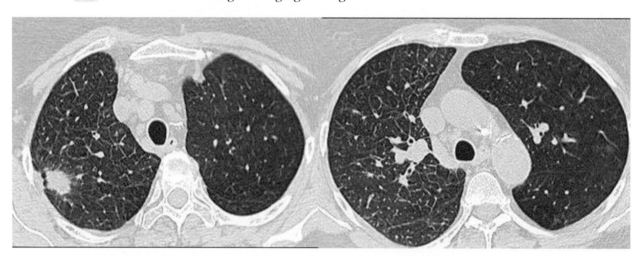

    A. Distortion of normal lung architecture
    B. Honeycombing
    C. Interstitial fibrosis
    D. Nodular interstitial thickening

34c The best next step to do is:
    A. Trial of antibiotics
    B. Trial of corticosteroid
    C. Oncology consult
    D. Wedge resection of lung nodule

34d The most common malignancy associated with lymphangitic carcinomatosis is:

    A. Bronchogenic adenocarcinoma

    B. Breast adenocarcinoma

    C. Gastric adenocarcinoma

    D. Colonic adenocarcinoma

35 Given the radiograph and the corresponding chest CT findings, what is the likely cause of interlobular septal thickening in this patient?

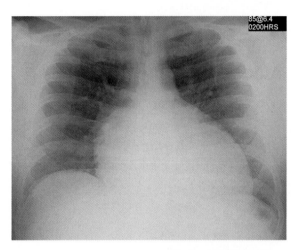 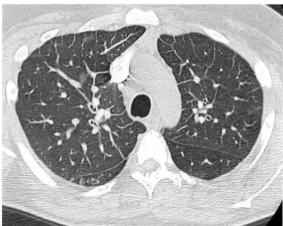

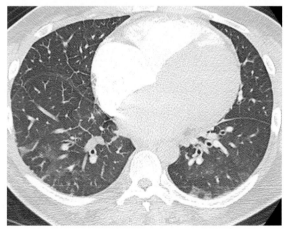

    A. Cardiogenic pulmonary edema

    B. Fibrotic interstitial lung disease

    C. Lymphangitic carcinomatosis

    D. Lymphangiectasia

Section 3: Diffuse Alveolar Disease and Inflammatory Conditions

36a What radiographic pattern best describes the CXR appearance?

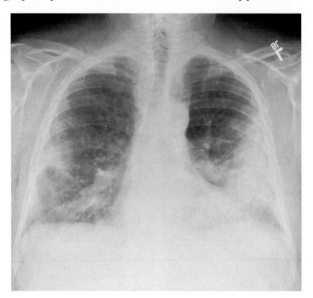

A. Reticular
B. Nodular
C. Pleural thickening
D. Consolidation

36b Chest CT on the same patient obtained 6 months later. Which of the following causes would best explain the imaging findings?

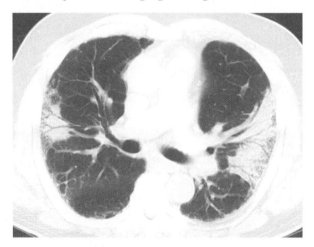

A. Lipoid pneumonia
B. Acute respiratory distress syndrome (ARDS)
C. Bacterial pneumonia
D. Pulmonary embolism

36c What is the preferential treatment for exogenous lipoid pneumonia?
A. Bronchoalveolar lavage
B. Removal of the offending agent
C. Corticosteroids
D. Broad-spectrum antibiotics

37a Which radiographic finding best supports characterizing the pulmonary opacities below as consolidation?

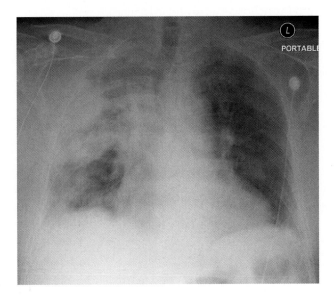

    A. Volume loss
    B. Outlines minor fissure
    C. Presence of "tram-track" opacities
    D. Peripheral distribution

37b A follow-up CT is obtained. Which lobe demonstrates the greatest degree of pulmonary consolidation?

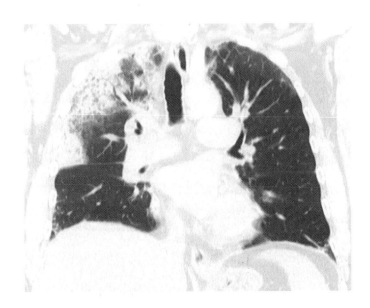

    A. Right middle lobe
    B. Left upper lobe
    C. Lingula
    D. Right upper lobe

37c Patient condition resolves spontaneously after 1 month and undergoes follow-up chest radiograph (left). Months later, the patient's symptoms return with repeat chest radiograph (right). What would be the most likely finding on pathology from bronchoscopic alveolar lavage?

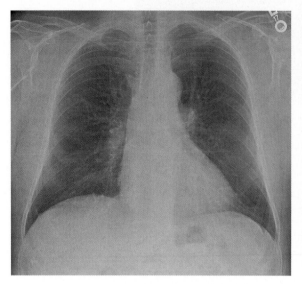 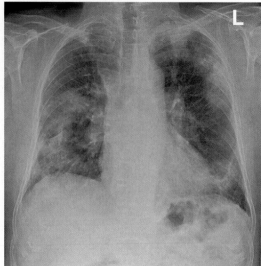

A. Poorly differentiated adenocarcinoma
B. Lipid-rich material
C. Lymphoma
D. Eosinophils

37d What characteristic finding best differentiates simple eosinophilic pneumonia from chronic eosinophilic pneumonia?

A. Pulmonary distribution
B. Time course
C. Symptoms
D. Blood eosinophilia

38a Bronchoalveolar lavage demonstrates lightly PAS-positive lipoproteinaceous material on the patient with the CT below. What is the most likely diagnosis?

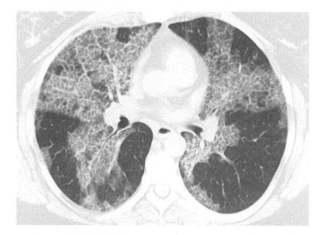

A. Exogenous lipoid pneumonia
B. Pulmonary alveolar proteinosis
C. *Pneumocystis jiroveci* pneumonia
D. Pulmonary edema

38b In idiopathic pulmonary alveolar proteinosis, which association would be most common?

    A. Smoking
    B. Obesity
    C. Female gender
    D. Air travel

39 Chest radiograph following blood product transfusion. The clinical team is worried about the possibility of transfusion-related acute lung injury (TRALI). How long after blood product transfusion does TRALI typically develop?

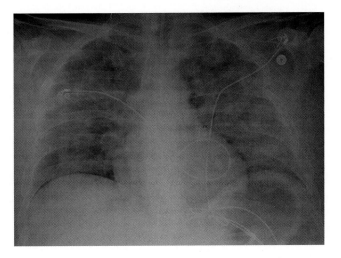

    A. Immediately
    B. 1 to 6 hours
    C. 12 to 24 hours
    D. 24 to 48 hours

40 Inspiratory and expiratory imaging of a nonsmoking patient is obtained. What is the likely diagnosis?

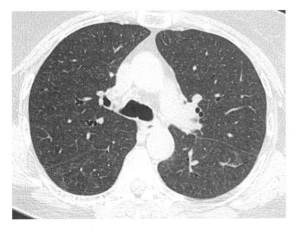 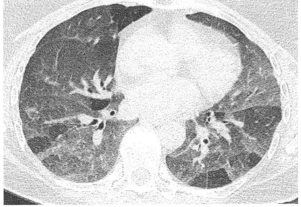

    A. Respiratory bronchiolitis
    B. Hypersensitivity pneumonitis
    C. Organizing pneumonia
    D. Eosinophilic pneumonia

41a What is the most likely etiology of these pulmonary opacities given corresponding symptoms and history of asthma, polyneuropathy, and sinus disease?

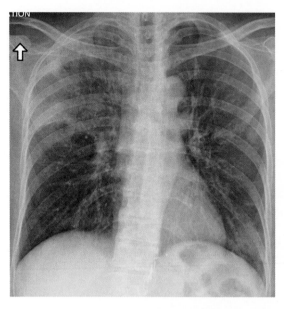
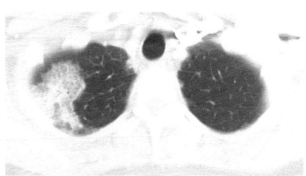

A. Churg-Strauss syndrome (eosinophilic granulomatosis with polyangiitis)
B. Organizing pneumonia
C. Granulomatosis with polyangiitis (Wegener granulomatosis)
D. Microscopic polyangiitis

41b What biomarker is most strongly associated with this disease?

A. cANCA
B. p-ANCA
C. Rheumatoid factor
D. Antiphospholipid antibodies

42 What is the likely diagnosis in this patient with a long-standing history of recurrent urinary tract infections?

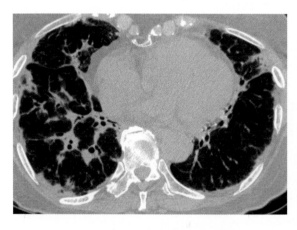
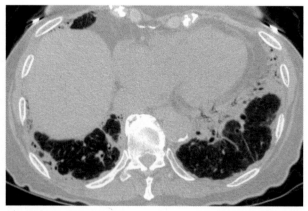

A. Organizing pneumonia
B. Septic emboli
C. Pulmonary hemorrhage
D. Usual interstitial pneumonia

43a What radiologic sign is present on this expiratory CT?

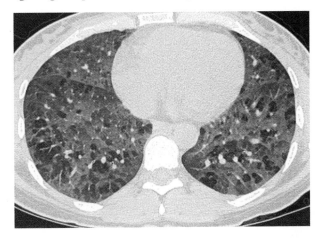

    A. Head cheese sign
    B. Comet tail
    C. Reverse halo
    D. Galaxy sign

43b With what disease is this sign most highly associated?

    A. Hypersensitivity pneumonitis
    B. Organizing pneumonia
    C. Eosinophilic pneumonia
    D. Desquamative interstitial pneumonia

44 This previously healthy 36-year-old male experienced acute-onset worsening shortness of breath after traveling to the mountains for a hiking trip. No fever or chills are present. What is the likely pathology?

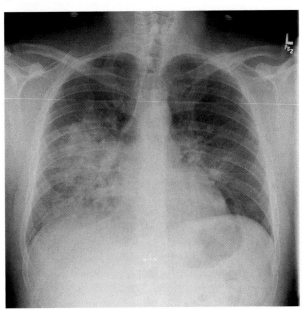

    A. Bronchopneumonia
    B. Non-cardiogenic pulmonary edema
    C. Pulmonary hemorrhage
    D. Cardiogenic pulmonary edema

45 Which of these radiologic signs is present?

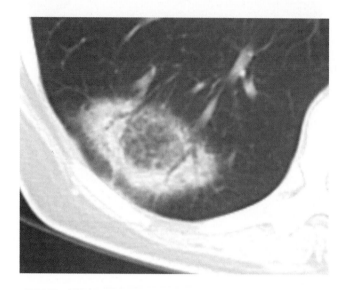

    A. Halo sign
    B. Reverse halo sign
    C. Galaxy sign
    D. Dependent viscera sign

46 What is the likely diagnosis given these inspiratory (left) and expiratory (right) CT images?

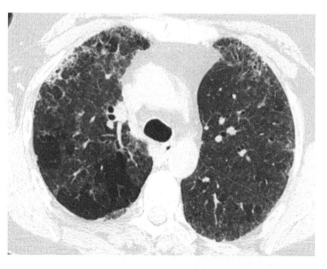
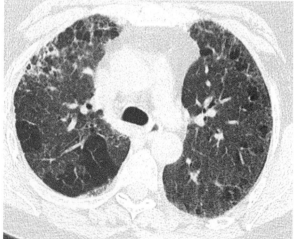

    A. Chronic hypersensitivity pneumonitis
    B. Idiopathic pulmonary fibrosis
    C. Sarcoidosis
    D. Progressive massive fibrosis

Section 4: Airway Disease

47a A 62-year-old female with chronic cough. What are the most salient imaging findings?

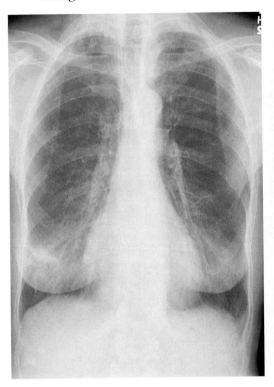 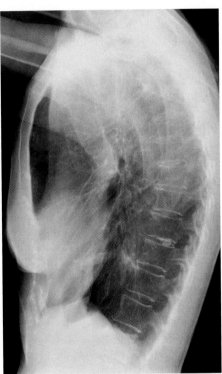

    A. Bronchiectasis and nodularity
    B. Airspace consolidation and scarring
    C. Pleural effusions and hyperinflation
    D. Emphysema and linear atelectasis

47b Which imaging finding is absent below?

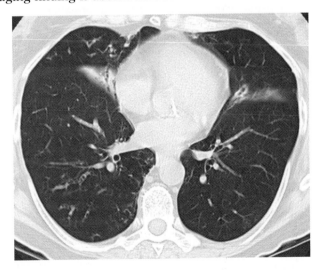

    A. Tree-in-bud nodularity
    B. Bronchiectasis with mucous plugging
    C. Air trapping
    D. Cavitation

47c What is the most likely diagnosis in this patient?

   A. Aspiration
   B. *Mycobacterium avium*-intracellulare (MAI)
   C. Allergic bronchopulmonary aspergillosis (ABPA)
   D. Cystic fibrosis

48a What type of anatomic variant is demonstrated on the image below?

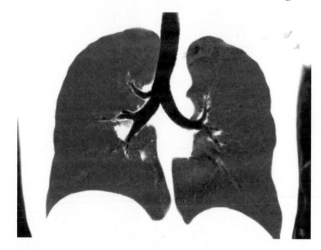

   A. Accessory right upper lobe bronchus
   B. Supernumerary right upper lobe bronchus
   C. Abnormal origin of the right upper lobe bronchus
   D. Abnormal segmental subdivision of the right upper lobe bronchus

48b What is the most specific term for the anatomic variant depicted?

   A. Tracheal bronchus
   B. Pig bronchus
   C. Cardiac bronchus
   D. Tracheal diverticulum

49a Inspiratory and dynamic expiratory CT images are provided. What is the diagnosis?

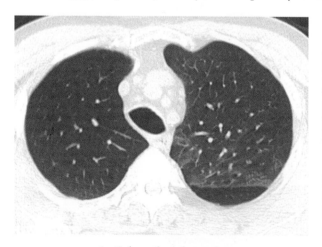
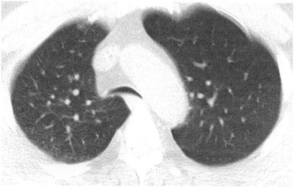

   A. Saber sheath trachea
   B. Tracheal diverticulum
   C. Tracheobronchitis
   D. Tracheomalacia

49b On inspiratory CT images, which is highly specific of tracheobronchomalacia?

    A. Saber-sheath trachea
    B. Lunate trachea
    C. Tracheal wall thickening
    D. Frown sign

50a Based on the imaging findings below, what would be the most likely diagnosis?

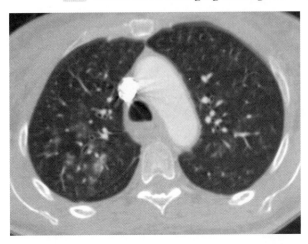
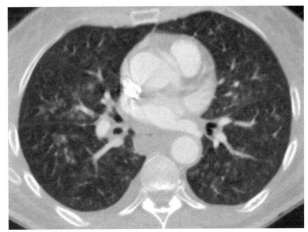

    A. Aspiration-related lung disease
    B. Lung contusions
    C. Endobronchial masses with postobstructive changes
    D. Cystic fibrosis

50b Which of the following are not considered imaging findings on CT of aspiration-related lung disease?

    A. Airway thickening and airway opacification
    B. Tree-in-bud nodularity with bilateral lower lobe distribution
    C. Centrilobular ground-glass opacities
    D. Randomly distributed lung nodules

51 The patient presents with shortness of breath. Based on the images below, which one of the following is the most likely diagnosis?

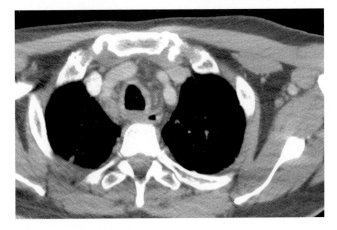

    A. Granulomatosis with polyangiitis
    B. Postintubation stenosis
    C. Tracheal neoplasm
    D. Tracheobronchopathia osteochondroplastica

52 What is the most likely diagnosis of the imaging findings below?

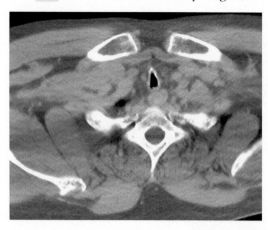
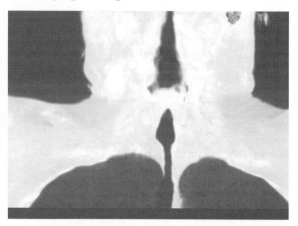

A. Postintubation tracheal stenosis secondary to prior tracheostomy
B. Granulomatosis with polyangiitis
C. Tracheobronchopathia osteochondroplastica (TBPO)
D. Squamous cell carcinoma

53a What imaging findings are present below?

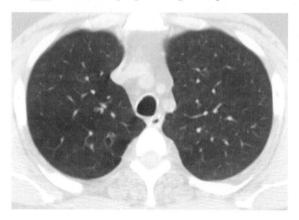
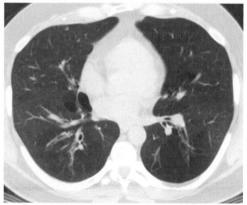

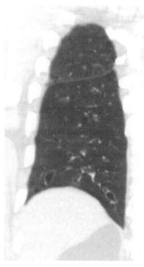
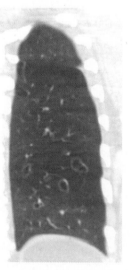

A. Bronchiectasis and mosaic attenuation pattern of the lungs
B. Lung cysts and mosaic attenuation pattern of the lungs
C. Bronchiectasis and tree-in-bud opacities
D. Lung cysts and nodules

53b Which one of the following is the most likely diagnosis?

    A. Cystic fibrosis

    B. Asthma

    C. Bronchiolitis obliterans

    D. Allergic bronchopulmonary aspergillosis

54a What imaging finding is present on this exam?

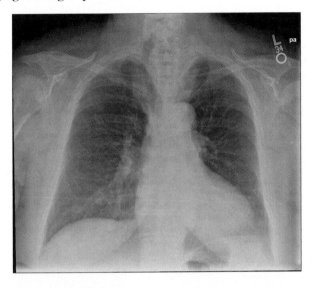

    A. Postintubation tracheal stenosis

    B. Bronchiectasis

    C. Tracheobronchomegaly

    D. Extrinsic compression of the trachea

54b Given the corresponding CT, what is the most likely diagnosis?

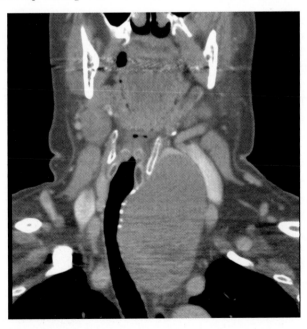

    A. Thyroid cyst/nodule

    B. Squamous cell carcinoma of the trachea

    C. Foregut duplication cyst

    D. Left common carotid artery aneurysm

55a What is the most common primary malignant neoplasm of the trachea?

    A. Squamous cell carcinoma
    B. Mucoepidermoid carcinoma
    C. Adenoid cystic carcinoma
    D. Carcinoid

55b What is the most common hematogenously spread metastatic lesion to involve the trachea?

    A. Thyroid cancer
    B. Esophageal cancer
    C. Lung cancer
    D. Melanoma

56a What is the likely diagnosis in this patient?

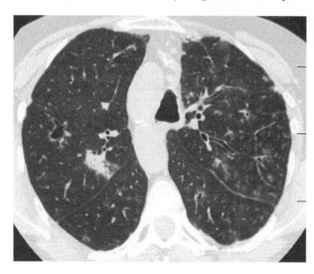 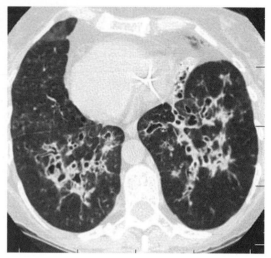

    A. Common variable immunodeficiency (CVID)
    B. Kartagener syndrome
    C. Sarcoid
    D. Diffuse panbronchiolitis

56b What percentage of patients with immotile cilia syndrome have situs inversus totalis?

    A. 10%
    B. 25%
    C. 50%
    D. 100%

57 Which of the following is the most important CT imaging feature for consideration of possible lung volume reduction surgery (LVRS) in the treatment of COPD?

    A. Predominantly upper lung distribution of emphysema
    B. Predominantly centrilobular emphysema
    C. Presence of large bullae
    D. Predominantly panlobular emphysema

58a In the setting of cystic fibrosis, what vessels are the typical source of hemoptysis?

    A. Pulmonary arteries
    B. Hypertrophied bronchial arteries
    C. Internal thoracic (mammary) arteries
    D. Intercostal arteries

58b What treatment is typically recommended for treatment of recurrent hemoptysis in the setting of bronchiectasis with hypertrophied bronchial arteries?

    A. Bronchial artery embolization
    B. Antimicrobial therapy
    C. Steroid therapy
    D. Surgical resection

59a Characterize the radiographic appearance:

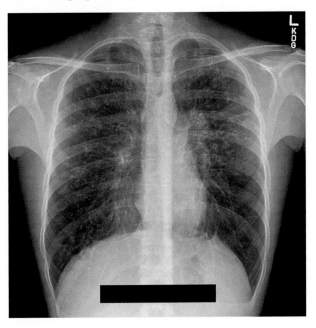

    A. Airway pattern, lower lobe predominant
    B. Nodular pattern, lower lobe predominant
    C. Consolidation, upper lobe predominant
    D. Airway pattern, upper lobe predominant

59b What is the most likely diagnosis on CT in this 27-year-old female (different patient)?

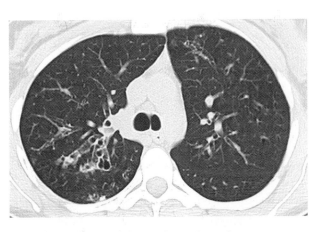 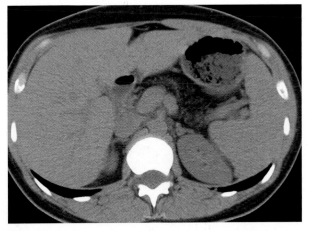

    A. Allergic bronchopulmonary aspergillosis
    B. Cystic fibrosis
    C. Kartagener syndrome
    D. Common variable immunodeficiency

60a Given this chest radiograph, what pattern of emphysema is most likely?

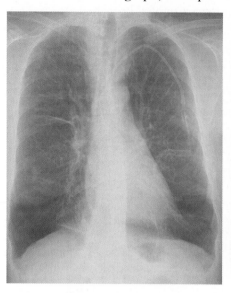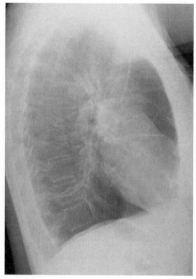

    A. Paraseptal
    B. Centrilobular
    C. Panlobular
    D. Cicatricial

60b Which of the following causes of emphysema is most likely?
    A. Alpha-1 antitrypsin deficiency
    B. Cigarette smoking
    C. HIV infection
    D. Marfan syndrome

60c Besides alpha-1 antitrypsin deficiency, which of the following is most associated with panlobular (panacinar) emphysema?
    A. Marfan syndrome
    B. Smoking
    C. IV methylphenidate abuse
    D. Malnutrition

61a Given the below CT images, what is the most likely diagnosis?

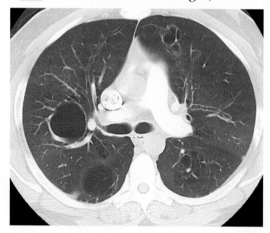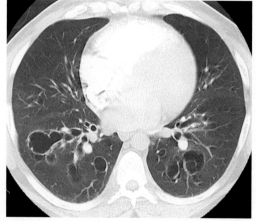

    A. Williams-Campbell
    B. Tracheobronchomegaly (Mounier-Kuhn)
    C. Ciliary dyskinesia
    D. Cystic fibrosis

61b In Williams-Campbell syndrome, what generations of bronchi are affected?

    A. 1 to 2

    B. 3 to 4

    C. 4 to 6

    D. 7-terminal

62 Given the below CT images, what is the most likely diagnosis?

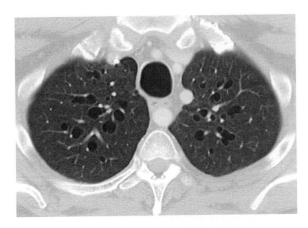 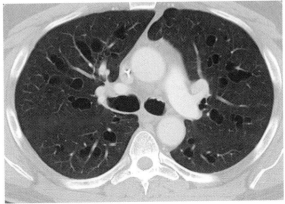

    A. Williams-Campbell

    B. Tracheobronchomegaly (Mounier-Kuhn)

    C. Ciliary dyskinesia

    D. Cystic fibrosis

63 Where is the foreign body located?

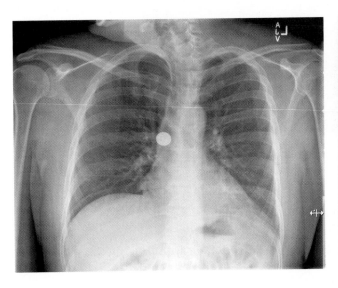 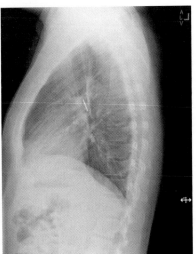

    A. Right mainstem bronchus

    B. Midthoracic esophagus

    C. Right pulmonary artery

    D. Superior right pulmonary vein

Section 5: Thoracic Manifestations of Systemic Disease

64a What is the most likely diagnosis given the constellation of findings?

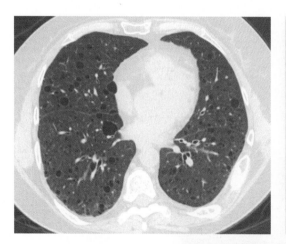
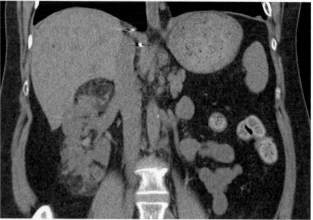

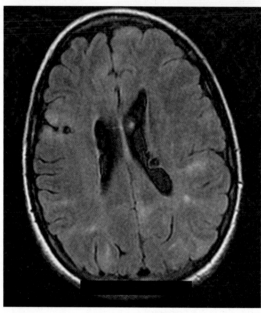

    A. Cystic lymphocytic interstitial pneumonia
    B. Pulmonary Langerhans cell histiocytosis
    C. Tuberous sclerosis
    D. Neurofibromatosis

64b Of the major criteria for tuberous sclerosis, which would be the least common?

    A. Subependymal giant cell tumors
    B. Lymphangioleiomyomatosis
    C. Renal angiomyolipomas
    D. Cardiac rhabdomyomas

65a What best explains the pulmonary opacities in this patient with chronic renal failure?

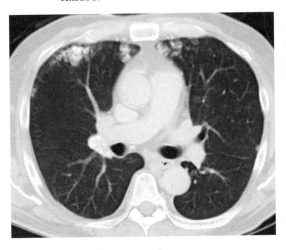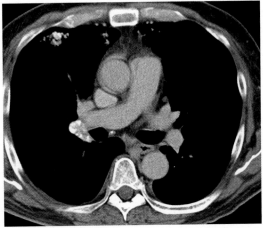

    A. Pulmonary edema
    B. Calcified metastases
    C. Pulmonary fibrosis
    D. Metastatic calcification

65b What percentage of patients who have undergone hemodialysis will have metastatic pulmonary calcification on autopsy?

    A. 10% to 25%
    B. 40% to 55%
    C. 60% to 75%
    D. 95% to 100%

65c Metastatic pulmonary calcification may accelerate in which clinical setting?

    A. Failed renal transplantation
    B. Starting dialysis
    C. Parathyroidectomy
    D. New renal transplantation

66a What is the pertinent finding on soft tissue kernel in this patient with cystic lung disease?

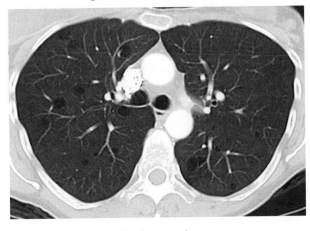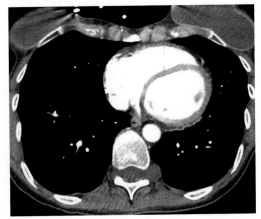

    A. Lymphadenopathy
    B. Intercostal artery aneurysm
    C. Paraspinal mass
    D. Pulmonary nodule

66b What is the most likely diagnosis?

    A. Lymphocytic interstitial pneumonia
    B. Birt-Hogg-Dube syndrome
    C. Langerhans cell histiocytosis
    D. Neurofibromatosis

67 What is the most common pulmonary manifestation of dermatomyositis–polymyositis interstitial lung disease?

    A. Usual interstitial pneumonia
    B. Nonspecific interstitial pneumonia
    C. Granulomatous lymphocytic interstitial lung disease
    D. Lymphoid interstitial pneumonia

68a The pulmonary pattern on radiograph is best be described as:

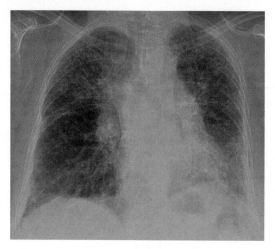

    A. Reticular
    B. Nodules
    C. Consolidation
    D. Bronchiectasis

68b The pulmonary CT pattern in this patient with rheumatoid arthritis is consistent with:

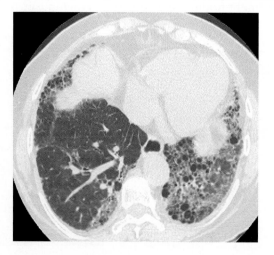

    A. Nonspecific interstitial pneumonia
    B. Usual interstitial pneumonia
    C. Bronchiolitis
    D. Organizing pneumonia

68c What is the most common CT pattern found in patients with rheumatoid arthritis?

    A. Nonspecific interstitial pneumonia
    B. Usual interstitial pneumonia
    C. Bronchiolitis
    D. Organizing pneumonia

69a The pulmonary pattern is:

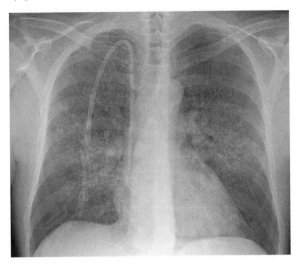

    A. Reticular
    B. Consolidation
    C. Cystic
    D. Nodular

69b Which cause of consolidation would support Goodpasture syndrome?

    A. Pulmonary edema
    B. Aspiration
    C. Alveolar proteinosis
    D. Pulmonary hemorrhage

70a What is the diagnosis?

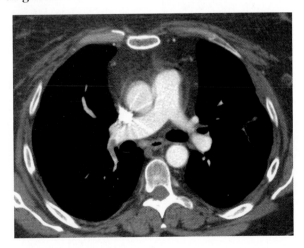

    A. Pulmonary artery hypertension
    B. Pulmonary embolism
    C. Pulmonary edema
    D. Pulmonary hemorrhage

70b Which of the following autoimmune disorders has the highest risk of pulmonary embolism?

    A. Sögren syndrome
    B. Systemic lupus erythematosus
    C. Systemic sclerosis
    D. Wegener granulomatosis

70c Which of the following is the most common thoracic complication of systemic lupus erythematosus?

    A. Pulmonary parenchymal disease
    B. Pulmonary artery hypertension
    C. Pleural effusion
    D. Lymphoma

71a What is the most common clinical circumstance associated with death in adult patients with sickle cell anemia?

    A. Cerebral vascular accident
    B. Myocardial infarction
    C. Aortic dissection
    D. Acute chest syndrome

71b What medical imaging finding on this CT is required to diagnose acute chest syndrome?

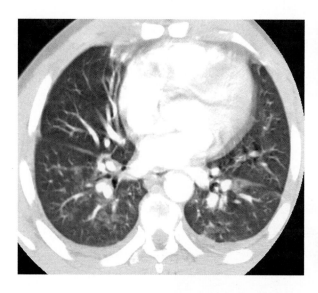 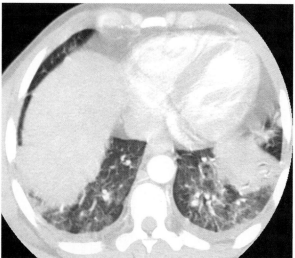

    A. Consolidation
    B. Pleural effusion
    C. Pulmonary embolism
    D. Cardiomegaly

72a Which systemic disease best correlates with the CT findings?

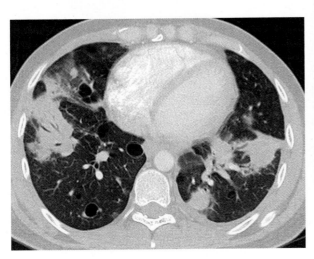
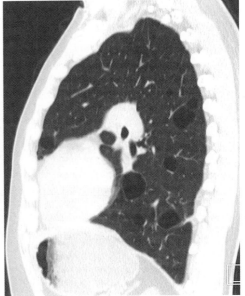

    A. Diabetes mellitus
    B. Granulomatosis with polyangiitis
    C. Hepatopulmonary syndrome
    D. Sögren syndrome

72b Chronic consolidation in the setting of Sögren syndrome raises concern for which complication?

    A. Lymphoma
    B. Sarcoidosis
    C. Alveolar proteinosis
    D. Lipoid pneumonia

73a What finding on the chest radiograph suggests granulomatosis with polyangiitis?

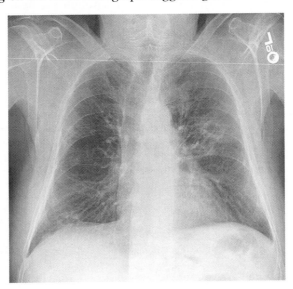

    A. Right apical cap
    B. Pulmonary cavitation
    C. Atherosclerotic aorta
    D. Deviated trachea

73b Cavitation of pulmonary nodules occurs in what percentage of granulomatosis with polyangiitis cases?

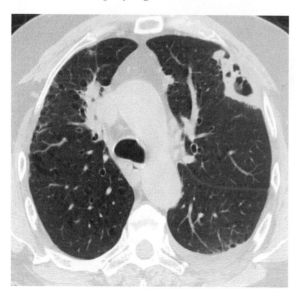 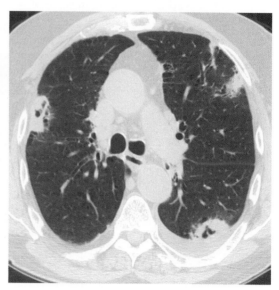

A. 5%
B. 25%
C. 50%
D. 85%

73c What system is the most likely to be involved in granulomatosis with polyangiitis?

A. Upper respiratory tract
B. Lungs
C. Kidneys
D. Liver

74a What percentage of cases with rheumatoid nodules demonstrate cavitation on CT?

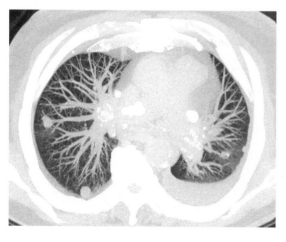 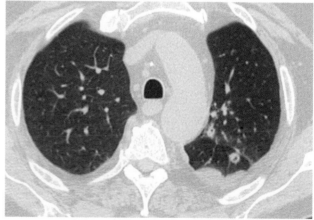

A. 0% to 10%
B. 25%
C. 50%
D. 90% to 100%

74b Given the mediastinal findings, what is a consideration in this patient with rheumatoid arthritis and history of coal mining?

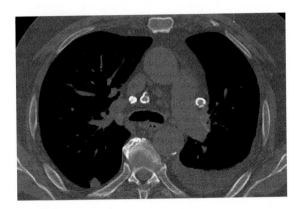

    A. Carney triad
    B. Caplan syndrome
    C. Sögren syndrome
    D. Heerfordt syndrome

75 What chest CT finding suggests hepatopulmonary syndrome in the setting of cirrhosis?

    A. Main pulmonary artery enlargement
    B. Pulmonary fibrosis
    C. Interstitial thickening and ground-glass opacities
    D. Dilated peripheral pulmonary vessels

76 What is the most likely diagnosis associated with this patient's chronic low lung volumes?

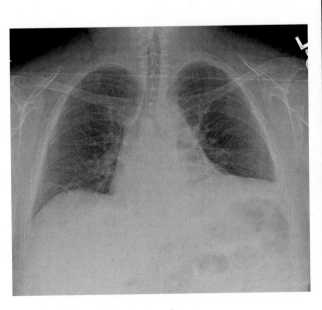 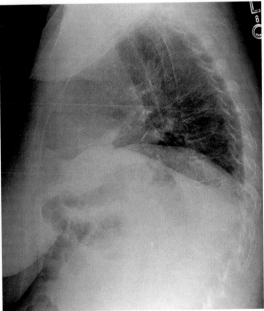

    A. Sögren syndrome
    B. Systemic sclerosis
    C. Systemic lupus erythematosus
    D. Granulomatosis with polyangiitis

77a These inspiratory and expiratory CT images are consistent with which disease?

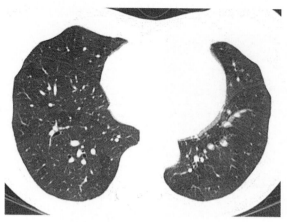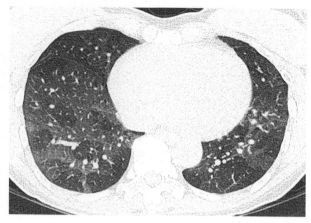

    A. Emphysema
    B. Nonspecific interstitial pneumonia
    C. Obliterative bronchiolitis
    D. Organizing pneumonia

77b Obliterative bronchiolitis is most commonly associated with which collagen vascular disease?

    A. Rheumatoid arthritis
    B. Systemic lupus erythematosus
    C. Scleroderma
    D. Mixed connective tissue disease

78a Which collagen vascular disease is most likely to cause the CT finding?

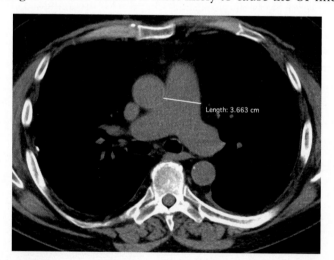

    A. Sögren syndrome
    B. Systemic sclerosis
    C. Polymyositis–dermatomyositis
    D. Systemic lupus erythematosus

78b What is the commonest pattern of lung parenchymal injury in systemic sclerosis?

    A. NSIP
    B. UIP
    C. Obliterative bronchiolitis
    D. Organizing pneumonia

Section 6: Atelectasis and Collapse

79a A 65-year-old woman presents with cough and an abnormal chest radiograph. Which radiologic sign is present?

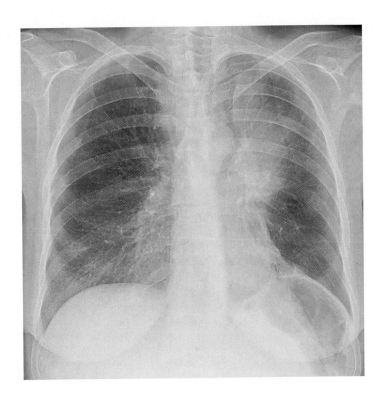

A. Flat waist sign
B. Luftsichel sign
C. S sign of Golden
D. Comet tail sign

79b What is the underlying abnormality?

A. Left upper lobe collapse
B. Lingular collapse
C. Pneumonia
D. Left lower lobe collapse

79c What is responsible for creating the air crescent or Luftsichel sign?

A. Left upper lobe bronchus
B. Superior segment of left lower lobe
C. Anterior segment of left upper lobe
D. Lingula

79d What is the most likely diagnosis?

A. Hamartoma
B. Foreign body
C. Mucus plug
D. Lung cancer

80a A 45-year-old intubated man undergoes chest radiography for sudden hypoxia (left). Comparison radiograph from hours later is also shown (right). What is likely responsible for the desaturation event?

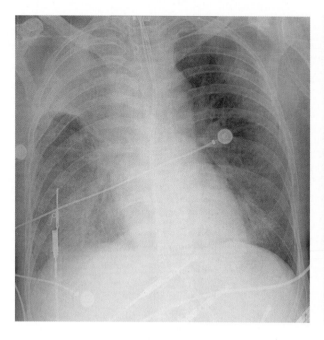 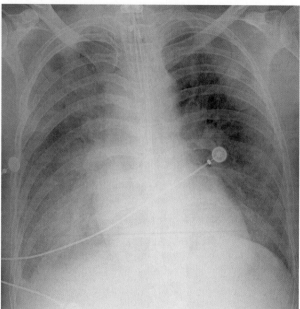

A. Pneumonia
B. Pulmonary edema
C. Enlarging pleural effusion
D. Right upper lobe atelectasis

80b What is a direct radiographic sign of volume loss?

A. Displacement of the minor fissure
B. Pulmonary opacity
C. Tracheal shift
D. Right hemidiaphragm elevation

80c What is the most likely cause for this patient's right upper lobe atelectasis?

A. Hamartoma
B. Foreign body
C. Mucus plug
D. Lung cancer

81 On follow-up radiograph, a shift in the location of a parenchymal abnormality due to changes in the degree of atelectasis is referred to as what radiologic sign?

A. "Shifting granuloma" sign
B. "Moving atelectasis" sign
C. "Changing places" sign
D. "Sliding nodule" sign

82a A 70-year-old man undergoes chest radiography for chest pain. What is the most significant abnormality?

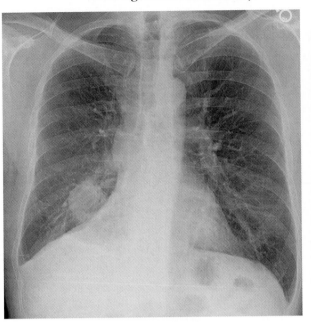 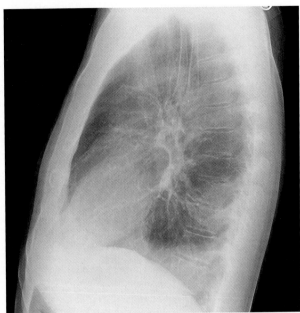

A. Pulmonary mass
B. Pulmonary nodule
C. Pleural effusion
D. Lobar collapse

82b A CT is obtained. What is the most likely diagnosis?

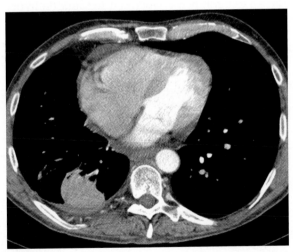

A. Rounded atelectasis
B. Lung cancer
C. Hamartoma
D. Pneumonia

82c Which of the following features is essential to diagnose rounded atelectasis?

A. Pleural plaque
B. FDG activity above mediastinal blood pool
C. Round mass
D. Volume loss of affected lobe

83a An intubated 50-year-old man has a daily portable chest radiograph. What is the most likely cause of the perihilar and basal lung opacities given no fever and a normal white blood cell count?

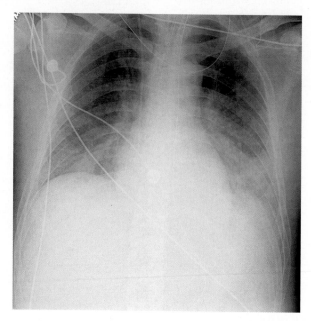

A. Pulmonary edema
B. Malignancy
C. Pleural effusions
D. Pneumonia

83b Four hours later, a radiograph was obtained for sudden hypoxia. What is the abnormality?

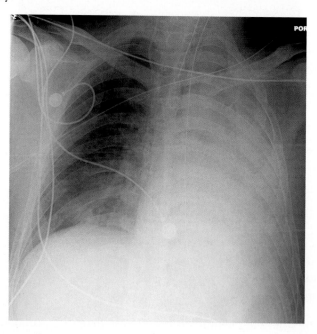

A. Increasing pulmonary edema
B. Pneumonia
C. Pneumothorax
D. Complete left lung atelectasis

83c What is the most likely cause of atelectasis?

    A. Carcinoid

    B. Foreign body aspiration

    C. Mucus plug

    D. Lung cancer

84a A 45-year-old woman with lupus undergoes CT for chest pain. What is the likely etiology of the opacity adjacent to the pleural effusion?

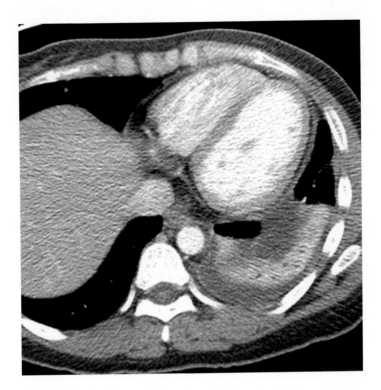

    A. Pneumonia

    B. Lung cancer

    C. Atelectasis

    D. Infarct

84b Which of the following types of atelectasis best characterizes the abnormality?

    A. Relaxation

    B. Adhesive

    C. Cicatricial

    D. Resorption

85 What best describes the role of prone imaging in the evaluation of possible diffuse lung disease by high-resolution CT (HRCT)?

    A. Differentiate honeycomb cyst formation from bronchiolectasis

    B. Separate dependent atelectasis from mild subpleural opacity

    C. Confirm the presence of lower lung traction bronchiectasis

    D. Distinguish round atelectasis from a pulmonary mass

86a A 68-year-old woman presents with progressive dyspnea and cough. PA and lateral radiographs are obtained. What is the abnormality?

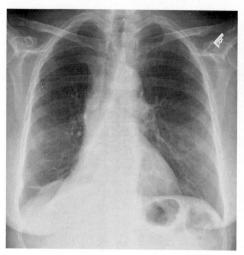 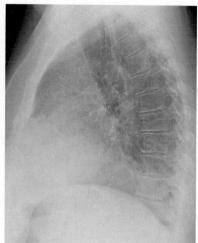

    A. Pneumonia
    B. AP window lymphadenopathy
    C. Loculated pleural effusion
    D. Atelectasis

86b Which lobe or lobes are collapsed?

    A. Right upper lobe
    B. Right lower lobe
    C. Right middle lobe
    D. Right lower and middle lobes

86c Which fissures are visible on the frontal radiograph?

    A. Right minor fissure only
    B. Right major fissure only
    C. Left major fissure only
    D. Right major and right minor fissures

86d A chest CT is obtained. What is the most likely diagnosis?

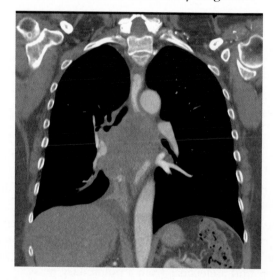

    A. Lung cancer
    B. Foreign body
    C. Mucus plug
    D. Carcinoid

87a A 55-year-old man presents with dyspnea to his primary care physician and undergoes chest radiography. What is the abnormality?

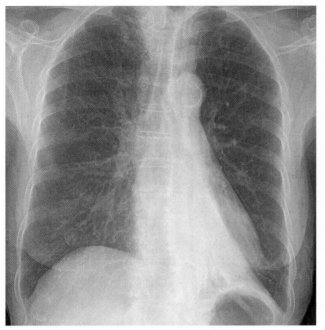
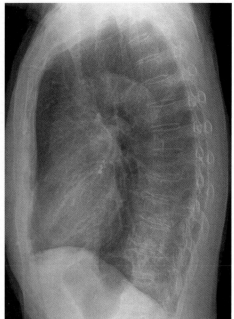

    A. Pneumonia
    B. Mediastinal mass
    C. Loculated pleural effusion
    D. Lobar atelectasis

87b Which sign may be seen with this condition?

    A. S sign of Golden
    B. Flat waist sign
    C. Comet tail sign
    D. Luftsichel sign

87c What sign is present on the lateral radiograph?

    A. Spine sign
    B. Doughnut sign
    C. Fat pad sign
    D. Comet tail sign

87d What is the likely etiology of lobar collapse in an adult who presents to his/her primary care physician?

    A. Lung cancer
    B. Foreign body
    C. Mucus plug
    D. Aspiration

88a A 48-year-old man presents with chronic cough to a pulmonologist who orders a chest radiograph. What is the abnormality?

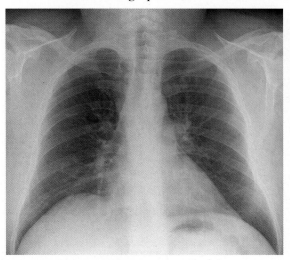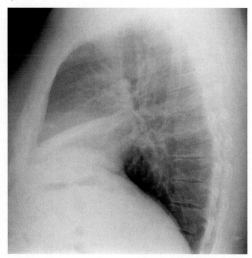

    A. Pneumonia
    B. Lobar atelectasis
    C. Lung mass
    D. Mediastinal lymphadenopathy

88b Which anatomic structure abuts the superior portion of the opacity on the lateral chest radiograph?

    A. Minor fissure
    B. Major fissure
    C. Intermediate stem line
    D. Right hilar vascular opacity

88c A CT is performed and reveals no centrally obstructing lesion. A review of the patient's abdominal CT from years earlier shows no interval change. What is the most common cause of this condition in adults?

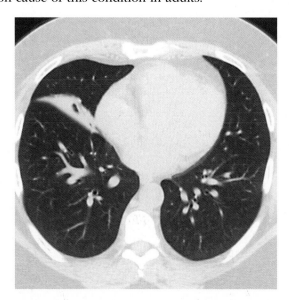

    A. Sarcoidosis
    B. Pneumoconiosis
    C. Benign tumor
    D. Nonobstructive inflammatory conditions

88d What is the most common cause of this condition in childhood?

    A. Cystic fibrosis

    B. Asthma

    C. Carcinoid tumor

    D. Foreign body aspiration

89a A 55-year-old man presents with dyspnea to his primary care physician and undergoes chest radiography. What is the abnormality?

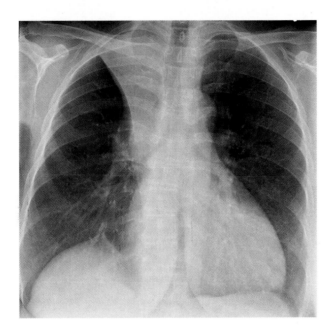

    A. Pneumonia

    B. Mediastinal mass

    C. Loculated pleural effusion

    D. Lobar atelectasis

89b What sign is present?

    A. S sign of Golden

    B. Flat waist sign

    C. Comet tail sign

    D. Luftsichel sign

89c What is the significance of the S sign of Golden?

    A. Central mass

    B. Foreign body

    C. Mucus plug

    D. Pneumonia

89d What is the density of the tumor?

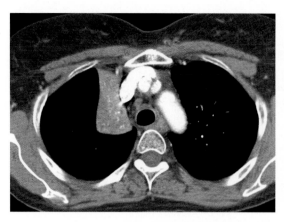 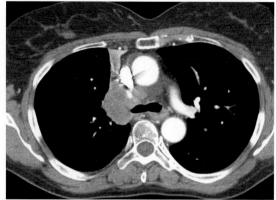

    A. Calcified
    B. Soft tissue
    C. Water
    D. Cavitary

90a An intubated premature infant with surfactant deficiency has a daily chest radiograph showing diffuse fine granular airspace opacities (left). Two hours later, a repeat radiograph (right) was performed for sudden desaturation. What is responsible for the imaging appearance?

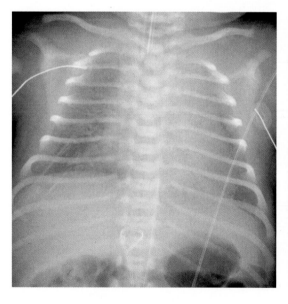 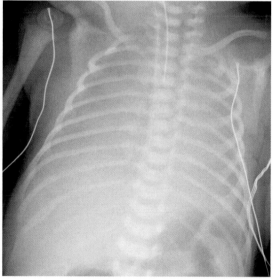

    A. Atelectasis
    B. Pulmonary edema
    C. Pneumonia
    D. Aspiration

90b Which of the following types of atelectasis best characterizes the abnormality?
    A. Relaxation
    B. Adhesive
    C. Cicatricial
    D. Resorption

Section 7: Pulmonary Physiology

91a A 67-year-old male with a 50 pack-year smoking history presents for evaluation of shortness of breath. Spirogram was done in the office and shows these results. What is the pattern described in the spirogram?

	ACTUAL	PREDICTED	% PREDICTED
FVC (L)	2.42	2.47	98
FEV$_1$ (L)	1.09	1.82	60
FEV$_1$/FVC (%)	45		

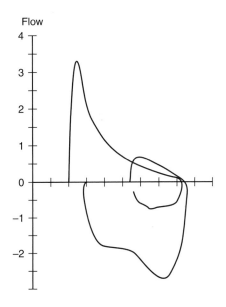

A. Airway obstruction
B. Variable intrathoracic obstruction
C. Restriction
D. Hyperinflation

91b What disease process most likely explains those findings?

A. Vocal cord dysfunction
B. Idiopathic pulmonary fibrosis
C. Chronic obstructive pulmonary disease
D. Tracheal stenosis

92a A 65-year-old male presents complaining of shortness of breath and cough. He has smoked 1 pack per day of cigarettes for the last 40 years. He worked for several years exposed to asbestos. Spirogram and lung volumes done in the office showed these results. What is the pattern described in the spirogram?

	ACTUAL	PREDICTED	% PREDICTED
FVC (L)	2.73	4.27	64
FEV₁ (L)	2.19	3.17	69
FEV₁/FVC (%)	80%		
TLC	4.67	6.49	72
RV	1.59	2.34	68
FRC	2.30	3.83	60

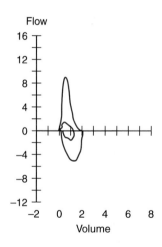

A. Airway obstruction
B. Variable intrathoracic obstruction
C. Restriction
D. Air trapping

92b What disease process most likely explains these findings?

A. Chronic obstructive pulmonary disease
B. Bronchiolitis obliterans
C. Asbestosis
D. Tracheal stenosis

93 A 32-year-old male undergoes pulmonary function testing as part of a pre-employment examination. He has no respiratory complaints. He has never smoked, but he had significant secondhand smoke exposure. The pulmonary function test shows these results. What disease process most likely explains these findings?

	ACTUAL	PREDICTED	% PREDICTED
FVC (L)	5.25	5.12	103
FEV$_1$ (L)	3.80	4.04	94
FEV$_1$/FVC (%)	72		
TLC (L)	6.69	6.83	98
RV (L)	1.52	1.69	90
FRC (L)	3.30	3.36	98
DLCO (mL/min/mm Hg)	18.8	19	99

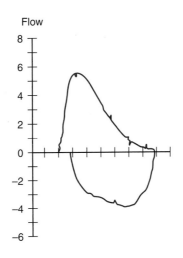

A. Pulmonary vascular disease.
B. No disease is apparent.
C. Chronic obstructive pulmonary disease.
D. Pulmonary fibrosis.

94a A 24-year-old male presents for evaluation to the clinic. He has had shortness of breath on exertion for the last 5 years but has progressed significantly in the last 3 months. He is a lifelong nonsmoker. On exam, he shows wheezing and oxygen saturation is 91% on ambient air. A spirogram with bronchodilator administration is performed with these results. What is the most accurate interpretation of this study?

	PRETREATMENT			POSTTREATMENT		
	ACTUAL	PREDICTED	% PREDICTED	ACTUAL	% PREDICTED	% CHANGE
FVC (L)	4.34	5.57	78	4.40	79	79
FEV₁ (L)	1.60	4.61	35	1.76	38	10
FEV₁/FVC (%)	37			40		

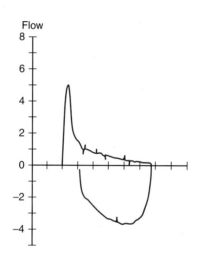

A. Moderate obstruction with reversibility
B. Moderate obstruction without reversibility
C. Severe obstruction with reversibility
D. Severe obstruction without reversibility

94b What is the most likely diagnosis?

A. Asthma
B. Pulmonary fibrosis
C. Primary pulmonary hypertension
D. Alpha-1 antitrypsin deficiency

95 A 25-year-old female presents for evaluation of dyspnea on exertion. She has smoked 1 pack per day for the last 5 years. She has seasonal allergies for which she takes loratadine. A spirogram with bronchodilator is done at the office. What is the most accurate description of this test?

	PRETREATMENT			POSTTREATMENT	
	ACTUAL	PREDICTED	% PREDICTED	ACTUAL	% CHANGE
FVC (L)	4.40	4.37	101	4.46	1
FEV$_1$ (L)	2.72	3.65	75	3.08	13
FEV$_1$/FVC (%)	62			69	

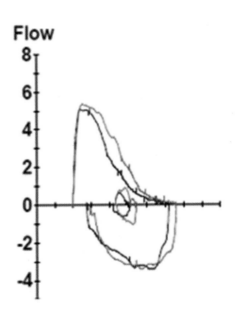

A. Airway obstruction without bronchodilator response
B. Restrictive pattern without bronchodilator response
C. Airway obstruction with bronchodilator response
D. Restrictive pattern with bronchodilator response

96 A 45-year-old female presents for evaluation of dyspnea and wheezing. She is a lifelong nonsmoker. She had a motor vehicle accident 3 years ago for which she required prolonged mechanical ventilation and a tracheostomy that was removed several weeks after her recovery. The spirogram and flow–volume loops are shown. What is the most accurate description of this test?

	ACTUAL	PREDICTED	% PREDICTED
FVC (L)	1.86	3.10	60
FEV$_1$ (L)	1.26	2.82	45
FEV$_1$/FVC (%)	68		

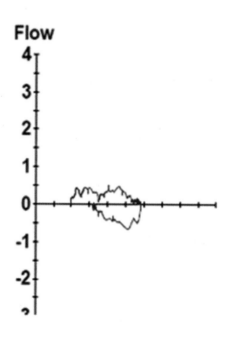

A. Variable intrathoracic obstruction
B. Fixed airway obstruction
C. Variable extrathoracic obstruction
D. Restriction

97 A 60-year-old female is seen in clinic for a 4-month history of shortness of breath and wheezing after climbing one flight of stairs. She has no chest pain or cough but has had intermittent hoarseness. What is the most likely diagnosis?

	ACTUAL	PREDICTED	% PREDICTED
FVC (L)	2.78	2.90	96
FEV$_1$ (L)	1.81	2.19	83
FEV$_1$/FVC (%)	65		

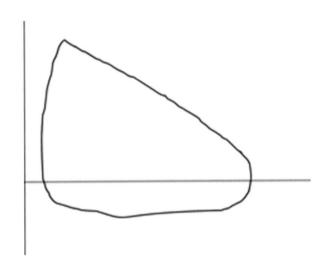

A. Vocal cord dysfunction
B. Tracheomalacia
C. Tracheal stenosis
D. Emphysema

98 A 65-year-old morbidly obese female is seen in clinic for shortness of breath. Spirogram shows the following flow–volume loop. What is the most likely diagnosis?

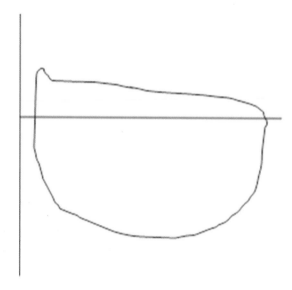

A. Vocal cord dysfunction
B. Tracheomalacia
C. Tracheal stenosis
D. Emphysema

99a A 50-year-old man with a 65 pack-year smoking history presents with cough. A selected CT image and pulmonary function test are provided. What is the most accurate description of the pulmonary function test? Where is the pulmonary function test?

	ACTUAL	PREDICTED	% PREDICTED
FVC (L)	1.90	3.06	62
FEV$_1$ (L)	1.10	2.61	42
FEV$_1$/FVC (%)	58		
TLC (L)	3.00	4.68	64
RV (L)	1.40	1.31	107
DLCO (mL/min/mm Hg)	10.4	26	40

A. Moderate airway obstruction and restriction
B. Moderate airway obstruction and hyperinflation
C. Severe airway obstruction and restriction
D. Severe airway obstruction and hyperinflation

99b What is the most likely diagnosis?

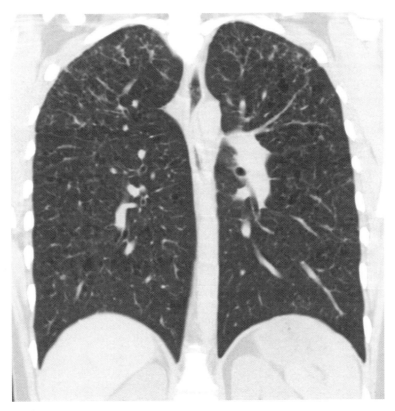

A. Chronic obstructive pulmonary disease
B. Idiopathic pulmonary fibrosis
C. Pulmonary Langerhans cell histiocytosis
D. Obliterative bronchiolitis

100a A 70-year-old male presents for evaluation of dyspnea on exertion. He has a 60 pack-year of smoking. His spirogram and lung volumes are shown. What is the most accurate description of this test?

	ACTUAL	PREDICTED	% PREDICTED
FVC (L)	2.06	4.58	45
FEV$_1$ (L)	0.90	3.60	25
FEV$_1$/FVC (%)	44		
TLC (L)	8.30	6.41	129
RV (L)	3.00	2.31	130
DLCO (mL/min/mm Hg)	12	24	50

A. Very severe airway obstruction, restriction, and air trapping
B. Very severe airway obstruction, hyperinflation, and air trapping
C. Very severe airway obstruction, restriction, and no air trapping
D. Very severe airway obstruction, hyperinflation, and no air trapping

100b What disease process is the most likely?

A. Chronic obstructive pulmonary disease

B. Idiopathic pulmonary fibrosis

C. Sarcoidosis

D. Primary pulmonary hypertension

ANSWERS AND EXPLANATIONS

Section 1: Infectious Pneumonia

1a **Answer D.**

1b **Answer B.**   The image provided is of a patient with an acute presentation of AIDS and respiratory failure due to a coinfection with cytomegalovirus (CMV) and *Pneumocystis jiroveci* (PJ).

However, differentiation between CMV and PJ pneumonia is challenging as both can manifest with ground-glass opacities, crazy paving, consolidation, as well as those signs mentioned above. For this reason, cultures and serum markers are important adjuncts to CT in the diagnosis of CMV and PJ pneumonia.

Different infections have typical CD4+ cell count levels in which they appear in HIV patients. PJ pneumonia is an AIDS-defining infection and appears at CD4+ counts <200 cells/mm^3. This is the same level at which other infections such as CMV pneumonia, mycobacterial infection, and toxoplasmosis appear. CD4+ counts below 50 cells/mm^3 are necessary for other infections such as invasive aspergillosis as well as central nervous system lymphoma. Other AIDS-related diseases such as Kaposi sarcoma are not related to CD4+ cell counts.

References: Jung AC, Paauw DS. Diagnosing HIV-related disease: using the CD4 count as a guide. *J Gen Intern Med* 1998;13:131–136.

Kanne JP, Yandow DR, Meyer CA. Pneumocystis jiroveci pneumonia: high-resolution CT findings in patients with and without HIV infection. *AJR Am J Roentgenol* 2012;198:W555–W561.

Kunihiro Y, Tanaka N, Matsumoto T, et al. The usefulness of a diagnostic method combining high-resolution CT findings and serum markers for cytomegalovirus pneumonia and pneumocystis pneumonia in non-AIDS patients. *Acta Radiol* 2014.

2 **Answer A.**   *Pseudomonas aeruginosa* pneumonia is a common cause of nosocomial pneumonia with a high mortality rate in critically ill patients. Bronchial wall thickening and pleural effusion are signs more common with *P. aeruginosa* than with CMV or *P. jiroveci*. Additionally, the dependent lung distribution makes aspiration-related pneumonia a distinct possibility in this setting. This patient is chronically ill, ventilated, and immunocompromised; this is a common context for *P. aeruginosa* pneumonia.

References: Okada F, Ono A, Ando Y, et al. Thin-section CT findings in Pseudomonas aeruginosa pulmonary infection. *Br J Radiol* 2012;85:1533–1538.

Omeri AK, Okada F, Takata S, et al. Comparison of high-resolution computed tomography findings between Pseudomonas aeruginosa pneumonia and Cytomegalovirus pneumonia. *Eur Radiol* 2014;24(12):3251–3259.

3a **Answer D.**

3b **Answer B.**   As is this case of hospital-acquired pneumonia, tree-in-bud opacities may be a manifestation of MRSA, for which there is no specific radiographic sign. Late-onset (>5 days after admission) hospital-acquired pneumonia should be treated initially with broad-spectrum antibiotics, including ones with efficacy treating MRSA and *Pseudomonas*.

More recently, methicillin-resistant *Staphylococcus aureus* (MRSA) pneumonia is increasing as a cause of community-acquired pneumonia in otherwise healthy children and adults. Some subsets of the population, such as those of low socioeconomic status, abusing intravenous drugs, or incarcerated, are at particular risk for community-acquired MRSA infections.

References: American Thoracic Society; Infectious Diseases Society of America. Guidelines for the management of adults with hospital-acquired, ventilator-associated, and healthcare-associated pneumonia. *Am J Respir Crit Care Med* 2005;171(4):388–416.

Morikawa K, Okada F, Ando Y, et al. Methicillin-resistant Staphylococcus aureus and methicillin-susceptible S. aureus pneumonia: comparison of clinical and thin-section CT findings. *Br J Radiol* 2012;85(1014):e168–e175.

Nguyen ET, Kanne JP, Hoang LM, et al. Community-acquired Methicillin-resistant Staphylococcus aureus pneumonia: radiographic and computed tomography findings. *J Thorac Imaging* 2008;23(1):13–19.

Rossi SE, Franquet T, Volpacchio M, et al. Tree-in-bud pattern at thin-section CT of the lungs: radiologic-pathologic overview. *Radiographics* 2005;25(3):789–801.

4 **Answer B.** A patient with the provided history and CT findings of a cavitary lesion and upper lung zone tree-in-bud opacities should be assumed to have *Mycobacterium tuberculosis* pneumonia until proven otherwise. Initiation of antimicrobial therapy before obtaining a good sputum sample might prevent effective culture of the organism and subsequent tailoring of therapy bases on drug sensitivities of the organism. A left bronchial intubation would not prevent infection of the right lung; infection is already present. This pattern is bilateral and upper lung zone predominant, which is not typical of aspiration. A bronchoscopy, which was performed in this case, can provide a good sample for culture. The sputum culture was positive for a strain of *M. tuberculosis* without significant drug resistance.

Reference: Jeong YJ, Lee KS. Pulmonary tuberculosis: up-to-date imaging and management. *AJR Am J Roentgenol* 2008;191(3):834–844.

5 **Answer A.** Present on the image is a pattern of uniform randomly distributed micronodules with some nodules contiguous with fissures and pleura. Radiographically, this distribution creates a miliary pattern. Although *C. immitis*, *P. jiroveci*, CMV, and *N. asteroids* can manifest nodules, the miliary pattern present on the image provided is typical of disseminated fungal or mycobacterial infection. The differential consideration would also include miliary pattern of metastasis, but clinical history can often assist with distinguishing the two. Also, a study of multiple pulmonary nodules in AIDS demonstrated that size <1 cm generally correlated with infection.

References: Edinburgh KJ, Jasmer RM, Huang L, et al. Multiple pulmonary nodules in AIDS: usefulness of CT in distinguishing among potential causes. *Radiology* 2000;214:427–432.

Walker CM, Abbott GF, Greene RE, et al. Imaging pulmonary infection: classic signs and patterns. *AJR Am J Roentgenol* 2014;202(3):479–492.

6a **Answer A.**

6b **Answer D.** The tricuspid valve is most commonly affected resulting in septic emboli. This is related to the inflow from the systemic venous system in the setting of sepsis, long-term indwelling catheter use, and IV drug abuse. The pattern of septic emboli is most frequently characterized by peripheral predominant, randomly distributed nodular areas of ill-defined consolidation. They may be wedge shaped. A "feeding vessel" sign has been described in associated as reflecting the vessel serving the infarcted territory, but this is only occasionally helpful in clinical practice. *Staphylococcus aureus* is the most commonly implicated organism.

References: Dodd JD, Souza CA, Müller NL. High-resolution MDCT of pulmonary septic embolism: evaluation of the feeding vessel sign. *AJR Am J Roentgenol* 2006;187(3):623–629.

Engelke C, Schaefer-Prokop C, Schirg E, et al. High-resolution CT and CT angiography of peripheral pulmonary vascular disorders. *Radiographics* 2002;22(4):739–764.

7a **Answer D.**

7b **Answer B.** *Legionella pneumophila* pneumonia is common in immunocompromised patients over 50 years of age. The dominant radiographic pattern in the image provided is consolidation surrounded by ground-glass opacities in a subsegmental distribution, which is typical of *L. pneumophila*. In a head-to-head comparison with streptococcal pneumonia, *L. pneumophila* pneumonia was unique in this CT pattern. Also in that study, CT imaging in 23 out of 35 patients with *L. pneumophila* pneumonia demonstrated pleural effusion, which is similar to other studies. Cavitation can occur in abscess formation associated with *Legionella* pneumonia, particularly in the immunocompromised patient, but is not common.

Reference: Yu H, Higa F, Hibiya K, et al. Computed tomographic features of 23 sporadic cases with Legionella pneumophila pneumonia. *Eur J Radiol* 2010;74(3):e73–e78.

8a **Answer B.**

8b **Answer C.**

8c **Answer A.** This is a culture-positive case of *M. abscessus*. *M. abscessus* is a fast-growing *Mycobacterium* that is frequently more aggressive than other nontuberculous mycobacterial infections and requires initial treatment with intravenous antimicrobial chemotherapy. A few studies have examined the specific CT appearance of *M. abscessus* as well as compared the CT appearance to *Mycobacterium avium* complex infections. The most common CT findings in *M. abscessus* include nodularity, tree-in-bud opacities, and bronchiectasis, seen in 80% to 90% of patients. In contrast to MAC, *M. abscessus* causes statistically significant less consolidation, thin-walled cavities, and discrete pulmonary nodules.

When specifically studying rapidly growing mycobacteria to include *M. abscessus* in patients with cancer, three distinct groups were identified. In the subgroup that developed pulmonary infection, *M. abscessus* was the most common rapidly growing *Mycobacterium*. Associated risk factors included underlying lung disease (70%), female gender (57%), and solid tumors (60%).

References: Han D, Lee KS, Koh WJ, et al. Radiographic and CT findings of nontuberculous mycobacterial pulmonary infection caused by Mycobacterium abscessus. *AJR Am J Roentgenol* 2003;181:513–517.

Okazaki A, Takato H, Fujimura M, et al. Successful treatment with chemotherapy and corticosteroids of pulmonary Mycobacterium abscessus infection accompanied by pleural effusion. *J Infect Chemother* 2013;19(5):964–968.

Redelman-Sidi G, Sepkowitz KA. Rapidly growing mycobacteria infection in patients with cancer. *Clin Infect Dis* 2010;51(4):422–434.

9 **Answer A.** In the setting of heart transplant, new nodules are more likely infectious than neoplastic, but both should always be considered in the appropriate context. In this case, there is a solid nodule with surrounding ground-glass, a "CT halo," sign. This sign is associated with angioinvasive infection, especially *Aspergillus*, which happens to be a very common cause of infection after transplant. CMV pneumonia much more commonly presents with a diffuse ground-glass appearance than an isolated discrete nodule. There are no features to suggest round atelectasis in this case although round atelectasis can present after surgery if there has been significant pleural irritation. Nocardia is also common after heart transplant, and *Nocardia* can mimic other infections. This is a biopsy-proven *Nocardia* nodule.

Post transplant lymphoproliferative disease (PTLD) should be considered for nodules and masses and normally occurs 4 to 6 months or later after transplantation. Nodules and masses prior to that timeframe are much more likely to be infectious. Also note that thoracic adenopathy is more highly associated with PTLD than either *Nocardia* or *Aspergillus*.

Reference: Knollmann FD, Hummel M, Hetzer R, et al. CT of heart transplant recipients: spectrum of disease. *Radiographics* 2000;20(6):1637–1648.

10 **Answer D.**   Predominant findings on the image provided are cylindrical bronchiectasis and bronchiolectasis in the lower lungs with small centrilobular nodules. Given a diffuse lower lung distribution, bronchiectasis is most commonly seen as the sequelae of prior infection or chronic aspiration. Cystic fibrosis, sarcoidosis, and allergic bronchopulmonary aspergillosis are upper lobe predominant. Other congenital syndromes are much less common such as ciliary dyskinesia or adult cystic fibrosis. There is no traction or interstitial change to suggest a fibrosing interstitial pneumonia to cause traction bronchiectasis. Follicular bronchiolitis and diffuse panbronchiolitis are considerations, but are extremely rare by comparison. Given the degree of bronchiectasis in this case, underlying immunodeficiency should be considered.

Reference: Cantin L, Bankier AA, Eisenberg RL. Bronchiectasis. *AJR Am J Roentgenol* 2009;193:W158–W171.

11 **Answer D.**   Commonly known as swine flu, H1N1 influenza A virus spread across the world in 2009 causing variable degrees of respiratory tract infection. While generally self-limited, a small subset of patients with H1N1 pneumonia progressed to more severe or fulminant disease. Occurring more often in those with underlying chronic disease, H1N1 virus also tended to affect a younger population relative to the common seasonal influenza pneumonia."Eighty-seven percent of deaths occurred in those under 65 years of age with children and working adults having risks of hospitalization and death 4 to 7 times and 8 to 12 times greater, respectively, than estimates of impact due to seasonal influenza covering the years 1976–2001" according to the final estimate of burden published by the CDC.

References: Marchiori E, Zanetti G, D'Ippolito G, et al. Swine-origin influenza A (H1N1) viral infection: thoracic findings on CT. *AJR Am J Roentgenol* 2011;196:W723–W728.

Shrestha SS, Swerdlow DL, Borse RH, et al. Estimating the burden of 2009 pandemic influenza A (H1N1) in the United States (April 2009–April 2010). *Clin Infect Dis* 2011;52(S1):S75–S82.

12 **Answer B.**   All of the answers are possible processes that can cause consolidation, but only one is the most likely based on the information provided. Consolidation is a very nonspecific finding in patients who have received lung transplants. Clinical information and especially the time since transplantation helps arrange the differential possibilities in a hierarchical fashion based on likelihood (see table in referenced article). In the intermediate time category of 1 week to 2 months, acute rejection, bronchial dehiscence, and candida infection are the most frequent concerns. However, in the 2- to 4-month category (termed primary late phase), infection due to CMV or *Aspergillus* is more frequent. Organizing pneumonia, primary disease recurrence (sarcoid in this case), chronic rejection, and posttransplant lymphoproliferative disorder are more common after 4 months (termed secondary late phase). Of note, in a study of CT findings in lung transplant recipients, sarcoidosis was found to be the most likely disease to recur posttransplant.

References: Collins J, Hartman MJ, Warner TF, et al. Frequency and CT findings of recurrent disease after lung transplantation. *Radiology* 2001;219:503–509.

Krishnam MS, Suh RD, Tomasian A, et al. Postoperative complications of lung transplantation: radiologic findings along a time continuum. *Radiographics* 2007;27(4):957–974.

13a   Answer A.

13b   Answer A.   The right upper lobe has three segments, the anterior, posterior, and apical segments. The anterior and posterior segments abut the minor fissure and either could be involved based on the frontal projection. However, the lateral projection confirms that a majority of the consolidation is located in both the anterior and posterior segments with sparing of the apical segment. The apicoposterior segment is a segment of the left upper lobe unless variant anatomy is present.

Streptococcus pneumoniae is the most common pathogen in the immunocompetent patient to present as a lobar pneumonia. Note that the term lobar is somewhat misleading as currently many patients do not fully progress to lobar pneumonia if treated appropriately early in the course of disease. Air bronchograms are common in this setting but not specific for infection. Of note, a bulging fissure sign is classically associated with *Klebsiella pneumoniae* (more frequent in alcoholics and nursing home residents) but may be present in others, including *Streptococcus* given the higher prevalence. *Proteus, Morganella,* and *Legionella* are also common pathogens to present in a lobar pattern. *Legionella* does typically rapidly progress to complete lobar consolidation.

References: Washington L, Palacio D. Imaging of bacterial pulmonary infection in the immunocompetent patient. *Semin Roentgenol* 2007;42(2):122–145.

Webb WR, Higgins CB. *Thoracic imaging*. Philadelphia, PA: Lippincott Williams & Wilkins, 2010.

14   Answer B.   Inhalational anthrax can present with hemorrhagic mediastinal adenopathy and edema, and in the correct setting, this finding can be quite specific. On noncontrast CT, the hemorrhage within the anthrax-induced adenopathy causes increased attenuation. Luckily, in the absence of a bioterrorism attack, it is a rare disease. The lymph node abnormality associated with tuberculosis is peripheral rim enhancement of larger lymph nodes; however, this finding can be seen in other diseases such as lymphoma, testicular cancer, and Whipple and Crohn disease. Tularemia is another possible bioterrorism agent but is characterized most frequently by rapid development of focal consolidation and hilar adenopathy (but no hemorrhagic adenopathy).

Reference: Ketai L, Tchoyoson Lim CC. Radiology of biological weapons—old and the new? *Semin Roentgenol* 2007;42(1):49–59. Review.

15a   Answer C.

15b   Answer A.   Multiorganism anaerobic infection is considered the most frequent cause of cavitation and lung abscess development. This is followed in frequency by *S. aureus* and *Pseudomonas*. Aspiration can be a frequent cause of multiorganism infection in the hospital and ICU setting, which includes an increased risk of anaerobic infection. Although postprimary tuberculosis is cavitary with a predilection for the upper lungs, the other findings of chronic TB are not identified such as upper lobe bronchiectasis and volume loss.

Depending on the clinical scenario, follow-up may be warranted in cases such as this to exclude an underlying neoplasm. Other considerations would include vasculitis.

References: Washington L, Palacio D. Imaging of bacterial pulmonary infection in the immunocompetent patient. *Semin Roentgenol* 2007;42(2):122–145.

Webb WR, Higgins CB. *Thoracic imaging*. Philadelphia, PA: Lippincott Williams & Wilkins, 2010.

16   Answer D.   EBV presents most commonly due to direct person-to-person transmission via the B lymphocytes lining the pharynx. It results most commonly in hepatosplenomegaly, lymphadenopathy, and pharyngitis. Correspondingly, the most common intrathoracic manifestation is enlarged lymph nodes. It can occasionally present as an interstitial pneumonia but this is rare. Understanding this presentation is important as other lymphoproliferative disorders are associated with EBV infection including Burkitt lymphoma, lymphoproliferative disease in HIV, and posttransplant lymphoproliferative disease.

Reference: Webb WR, Higgins CB. *Thoracic imaging*. Philadelphia, PA: Lippincott Williams & Wilkins, 2010.

17 **Answer A.** Community-acquired bacterial pneumonia remains the most common cause of infectious pneumonia even in the immunosuppressed. This is frequently bronchopneumonia or lobar pneumonia depending on the pathogen, and recurrent pneumonias are considered an AIDS-defining illness. TB is possible and should be a consideration, especially if significant adenopathy is present. Viral pneumonias are much more likely to present with an interstitial pattern than lobar consolidation.

Reference: Oh YW, Effmann EL, Godwin JD. Pulmonary infections in immunocompromised hosts: the importance of correlating the conventional radiologic appearance with the clinical setting. *Radiology* 2000;217(3):647–656.

18 **Answer C.** This is a case of B-cell lymphoma in the setting of AIDS. Extranodal lymphoma is more common in HIV than in nonimmunosuppressed patients. Additionally, doubling time can be quite rapid, which limits the use of doubling time for distinguishing this from infection. Both septic emboli and angioinvasive fungal disease would likely present much more acutely with dyspnea and pulmonary symptoms than the constitutional symptoms here. Note that there are CT halos surrounding several of the nodules, but in this case, these are not related to angioinvasive aspergillosis. Kaposi sarcoma is the most common AIDS-related neoplasm and classically presents with a more bronchovascular appearance. In the past, gallium scans were used to help distinguish the two (uptake is positive in lymphoma), but this is typically accomplished with biopsy today. Organizing pneumonia is more likely to present with peripheral airspace disease that is less nodular than shown. The reverse halo sign (not the halo sign) is associated with organizing pneumonia.

Reference: Marchiori E, Müller NL, Soares Souza A, et al. Pulmonary disease in patients with AIDS: high-resolution CT and pathologic findings. *AJR Am J Roentgenol* 2005;184(3):757–764.

19a **Answer A.**

19b **Answer C.** The appearance shown is typical of varicella pneumonia, which frequently presents as diffuse, ill-defined pulmonary nodules. This diagnosis is most likely when combined with the history of skin lesions, typical for the chickenpox rash. Chickenpox demonstrates an approximate rate of pneumonia of 10% to 20% (more common than pneumonia associated with zoster/shingles). Risk of pneumonia increases with immunodeficiency, pregnancy, and lymphoma/leukemia. Onset is generally 2 to 3 days after appearance of the typical skin lesions. Healed varicella pneumonia frequently demonstrates diffuse tiny pulmonary calcified nodules. Note that the morbidity and mortality of adult-onset chickenpox are considerably higher than in childhood. Although respiratory bronchiolitis and hypersensitivity pneumonitis can present with upper lung predominant centrilobular nodules, there is no specific association with chickenpox and either of these diagnoses.

Reference: Kim JS, Ryu CW, Lee SI, et al. High-resolution CT findings of varicella-zoster pneumonia. *AJR Am J Roentgenol* 1999;172(1):113–116.

Section 2: Diffuse Lung Disease

20a Answer B.

20b Answer C.

20c Answer C.   Clinical scenario, Garland triad (right upper paratracheal and bilateral hilar lymphadenopathy with preserved cardiac borders), and upper/midlung predominant opacities favors thoracic sarcoidosis.

Clinical staging is based on chest radiograph pattern. 5-part "Scadding" classification system exists: 0—normal chest x-ray (5% to 15%); I—lymphadenopathy (LN) with clear lungs (50%); II—LN and pulmonary disease, 25% to 30%; III—isolated pulmonary disease (15%); and IV—lung fibrosis (10% to 15%). Definite diagnosis requires presence of noncaseating epithelioid cell granulomas in more than 1 organ or positive Kveim-Siltzbach skin test.

High-resolution CT is helpful in distinguishing active interstitial inflammation from irreversible fibrosis, assessment of atypical features, and differential diagnosis. Typical parenchymal manifestations are seen in 60% to 70% of cases: bilateral hilar enlargement, perilymphatic micronodularity along bronchovascular bundles and fissures (patchy, upper, and midlung predominant), perihilar opacities, and fibrotic changes. Other pulmonary parenchymal findings, isolated mediastinal lymphadenopathy, pleural/airway involvement, honeycombing, and mycetoma are considered atypical. Perilymphatic nodularity may improve, stabilize, or progress into fibrosis. FDG uptake in thoracic sarcoidosis is nonspecific, variable in intensity, and most predominant in involved lymph nodes, parenchymal nodules, and opacities.

Half of the patients are asymptomatic in stages I to II. Pulmonary function worsens with an increasing stage, but radiologic staging does not correlate well with severity of pulmonary function abnormalities. Often, radiographic abnormalities appear worse than the degree of functional impairment. Spontaneous remission occurs in 60% to 90% in stage 1, 40% to 70% in stage 2, 10% to 20% in stage 3, and 0% in stage 4 disease.

Treatment may not be indicated in stage I alone. Oral steroids are used as first-line therapy beyond stage I and before end-stage fibrosis with associated improved radiologic findings during the treatment. Cytotoxic drugs and immunomodulators may be considered for complicated or severe refractory sarcoidosis. Lofgren syndrome (fever, polyarthritis, erythema nodosum, and bilateral hilar lymphadenopathy) has spontaneous remission rate more than 85%. Steroids are not usually required. Recurrence of disease in a pulmonary allograft after lung transplantation is 47% to 67%, but frequently not clinically significant.

References: Criado E, Sanchez M, Ramirez J, et al. Pulmonary sarcoidosis: typical and atypical manifestations at high-resolution CT with pathologic correlation. *Radiographics* 2010;30(6):1567–1586.

Prabhakar HB, Rabinowitz CB, Gibbons FK, et al. Imaging features of sarcoidosis on MDCT, FDG PET, and PET/CT. *AJR Am J Ronetgenol* 2008;190(Suppl): S1–S6.

Wu JJ, Rashcovsky Shiff K. Sarcoidosis. *Am Fam Physician* 2004;70(2):312–322.

21a Answer D.

21b Answer A.

21c Answer C.   Frontal chest radiograph shows upper and midlung predominant bilateral reticular opacities and scattered cystic lesions in the background of mildly increased lung volumes. These features could be seen in pulmonary Langerhans cell histiocytosis (PLCH), lymphangioleiomyomatosis, and emphysema. There is no evidence of honeycombing or decreased lung volumes, as seen in idiopathic pulmonary fibrosis. Postradiation changes could be silent on radiograph, manifest with alveolar opacities (postradiation pneumonitis), or fibrotic features (volume loss, distortion of pulmonary architecture).

Upper and midlung predominant centrilobular micronodules and thin-walled, bizarre-shaped cavitary lesions sparing the costophrenic angles are hallmarks of smoking-related PLCH. Upper and midlung predominant micronodules could be seen in upper respiratory viral infection or respiratory bronchiolitis related to smoking but have no association with cystic lesions. Vegetations on cardiac valves (usually tricuspid) could lead to septic emboli but shows a predilection to the lower lungs, migratory character, and foci of peripheral consolidation with frequent cavitation. Hypersensitivity pneumonitis (HP) caused by exposure to inhaled antigens presents with centrilobular micronodules and ground-glass opacities, but cysts seen in HP are distinct from the thin-walled cavitary lesions of PLCH.

PLCH lesions evolve from early bronchiolocentric multicellular dense infiltrates with Langerhans cells (with characteristic Birbeck granules) into a predominantly fibroblast-containing lesion with bronchiole dilatation (midphase) followed by end-stage fibrotic stellate scars with paracicatricial airspace enlargement.

Presence of Langerhans cells within bronchial mucosa or alveolar parenchyma is not specific for PLCH and could be seen in COPD, lung cancer, and other interstitial lung diseases. More definite diagnosis of PLCH requires correlation of smoking history, radiologic features, and combination of nodular and cystic lesions on light microscopy containing aggregates of Langerhans cells. TGF-beta is an essential factor in the development of Langerhans cells, sustained chronic inflammation, and airway-centered fibrosis.

Pneumothorax is seen in approximately 15% of PLCH cases (predominantly unilateral), is associated with worse outcome, and does not seem to benefit from steroid use but may require surgical management or mechanical pleurodesis. Steroids may be beneficial in selected cases for parenchymal stabilization or complicating pulmonary hypertension, but smoking cessation is the most important factor in disease stabilization (up to 50%), or even regression in early stages (25% of cases).

References: Abbott GF, Rosado-de-Christenson ML, Franks TF. From the archives of the AFIP pulmonary Langerhans cell histiocytosis. *RadioGraphics* 2004;24:821–841.

Caminati A, Harari S. Smoking-related interstitial pneumonias and pulmonary Langerhans cell histiocytosis. *Proc Am Thorac Soc* 2006;3(4):299–306.

Kim HJ, Lee KS, Johkoh T, et al. Pulmonary Langerhans cell histiocytosis in adults: high-resolution CT—pathology comparisons and evolutional changes at CT. *Eur Radiol* 2011;21:1406–1415.

22a **Answer: D.**

22b **Answer: A.** Frontal chest radiograph demonstrates at least moderate-sized right-sided pneumothorax (best seen overlying the diaphragm as a thin linear opacity), reticular pattern, and bilateral scattered cystic lesions. The presence of right-sided pneumothorax in a symptomatic patient requires an emergent notification of a referring physician for possible chest tube placement. After stabilization, CT of the chest would aid in the evaluation for additional findings and cause of the pneumothorax.

Bilateral scattered thin-walled small cystic lesions without zonal predilection in female patient with hepatic and renal fat-containing masses are most suggestive of LAM in a patient with tuberous sclerosis (TS)—LAM–TS complex.

In LAM, thin-walled uniform round or oval cysts result from air trapping due to smooth muscle–like cell proliferation along the bronchioles, blood vessels, and lymphatics. Cysts frequently enlarge as the disease progresses. Pneumothorax is seen up to 50% of the patients, sometimes with associated chylous effusion (10% to 20%). Lungs are hyperinflated due to air trapping in half of the patients. Reticular pattern is common on CXR (up to 90%) and results from summation of thin-walled cystic lesions. Hilar and abdominal lymphadenopathy is frequent, caused by proliferation of abnormal smooth muscle cells along lymphatic vessels.

The disease is seen in symptomatic females of childbearing age that present with dyspnea (70%), pneumothorax (50%), or chylous pleural effusion (28%). Chyloptysis and hemoptysis are also seen due to obstruction of pulmonary blood and lymphatic vessels by LAM cells.

Characteristic LAM findings in females with tuberous sclerosis (TS) are seen only in 30% of the cases with overall gender-free occurrence of LAM in TS not exceeding 1%. Interestingly, a greater number of cystic lesions and likelihood of pneumothorax and chylous effusions are seen in sporadic LAM as opposed to LAM–TS complex.

Smoking can contribute to distal airway damage, exacerbating air trapping, and chance of pneumothorax. Additionally, pregnancy is associated with estrogen and progesterone swings, each negatively affecting the course of the disease. LAM recurrence in transplanted lung (presumably due to migration or in vivo metastasizing from native to donor lung) is rare.

The main differentials based on imaging are as follows: (1) PLCH—bizarre-shaped cysts with upper/midlung predominance, interspersed with centrilobular nodules in a smoking host; (2) LIP—most often in autoimmune disorders and AIDS, could manifest solely with lower lung predominant thin-walled cysts in perivascular distribution; and (3) *P. jiroveci* pneumonia—scattered cystic lesions in an immunocompromised host.

References: Abbott GF, Rosado-de-Christenson ML, Frazier AA, et al. Lymphangioleiomyomatosis: radiologic-pathologic correlation. *Radiographics* 2005;25:803–828.

Avila NA, Dwyer AJ, Moss J. Imaging features of lymphangioleiomyomatosis: diagnostic pitfalls. *AJR Am J Roentgenol* 2011;196(4):982–986.

Seaman DM, Meyer CA, Gilman MD, et al. Diffuse cystic lung disease at high-resolution CT. *AJR Am J Roentgenol* 2011;196(6):1305–1311.

22c **Answer: A.**

22d **Answer: B.**

23a **Answer C.**

23b **Answer D.**

23c **Answer B.**

23d **Answer B.** On radiographs, bilateral partially cavitating nodules and background of bronchiectases are seen. Elevation of right hemidiagram with partial atelectasis (best seen on lateral view) is responsible for the right lung base opacity and lateral silhouetting of the hemidiagram on frontal projection. There is no radiographically detectable lymphadenopathy, hydrostatic edema, right-sided pleural effusion, or honeycombing.

Polypoid long segment intraluminal tracheal mass and bilateral cavitary parenchymal lesions are present on CT. Distribution of lesions suggests gravitational effect. Chronic atelectasis and postobstructive consolidation with extensive bronchiectases within the right middle lobe are evident.

The most likely diagnosis here is recurrent tracheobronchial papillomatosis with pulmonary involvement. Incidence of recurrent laryngeal papillomatosis is 4.3 and 1.8 per 100,000 in children and adults in United States, respectively. The younger the age, the higher the likelihood of distal spread and severity of the disease. It is caused by human papillomavirus (most common HPV-6 and HPV-11). Children acquire the disease during birth by direct contact with mother's genital lesions. Adults develop the disease due to either reactivation of latent virus or new infection after sexual oral contact.

The most common site of involvement is larynx with only 5% of patients having tracheal involvement and <1% demonstrating pulmonary disease. Extralaryngeal spread of the infection totals 30% and 16% in pediatric and adult groups, respectively.

Tracheobronchial papillomatosis can present either as a focal mass or as diffuse cobblestone changes of mucosa. Nodular appearance of bronchi can be seen. Pulmonary papilloma lesions begin as asymptomatic, noncalcified, peripheral nodules that tend to enlarge and undergo central cavitation/liquefaction and necrosis, often with an air fluid level. A dependent distribution is common. Calcification is not characteristic.

No definite cure exists. The rate of malignant transformation into squamous cell carcinoma is 14% regardless of the age but is usually associated with irradiation in kids and smoking in adults and more frequently seen in HPV-16 and HPV-18 infection.

In assessment of large airway lesions, conventional chest radiography still remains the initial imaging test; however, it has a low sensitivity. MDCT is the test of choice for identification, localization, extent, and complications. Stenosis and/or malacia could be assessed with CT dynamic imaging of large airways; MRI would be inferior with unnecessary labor and cost involved. Virtual bronchoscopy is superior to conventional bronchoscopy for infection spread and mapping the extent of the process more safely.

References: Hammoud D, Haddad BE. Squamous cell carcinoma of the lungs arising in recurrent respiratory papillomatosis (case report). *Resp Med* 2010;3(4):270–272.

Marchiori E, Neto CA, Meirelles GS, et al. Laryngotracheobronchial papillomatosis: findings on computed tomography scans of the chest. *J Bras Pneumol* 2008;34(12):1084–1089.

Ngo AV, Walker CM, Chung JH, et al. Tumors and tumorlike conditions of the large airways. *AJR Am J Roentgenol* 2013;201:301–313.

24a **Answer A.**

24b **Answer B.**

24c **Answer C.** The important observation from the chest radiograph is preserved lung volumes, which opposes idiopathic pulmonary fibrosis (low lung volumes). Bilateral mid- and lower lung predominant reticular opacities warrant correlation with chest CT. There are no definite masses to warrant immediate biopsy or PET/CT (both of which should probably only be done after diagnostic CT regardless).

The key CT findings here are perilymphatic cystic lesions and several small peripheral opacities. The constellation of clinical and imaging information is most suggestive of LIP in settings of Sögren disease. Other parenchymal findings that can be seen are poorly defined centrilobular and subpleural nodules and thickened peribronchovascular bundles and interlobular septa.

The most helpful finding in differential diagnosis is presence of thin-walled perivascular cysts (in 80%) that are believed to result from partial airway obstruction by peribronchiolar cellular deposits. Nodules may represent lymphoproliferative foci or amyloid deposits and may calcify. Mediastinal/hilar lymphadenopathy is occasionally seen. Pleural effusions are rare.

LIP is seen in 1% of patients with Sögren syndrome. Twenty-five percent of patients with LIP have Sögren syndrome. Females are affected more often than males (2:1), especially in the fourth to sixth decades of life. The disease is rarely isolated and can be seen in other autoimmune disorders. LIP in children is considered an AIDS-defining illness. Of note, improvement of radiologic findings correlates with immune status decline in this group. Eighty percent of adult patients with LIP have serum dysproteinemias (most common, IgM). Histopathologically, the infiltrates are consisted of polyclonal lymphocytes mixed with plasma cells.

The onset is usually insidious with mild hypoxemia, cough, and progressive respiratory distress over period of several years. Tissue diagnosis requires thoracoscopic or open lung biopsy. The course of the disease is unpredictable. Improvement or resolution of symptoms is seen in 50% to 60% of patients treated with corticosteroids and/or cytostatics. Thirty-three to fifty percent of patients succumb within 5 years of diagnosis, from infection due to either immunosuppression or lung fibrosis related to treatment of underlying disorder. Five percent of cases progress into low-grade B-cell lymphoma. Radiologically, cysts are seen only in 2% of patients with lymphoma, whereas air–space consolidation and nodules larger than 1 cm are more common in patients with lymphoma (66% and 41%) than LIP (18 % and 6%). Pleural effusions can be seen in up to 25% of malignant lymphoma but would be very unusual in LIP.

References: Johkoh T, Muller N, Pickford HA, et al. Lymphocytic interstitial pneumonia: thin-section CT findings in 22 patients. *Radiology* 1999;212:567–572.

Lynch DA, Travis WD, Muller NL, et al. Idiopathic Interstitial Pneumonias: CT features. *Radiology* 2005;236:10–21.

Mueller-Mang C, Grosse C, Schmid K, et al. What every radiologist should know about idiopathic interstitial pneumonias. *RadioGraphics* 2007;27:595–615.

Swigris JJ, Berry GJ, Raffin TA, et al. Lymphoid interstitial pneumonia: a narrative review. *Chest* 2002;122(6):2150–2164.

25a **Answer B.**

25b **Answer A.**   Images show upper and midlung extensive bilateral cavitary/cystic lesions with various degree of wall thickness and septations within areas of ground-glass opacities. Lesions are intraparenchymal and peribronchial rather than perivascular. There is no centrilobular emphysema, pulmonary edema, or peripheral fibrosis.

Given the history and imaging findings, the most likely diagnosis is chronic *Pneumocystis jiroveci* pneumonia. The main imaging manifestations of chronic *P. jiroveci* pneumonia include interlobular thickening, bronchiectasis, and a variable degree of fibrosis.

PLCH is upper lung predominant but does not usually manifest as such large cysts. Septic emboli demonstrate more randomly distributed peripheral nodular opacities with variable degrees of cavitation rather than the central and upper lung predominant abnormality shown. Cysts in LAM are more diffusely distributed and thin walled.

P. jiroveci pneumonia is the most common OPPORTUNISTIC infection among people with HIV/AIDS. However, the most common infection among patients with HIV/AIDS is bacterial pneumonia (20- to 40-fold increase).

Approximately 1/3 of patients have normal radiographic findings on initial evaluation and radiologic abnormalities lag behind the symptoms in acute phase. Classic appearance is bilateral perihilar or interstitial opacities (reticular, reticulonodular, or ground glass). If no treatment is given, progressive alveolar consolidation may occur over several days. With treatment, the disease has a tendency to improve within a couple of weeks, with some patients developing irreversible coarse reticular opacities due to fibrosis.

The first-line treatment is generally trimethoprim–sulfamethoxazole. Corticosteroids given within 72 hours from the onset of the disease are found to improve survival. Patients with HIV and PJP infection have higher survival rates than patients without HIV (86% to 92% vs. 51% to 80%, respectively), likely due to decreased inflammatory response in patients with HIV.

The primary CT finding in the acute phase is geographic ground-glass attenuation (90% of cases). This finding has high predictive value in a patient with HIV in the appropriate clinical scenario and, by itself, sufficient enough to start an empirical treatment. Atypical manifestations are seen in 10% of cases and include isolated focal or asymmetric dense consolidation, adenopathy, and various size nodules that may cavitate or calcify. Pneumothorax is seen in 50% of cases. Up to 38% of patients have thin-walled cystic lesions that are believed to represent pneumatoceles, usually multiple with upper lobe predilection. The cysts usually resolve within a year following treatment but may persist permanently.

As stated before, the majority of HIV/AIDS–infected patients demonstrate CD4 T lymphocyte count <200 to 100 cells/mm^3 with only 10% to 15% patients having T-helper count >200 cell/mm^3.

References: Allen CA, Al-Jahdali HH, Irion KL, et al. Imaging manifestations of HIV/AIDS. *Ann Thorac Med* 2010;5(4):201–216.

David MH, David AL, McAdams HP, et al. *Imaging of Diseases of the Chest*. Philadelphia, Pa: Elsevier Mosby; 2009.

Kanne JP, Yandow DR, Meyer CA. Pneumocystis jiroveci pneumonia: high-resolution CT findings in patients with and without HIV infection. *AJR Am J Roentgenol* 2012;198:W555–W561.

Kim KL, Kim CW, Lee MK, et al. Imaging of occupational lung disease. *Radiographics* 2001;21(6):1371–1391.

26a **Answer C.**

26b **Answer A.**

26c **Answer C.** The most significant findings in this case are bilateral small pulmonary nodules (most abundant in upper and midlungs) in a perilymphatic distribution. Some of the nodules coalesce in the upper lobes and form elongated opacities with distortion of pulmonary architecture. Differential considerations include pneumoconiosis or sarcoidosis, but given the history of foundry work, pneumoconiosis is more likely. Kerley B lines are represented by short thick lines perpendicular to pleura in lower lungs and can be seen in pneumoconiosis, but occur most commonly in interstitial edema. Healed varicella classically presents with scattered miliary calcified pulmonary nodules; distortion of pulmonary architecture is not characteristic. Granulomatosis with polyangiitis would not produce this constellation of findings. Calcified pleural plaques are seen in asbestos exposure. In silicosis, calcification of mediastinal lymph nodes ("eggshell" calcifications) is present in 5% of cases. The latter is not specific and could be observed in other conditions such as sarcoidosis and histoplasmosis.

Classic silicosis is a chronic form of silicosis that occurs due to inhalation of lower dose dust containing crystalline silicon dioxide. Disease usually manifests after 10 to 20 years of exposure. When changes occur within 10 years from exposure, the form is called accelerated. On CT, 1- to 10-mm nodules are present in a perilymphatic distribution. Geographic and confluent ground-glass opacities with interlobular septal thickening in silica exposure are features of acute silicosis and silicoproteinosis due to inhalation of large quantity of particles. Patients present with progressive dyspnea, with frequently fatal outcome usually within 1 year. Besides silica particles deposition, alveolar filling with acid-Schiff–positive proteinaceous material is seen, similar to that in alveolar proteinosis, explaining imaging findings.

In the complicated form of chronic silicosis, opacities initially form in upper and midlungs and gradually migrate toward the hila, distorting architecture and producing adjacent cicatricial emphysema as they evolve into perihilar confluent soft tissue conglomerates (progressive massive fibrosis), which may partially calcify. Internal foci of low attenuation could be observed due to necrosis of mass-like tissue. Occasionally, cavitations with or without pleural thickening could develop, which should raise a suspicion of mycobacterial infection. Susceptibility to TB in silicosis is increased in 2 to 30 times.

Coal worker's pneumoconiosis (CWP) and silicosis are distinct entities, despite similar imaging findings and inhalational exposure to inorganic dust. In CWP, workers are exposed to washed coal, which is nearly free of silica or mixed with smaller amount of kaolin, mica, or silica. CWP is seen in coal miners, whereas silicosis has wider range of professional exposure (sandblasters, miners, tunnelers, potters, glassmakers, foundry/quarry/dental/construction workers). Clinically, patients with CWP and PMF tend to do better than patients with silicosis and PMF, and the first group has more frequent mismatch between clinical severity and imaging findings.

References: Chong S, Lee KS, Chung MJ, et al. Pneumoconiosis: comparison of imaging and pathologic findings. *Radiographics* 2006;26(1):59–77.

Cox CW, Rose CS, Lynch DA. State of the art: imaging of occupational lung disease. *Radiology* 2014;270(3):681–696.

Hansell DM, Armstrong P, Lynch DA. Inhalational lung disease. Pneumoconiosis. In: *Imaging of diseases of the chest*, 4th ed. Elsevier Mosby:440–449.

27a Answer A.

27b Answer A.

27c Answer C.

27d Answer A.

27e Answer C. On radiographs, well-defined bizarre-shaped dense opacities are different in appearance on the lateral view indicating extraparenchymal origin. In contrast, parenchymal lesions have smudgy or less defined margins and, if seen on both frontal and lateral radiographs, do not drastically change their appearance between projections. The density of opacities higher than bone implies calcium with linear coarse calcifications seen on diaphragmatic and pericardial surfaces. The appearance is nearly pathognomonic of prior asbestos exposure and represents advanced calcified pleural plaques.

The most common manifestation of asbestos exposure is in the pleura with unilateral reactive pleural effusion (latency of 10 years, from chronic irritation by asbestos fibers). Calcium deposition on parietal pleura is detected in 25% on CXR and 60% on CT, most commonly between fourth and eighth ribs, after

20 years. Visceral pleural calcifications could occur in interlobar fissure. Dense white edge of the plaques is called a rolled edge. When a plaque is soft, it is seen as an irregular, smooth elevation of pleura with single indistinct margin (since it blends with normal pleura). Round atelectasis, either solitary or multifocal, is not unique but common among patients with asbestos exposure and pleural thickening.

The earliest parenchymal change in asbestosis is curvilinear subpleural lines in the lower lungs. These could be subtle and obscured by dependent atelectasis. Therefore, prone images are pivotal to early diagnosis. Later, parenchymal bands and fibrosis with honeycombing and bronchiectases can occur (seen on provided CT images).

Asbestosis spreads centrifugally from terminal bronchioles and alveolar ducts. As in the case here, it has lower and basal lung predilection. Histologically, it is indistinguishable from usual interstitial pneumonia. The fibrosis tends to progress despite exposure removal. None of the features of fibrosis in asbestosis are specific. Fibrosis related to drug reaction more frequently manifests with organizing pneumonia or NSIP pattern and would not result in bilateral pleural plaques. ARDS-related fibrosis has anterior upper/midlung predominance, possibly related to anterior lung barotrauma or hyperoxygenation in a mechanically ventilated host. IPF diagnosis requires excluding other causes of pulmonary fibrosis, and the presence of pleural plaques in these cases strongly points to prior asbestos exposure.

The diagnosis of asbestosis requires occupational history or potential environmental exposure, clinical findings (unresolving lower lung crackles, clubbing, dyspnea), abnormal pulmonary function tests (reduced vital and diffusion capacity), and radiologic findings. One of the indications for HRCT is identification of asbestosis in symptomatic workers with normal parenchyma on chest radiographs. Other indications for CT use are as follows: identification of pulmonary fibrosis as distinct from emphysema and diffuse pleural disease, detection of pulmonary fibrosis for compensation purpose when chest radiograph does not support abnormal pulmonary function tests, and further workup of suspected pleural or parenchymal mass. When the appearance is classic and no worrisome radiographic/clinical findings are present, HRCT is not needed.

Lung cancer and mesothelioma are estimated to occur in 20% to 25% of patients with heavy exposure to asbestos. Asbestos-related lung cancer manifests as either adenocarcinoma or squamous cell carcinoma, with up to 100× increased incidence in asbestos-exposed smokers over nonsmoking unexposed patients. Pleural mesotheliomas, on the other hand, do not demonstrate clear association with smoking but with type of asbestos particles, occurring mostly due to crocidolite deposition. Malignant pleural mesothelioma is a spectrum of asbestos-related disease and characterized by nodular or diffuse pleural thickening (thickness >1 cm). Small pleural effusions could be present. The disease has a 10% lifetime occurrence in asbestos workers (with latency of 30 years or more) and could also occur in their household members or residents living near asbestos mines and plants.

References: Chong S, Lee KS, Chung MJ, et al. Pneumoconiosis: comparison of imaging and pathologic findings. *Radiographics* 2006;26(1):59–77.

Hansell DM, Armstrong P, Lynch DA. Inhalational lung disease pneumoconiosis. In: *Imaging of diseases of the chest*, 4th ed. Elsevier Mosby:458–462.

Kim KL, Kim CW, Lee MK, et al. Imaging of occupational lung disease. *Radiographics* 2001;21(6):1371–1391.

Webb WR, Muller NL, Naidich DP. Pneumoconiosis. Occupational and environmental lung disease, (Chapter 9). In: *High-resolution of the lung*, 4th ed. Philadelphia, PA: Lippincott Williams & Wilkins, 2014:302–318.

28a **Answer C.**

28b **Answer A.**

28c **Answer A.** On CT, rapid progression in bilateral cystic disease is evident. Some of the lesions are clearly subpleural, responsible for pneumothorax. Thickened bronchovascular bundles, foci of parenchymal consolidation, scattered ill-defined various size nodules, and pleural effusions are seen on follow-up. Given the history, cystic or cavitary metastasis is the most likely diagnosis. The rest of the provided choices are unlikely: (1) Emphysema classically lacks walls; (2) pulmonary Langerhans cell histiocytosis manifests with smoking-related small and bizarre-shaped cysts, centrilobular micronodules, and no pleural effusions or interstitial thickening; and (3) Birt-Hogg-Dube syndrome is an autosomal dominant disease with lower lung predominant thin-walled large septated cysts, positive dermatologic findings (fibrofolliculomas), and renal tumors.

All of the above could present with secondary pneumothorax, which accounts only for 20% of all pneumothoraces. Most commonly, pneumothorax is due to COPD, followed by cystic fibrosis and cystic lung diseases. Ten to fifty percent of pneumothoraces are radiographically occult. Earliest accumulation of air in pneumothorax on supine radiographs is anteromedial (increased definition of cardiac/mediastinal contours and outlining of medial diaphragm under cardiac silhouette).

Multiple variable size peripheral round nodules and thickened interstitium are typical manifestations of lung parenchymal metastatic disease. Atypical features include the rest of included choices as well as calcification, perinodular ground-glass attenuation, tumor embolism, endobronchial metastasis, dilated vessels within a mass, and a sterilized metastasis (PET-negative CT-persistent nodule, histologically represented by necrotic or fibrotic cells with no viable tumor cells).

Incidence of cavitation is higher in primary bronchogenic carcinoma than in metastatic disease, 9% versus 4%, respectively. Cavitary primary lung carcinomas are represented by squamous cell and adenocarcinomas. Among secondary lung malignancies, 70% of cavitary mets are represented by squamous cell carcinomas (most common, head and neck origin). Urogenital transitional cell carcinomas, colorectal carcinomas, melanoma, and sarcoma metastases are also known for cystic transformation. This may relate to creation of a check-valve mechanism and peripheral tumor necrosis with rupture into pleural cavity.

References: Lee KH, Lee JS, Lynch DA, et al. The radiologic differential diagnosis of diffuse lung diseases characterized by multiple cysts or cavities (pictorial essay). *J Comput Assist Tomogr* 2002;26(1):5–12.

Seo JB, Im JG, Goo JM, et al. Atypical pulmonary metastases: spectrum of radiologic findings. *RadioGraphics* 2001;21:403–417.

Tateishi U, Hasegawa T, Kusumoto M, et al. Metastatic angiosarcoma of the lung: spectrum of CT findings. *AJR AM J Roentgenol* 2003;180:1671–1674.

29a **Answer B.**

29b **Answer B.**

29c **Answer B.** UIP-related fibrosis has peripheral and basal predilection with key findings of subpleural reticulations and honeycombing. Conglomerate mass-like fibrosis, peribronchovascular and subpleural nodularity, and upper and midvolume loss with hilar retraction are not the features of UIP and IPF but could be seen in advanced stages of sarcoidosis, chronic beryllium disease, and other pneumoconioses. However, beryllium exposure is specifically associated with ceramics manufacture, nuclear weapon production, and aerospace industry and is seen in up to 16% of workers in some studies.

The pathologic hallmark of chronic berylliosis is noncaseating granulomas indistinguishable from granulomas in sarcoidosis. It is thought to result from initial macrophage-initiated response to inhaled beryllium that is presented to CD4 T cells initiating chronic inflammation. The pathologic and imaging findings are indistinguishable to those in sarcoidosis. Therefore, the presence of noncaseating granulomas is not characteristic. Mononuclear cellular infiltrate with documented exposure and positive beryllium lymphocyte proliferation testing are generally considered adequate to establish a diagnosis. The latter test is positive in 90% with chronic disease (highest sensitivity is from bronchial lavage). Clinical findings are similar to those in sarcoidosis including extrathoracic manifestations with skin lesions (most frequent). Lymphadenopathy, (up to 40%), hypercalcemia, hepatosplenomegaly, and renal calcinosis are also reported.

According to workplace standards, maximum permissible level of beryllium is 2 mcg/m^3 over 8-hour period, with a peak level of 25 mcg/m^3. Any potential exposure to beryllium dust or fumes is enough to raise practical concern for chronic disease.

References: Hansell DM, Armstrong P, Lynch DA. Inhalational lung disease pneumoconiosis. In: *Imaging of diseases of the chest*, 4th ed. Elsevier Mosby:465–466.

Sharma N, Patel J, Mohammed TL. Chronic beryllium disease: computed tomographic findings. *J Comput Assist Tomogr* 2010;34(6):945–948.

Cox CW, Rose CS, Lynch DA. State of the art: imaging of occupational lung disease. *Radiology* 2014;270(3):681–696.

Webb WR, Muller NL, Naidich DP. Pneumoconiosis. Occupational and environmental lung disease, (Chapter 9). In: *High-resolution of the lung*. 4th ed. Philadelphia, PA: Lippincott Williams & Wilkins, 2014:329–330.

30a **Answer C.**

30b **Answer B.**

30c **Answer C.**

30d **Answer D.** The radiographic images show bilateral basal and posterior predominant reticular pattern. No cardiomegaly, lymphadenopathy, or pleural effusions are identified. Decreased lung volumes and relatively symmetric posterior basal predominant reticulations suggest that this is related to the presence of lung fibrosis.

On the CT images, there is peripheral and lower lung predominant reticular abnormality with development of significant honeycomb cyst formation over time. This is classic for the UIP pattern of fibrosing interstitial pneumonia. The pattern of fibrosis in NSIP demonstrates more ground-glass abnormality (especially in a bronchovascular pattern) and more traction bronchiectasis. Honeycomb cyst formation can be seen in NSIP but is generally a very late finding indicative of end-stage fibrosis. Organizing pneumonia is characterized by peripheral and lower lung predominant consolidation and ground glass. LIP is characterized by lower lung predominant cysts in a perivascular distribution rather than the subpleural honeycomb cysts found here.

A number of conditions could present with features of UIP (connective tissue disease such as rheumatoid arthritis, chronic hypersensitivity pneumonitis, or drug toxicity). It is crucial to exclude any of these identifiable causes to diagnosis idiopathic pulmonary fibrosis (IPF) and guide optimal treatment. IPF has a considerably worse prognosis compared to other causes of fibrosing interstitial pneumonia.

References: Hobbs S, Lynch D. The idiopathic interstitial pneumonias: an update and review. *Radiol Clin North Am* 2014;52(1):105–120.

Lynch DA, Travis WD, Muller NL, et al. Idiopathic interstitial pneumonias: CT features. *Radiology* 2005;236:10–21.

Webb WR, Muller NL, Naidich DP. The idiopathic interstitial pneumonias (Chapter 4). In: *High-resolution of the lung*. 4th ed. Philadelphia, PA: Lippincott Williams & Wilkins, 2014:177–189.

Souza CA, Müller NL, Flint J. Idiopathic pulmonary fibrosis: spectrum of high-resolution CT findings. *AJR Am J Roentgenol* 2005;185:1531–1539.

31a   Answer A.

31b   Answer A.

31c   Answer B.

31d   Answer D.   CT images show advanced traction bronchiectases, most abundant in the lower lungs, with relative subpleural sparing in the dorsal lower lobes but extension into cardiophrenic angles. Similarly, bilateral peripheral ground-glass opacities demonstrate relative sparing of the most peripheral lung. Patchy consolidation and small pleural effusion are seen on the left. The imaging findings are most indicative of fibrotic nonspecific interstitial pneumonia (NSIP). Multifocal consolidation on the left could represent foci of organizing pneumonia.

NSIP is chronic interstitial lung disease that accounts for 40% of pathologically proven interstitial lung diseases. The most common etiologies include connective tissue diseases, drug exposure, hypersensitivity pneumonitis, and occupational exposure.

The primary findings of NSIP include (1) extensive ground-glass opacities with absent or mild reticulation, (2) traction bronchiectases, (3) absent or minimal honeycombing, (4) basal predominance, and (5) subpleural sparing. Among these criteria, ground-glass opacities with minimal or absent reticulation is considered the cellular type of NSIP. Remainder of the findings corresponds to fibrotic NSIP. CT features of NSIP can overlap with organizing pneumonia and desquamative interstitial pneumonia; in these cases, surgical biopsy should be performed with sampling of more than one lobe.

Fibrotic NSIP carries worse survival than cellular NSIP, 6 to 14 years versus complete improvement in nearly all cases. However, fibrotic NSIP is not as poor a prognosis as IPF (2.5 to 3.5 years average survival from initial diagnosis). Idiopathic NSIP has at least an 80% 5-year survival.

Response to corticosteroids and cytotoxic agents is nonuniform in NSIP and depends on the type. Cellular NSIP frequently responds to corticosteroids but is the more rare type of NSIP. Fibrotic NSIP has a worse response to the corticosteroids and cytotoxic agents.

References: Lynch DA, Travis WD, Muller NL, et al. Idiopathic interstitial pneumonias: CT features. *Radiology* 2005;236:10–21.

Poletti V, Romagnoli M, Piciucchi S, et al. Current status of idiopathic nonspecific interstitial pneumonia. *Semin Respir Crit Care Med* 2012;33:440–449.

Silva CI, Muller NL, Hansell DM, et al. Nonspecific interstitial pneumonia and idiopathic pulmonary fibrosis: changes in pattern and distribution of disease over time. *Radiology* 2008;247(1):251–259.

Webb WR, Muller NL, Naidich DP. The idiopathic interstitial pneumonias (Chapter 4). In: *High-resolution of the lung.* 4th ed. Philadelphia, PA: Lippincott Williams & Wilkins, 2014:189–198.

32a **Answer B.**

32b **Answer A.** Bilateral extensive ground-glass opacities (GGO) are present. Appearance is nonspecific, and biopsy would be required for definitive diagnosis. Differential considerations would include hypersensitivity pneumonitis (exposure to an extrinsic allergen), desquamative interstitial pneumonia (history of smoking), and nonspecific interstitial pneumonia. In this patient, hypersensitivity pneumonitis is less likely in the setting of smoking (one of the few diseases actually prevented by smoking). Usual interstitial pneumonia manifests with subpleural reticulations, intralobular lines, and honeycombing, which are not seen. Pulmonary edema manifests first as vessel distension and interlobular septal thickening, which are not seen in this case.

Imaging features of DIP include bilateral confluent or patchy ground-glass opacities, frequently with small parenchymal cysts in the areas of ground glass. Mild reticulation could be present owing to minimal septal fibrosis.

Even though DIP, like RB–ILD (respiratory bronchiolitis–interstitial lung disease), is predominantly a smoking-related illness, distribution of findings is different: diffuse or geographic areas of ground-glass opacities with lower lung predominance in DIP and upper lung predominant ground-glass nodules in RB–ILD. Some authors believe that RB-ILD and DIP represents continuum in smoking-related injury. Pathologically, RB–ILD is centrilobular peribronchiolar pathologic process whereas DIP represents intra-alveolar accumulation of macrophages with some giant cells. The term "desquamative" is a misnomer and originates from a prior belief that pneumocyte desquamation was occurring.

Desquamative interstitial pneumonia (DIP) can be seen in up to 40% in nonsmoking population in association to exposure to inhaled occupational inorganic particles (beryllium, aluminum, diesel fumes) and aflatoxin. drugs (nitrofurantoin, busulfan), viral illnesses, and autoimmune disease. However, the usual occurrence is in smoking males (male: female ratio is 2:1), 40 to 60 years old, who present with exertional dyspnea and/or mild nonproductive cough. On physical exam, basal crackles and cyanosis are frequently seen. The most frequent abnormal pattern on pulmonary functional test is a restrictive pattern. Severe obstruction on spirometry (FEV1 <70%) is not characteristic and, when present, likely reflects concomitant chronic bronchitis or emphysema.

Survival from DIP is estimated to be between 68% and 98%. Smoking cessation (or removal of an offending agent in nonsmoking–related DIP) is pivotal. About 20% of patients show spontaneous improvement with cessation of exposure. A large number of patients require corticosteroids. Without treatment, 60% patients deteriorate clinically. About 25% of patients will progress despite the treatment.

References: Attili A, Kazerooni E, Gross BH, et al. Smoking-related interstitial lung disease: radiologic-clinical-pathologic correlation. *Radiographics* 2008;28:1383–1398.

Godbert B, Wissler M, Vignaud J. Desquamative interstitial pneumonia: an analytic review with an emphasis on aetiology. *Eur Respir Rev* 2013;22(128): 117–123.

Hobbs S, Lynch D. The idiopathic interstitial pneumonias: an update and review. *Radiol Clin North Am* 2014;52(1):105–120.

33a **Answer B.**

33b **Answer C.**

33c **Answer B.**

33d **Answer D.**   Radiographic images show extensive bilateral patchy consolidation. Small left-sided pleural effusion, small right apical pneumothorax, and subcutaneous air within upper chest/lower neck are present. Several thin vertical lucencies within the upper mediastinum are suspicious for mild pneumomediastinum. Please note that the patient is intubated. The cardiac silhouette is not enlarged on this portable chest radiograph. The lung volumes are normal. The appearance would be highly unlikely to represent cardiogenic edema. No architectural distortion and characteristic apicobasal and peripheral gradients are present. Presence of pneumothorax and subcutaneous air and suspicion for mild pneumomediastinum raise a question of barotrauma in a mechanically ventilated patient, which is frequently seen in causes of noncardiogenic edema or ARDS. Aspiration tends to be either central (perihilar) or lower lung predominant and not as diffuse as this process is but can transition to ARDS. Similarly, lobar pneumonia refers to infection in a single lobe and this process is clearly diffuse.

This is a case of acute interstitial pneumonia (AIP). AIP is an idiopathic condition that is histologically and radiographically similar to acute respiratory distress syndrome. The latter could be caused by multiple factors that include but not limited to viral infection, aspiration, sepsis, shock, trauma, or drug reaction. On CT, bilateral ground-glass opacities are present with gradual appearance of more dense foci of consolidation in dependent distribution. Note the relative absence of septal thickening normally seen in pulmonary edema. Bilateral pleural effusions are evident. The underlying pathology is that of diffuse alveolar damage (DAD). In the acute phase, a combination of airspace exudates, noncardiogenic interstitial edema, inflammation, and alveolar collapse in the dependent portions of the lungs is seen. The organizing phase of ARDS is first seen in the beginning of the 2nd week after an insult and depends on the ability of denuded alveoli and exposed epithelial membranes to reorganize and repair, resulting in increased consolidation. Upper and anterior lung predominant fibrosis results from this fibroproliferative phase. Anterior fibrosis is thought to result from barotrauma and oxygen toxicity in mechanical ventilation to the anterior lungs, whereas the dorsal lungs are relatively protected by the gravity-dependent atelectasis and consolidation.

References: Webb WR, Muller NL, Naidich DP. The idiopathic interstitial pneumonias (Chapter 4). In: *High-resolution of the lung*, 4th ed. Philadelphia, PA: Lippincott Williams & Wilkins, 2014:206–209.

Lynch DA, Travis WD, Muller NL, et al. Idiopathic interstitial pneumonias: CT features. *Radiology* 2005;236:10–21.

Kligerman SJ, Franks TJ, Galvin JR. From the radiologic pathology archives: organization and fibrosis as a response to lung injury in diffuse alveolar damage, organizing pneumonia, and acute fibrinous and organizing pneumonia. *Radiographics* 2013;33(7):1951–1975.

34a **Answer C.**

34b **Answer D.**

34c **Answer C.**

34d **Answer A.** Frontal chest radiograph shows unilateral (right) reticular and reticulonodular pattern. Differential considerations favor lymphangitic carcinomatosis (LC) or atypical infection (viral pneumonia). Subsequent CT images show unilateral variable (smooth and nodular) septal thickening, thickening of centrilobular core structures, and preservation of normal lobular architecture. Spiculated lung lesion with adjacent pleural reaction is present. The unilateral process and presence of spiculated lesion make lymphangitic carcinomatosis the most likely diagnosis. Emphysema would manifest as hyperinflation and upper lung lucency. Pulmonary edema is generally. a bilateral process.

When unilateral and seen in the presence of an upper lung suspicious lesion, it is often due to bronchogenic carcinoma (as in the case here). Secondary malignancies associated with LC are adenocarcinomas especially those originating from the breast, stomach, colon, and prostate. However, these have bilateral findings in 80% to 90% of the time. Lymphangitic carcinomatosis generally indicates stage IV disease and wedge resection would not address the more extensive disease.

Radiographic findings in lymphangitic carcinomatosis are negative in half of the cases. The remainder shows reticular or reticulonodular pattern. On CT, reticular pattern corresponds to thickening of interlobular septa that is most frequently nodular or beaded in appearance.

Pathogenesis most commonly reflects initial hematogenous dissemination to the lungs with subsequent invasion or the interstitium and lymphatics. The tumor spreads from the peripheral lung centrally via the interstitium around the lymphatics. In a minority of patients, the spread occurs retrograde from tumor-laden hilar lymph nodes. LC is associated with poor prognosis, with demise frequently seen within 6 months.

References: Johkoh T, Ikezoe J, Tomiyama N, et al. CT findings in lymphangitic carcinomatosis of the lung: correlation with histologic findings and pulmonary function tests. *AJR Am J Roentgenol* 1992;158:1217–1222.

Prakash P, Kalra MK, Sharma A, et al. FDG PET/CT in assessment of pulmonary lymphangitic carcinomatosis. *AJR Am J Roentgenol* 2010;194:231–236.

Scheafer-Prokop C, Prokop M, Fleischman D, et al. High-resolution CT of diffuse interstitial lung disease: key findings in common disorders. *Eur Radiol* 2001;11:373–392.

35 **Answer A.** The chest radiograph demonstrates significant enlargement of the cardiac silhouette. This could be related to cardiomegaly or pericardial effusion but is confirmed as cardiomegaly on the CT. Additionally, the interlobular septal thickening is smooth, diffuse, and bilateral with a mild degree of lower lung ground-glass opacity as well. The appearance is classic for cardiogenic interstitial pulmonary edema. Pleural effusions are common and more often right-sided if small.

Lymphangitic carcinomatosis would be more likely to present with nodular thickening. Similarly, there is no architectural distortion to suggest an underlying fibrotic lung disease. Lymphangiectasia is frequently fatal in infancy but can be seen in adults. The interlobular septal thickening in those cases is generally accompanied by pleural thickening and significant mediastinal abnormality such as lymphangiomas (not seen here). Other mimics of smooth interlobular septal thickening would include sarcoidosis, Niemann-Pick, and lymphangiomatosis (not to be confused with lymphangioleiomyomatosis).

Reference: Oikonomou A, Prassopoulos P. Mimics in chest disease: interstitial opacities. *Insights Imaging* 2013;4(1):9–27.

Section 3: Diffuse Alveolar Disease and Inflammatory Conditions

36a **Answer D.**

36b **Answer A.**

36c **Answer B.**   Initial presentation on chest radiograph is consistent with consolidation supported by the homogeneous opacities with air bronchograms. The peripheral distribution could raise concern for pleural thickening although the poorly defined inner margins, outlining of the horizontal fissure, and air bronchograms contradict a pleural-based process. Interstitial opacities, such as reticular and nodular patterns, can be peripheral, but would not produce the homogenous opacities, air bronchograms, or clear outline of the fissure.

Of the options provided, only lipoid pneumonia would produce a static consolidation for 6 months. Although many frequently think of lipoid pneumonia only in the case of low (fat)-density alveolar consolidation, that is not always seen. As the name implies, ARDS is an acute process and one would expect signs of respiratory distress, such as intubation, before suggesting the diagnosis radiographically. Incomplete treatment of bacterial pneumonia could produce a persistent consolidation, but the static nature in this case suggests against it as one would expect progression over time. Infectious pneumonia can convert into an organizing pneumonia, but this is not given as an option. Finally, pulmonary embolism can produce peripheral consolidation due to infarct, but again, the static nature excluded this diagnosis at 6 months. Additionally, hemorrhage as the cause of consolidation in pulmonary infarcts tends to fill the airways, causing a notable absence of air bronchograms.

In terms of treatment, Gondouin et al. reported a multicenter case study of exogenous lipoid pneumonia including 44 patients. In this study, and in others, corticosteroids and bronchoalveolar lavage demonstrated no significant benefit in the treatment of lipoid pneumonia. As the disease is not infectious, antibiotics have no use in the treatment, but patients often fail antibiotics early due to a presumed infectious etiology at initial presentation. Of the 44 cases studied by Gondouin, 13 improved with removal of offending agent, 7 stabilized, and 5 patients experienced ongoing progression and deterioration to include pulmonary fibrosis, recurrent infection, and *Aspergillus*-related complication.

Reference: Gondouin A, et al. Exogenous lipid pneumonia: a retrospective multicentre study of 44 cases in France. *Eur Respir J* 1996;9:1463–1469.

37a **Answer B.**

37b **Answer D.**

37c **Answer D.**

37d **Answer B.**   The initial chest radiograph demonstrates a right upper lobe predominant consolidation that outlines the minor fissure. Classic findings of consolidation on chest radiograph include poorly defined margins, air bronchograms, contained by fissures, and maintained lung volume. While these opacities do prove to be peripherally predominant, this characteristic does not help categorizes these opacities as consolidation. Volume loss is not significant on this initial chest radiograph, nor is it a finding of consolidation. Finally, "tram-track" opacities are an axial interstitial finding relating to thickening of the bronchial wall and therefore not a finding of consolidation.

Localizing pulmonary disease can be a challenge on single CT images, and therefore, understanding the relationship with fissures can be helpful. The anatomic position on CT is the same as chest radiograph with the patient position facing the viewer with the patient's right on the left side of the image. That places the consolidations on the provided CT in the patient's right lung. The consolidation along the superior aspect of the minor fissure localizes the findings to the right upper lobe. Interestingly, this patient also has an accessory left horizontal fissure.

When the disease recurs, it demonstrates a classic distribution for eosinophilic pneumonia with peripheral patchy consolidations, often with an upper lobe predominance. This appearance has been described as the "photographic negative on pulmonary edema." Bronchoalveolar lavage revealing eosinophils in the setting of pulmonary consolidation is diagnostic of eosinophilic pneumonia, and secondary causes such as infection or drug toxicity should be excluded. The spontaneous resolution and disease recurrence removes neoplastic etiologies from the differential, such as bronchogenic carcinoma or lymphoma. Lipid-rich pneumonias such as lipoid pneumonia and alveolar proteinosis can cause chronic consolidation, but the recurrent pattern and peripheral upper lobe distribution would favor eosinophilic pneumonia.

Initial time course of disease in this patient, spontaneously resolving after 1 month, is consistent with simple eosinophilic pneumonia, also known as Loeffler syndrome, and helps differentiate from chronic eosinophilic pneumonia, which generally requires steroid treatment and/or identification of an underlying process. Simple eosinophilic pneumonia also typically causes "shifting consolidations," where chronic eosinophilic pneumonia will produce more static homogenous consolidations. Otherwise, both of these types of eosinophilic lung disease may produce similar peripheral consolidations, symptoms, and blood eosinophilia.

References: Jeong YJ, et al. Eosinophilic lung diseases: a clinical, radiologic, and pathologic overview. *Radiographics* 2007;27:617–639.

Webb WR, Higgins CB. *Thoracic imaging.* Philadelphia, PA: Lippincott Williams & Wilkins. 2010.

38a **Answer B.**

38b **Answer A.** Because the "crazy-paving" sign has a differential diagnosis to include infection, pulmonary edema, malignancy, lipoid pneumonia, and pulmonary hemorrhage, bronchoalveolar lavage plays an important role in identifying PAS-positive lipoproteinaceous material diagnostic of pulmonary alveolar proteinosis. BAL also serves a therapeutic function as serial lavage is generally curative, at least temporarily. Initial lavage may reveal a thick milky fluid, which clears on repeat lavage. Exogenous lipoid pneumonia resulting from aspiration of lipid-rich material is generally diagnosed clinically by identifying the aspirated material rather than BAL, which may have few pathologic findings as the lipid is removed in the fixation of the fluid.

Approximately 75% of patients with idiopathic pulmonary alveolar proteinosis are smokers. When corrected for smoking, gender, weight, and activities such as air travel have no significant association with the disease.

References: Frazier AA, Franks TJ, Cooke EO. From the archives of the AFIP: pulmonary alveolar proteinosis. *Radiographics* 2008;28:883–899.

Michaud G, Reddy C, Ernst A. Whole-lung lavage for pulmonary alveolar proteinosis. *Chest* 2009;136:1678–1681.

39 **Answer B.** TRALI is a serious and potentially life-threatening complication of blood product transfusion. The mechanism is not entirely understood, but the clinical presentation is similar to that of ARDS and noncardiogenic edema. Onset is most frequently within 1 to 2 hours with most cases manifesting under 6 hours. Resolution normally occurs within 2 to 4 days with supportive measures. Separating this disease process from fluid overload related to the transfusion (transfusion-associated circulatory overload—TACO) is critical as the use of diuretics should be avoided in TRALI. This was a case of TRALI. Note the lack of features to support cardiogenic edema and TACO including normal cardiac size, lack of effusions, and lack of a more diffuse or lower lung gradient.

Reference: Carcano C, Okafor N, Martinez F, et al. Radiographic manifestations of transfusion-related acute lung injury. *Clin Imaging* 2013;37(6):1020–1023.

40 **Answer B.** On inspiratory exam, there is a diffuse centrilobular ground-glass nodularity. In isolation, the differential diagnosis would include both hypersensitivity pneumonitis and respiratory bronchiolitis. However, the presence of significant geographic and lobular air trapping on expiratory exam is more suggestive of subacute hypersensitivity pneumonitis. Respiratory bronchiolitis is also strongly associated with smoking, and smoking is actually mildly protective against hypersensitivity pneumonitis.

HP is an interstitial lung disease related to inhalation of organic particles and a resulting diffuse granulomatous process. Acute HP is characterized by near immediate onset after antigen exposure in a patient who has been previously sensitized. Subacute HP results from more continuous exposure to low doses of the antigen and can eventually progress to chronic disease if the antigen is not removed. The antigen can vary, with typical causes including molds and birds, but upward of 40% of patients do not have an identifiable antigen.

The commonest CT imaging appearance of subacute HP is upper lung predominant centrilobular ground-glass nodules. Air trapping and mosaic attenuation is a frequent-associated feature. In some cases, only air trapping or a normal CT exam may be present. Occasionally, superimposed organizing pneumonia with consolidation can be identified as can pulmonary cysts or emphysema. Chronic HP can demonstrate similar findings, but with an increasing degree of reticular abnormality and fibrosis (which can be either NSIP or UIP pattern).

References: Cox CW, Rose CS, Lynch DA. State of the art: imaging of occupational lung disease. *Radiology* 2014;270(3):681–696.

Silva CI, Churg A, Müller NL. Hypersensitivity pneumonitis: spectrum of high-resolution CT and pathologic findings. *AJR Am J Roentgenol* 2007;188(2):334–344.

41a **Answer A.**

41b **Answer B.** Churg-Strauss syndrome, now called eosinophilic granulomatosis with polyangiitis, demonstrates a triad of eosinophilia, necrotizing vasculitis, and asthma. The rheumatologic guidelines for diagnosis include having at least four of the following six findings: (1) asthma, (2) mono- or polyneuropathy, (3) migratory pulmonary opacities, (4) paranasal sinus disease, (5) extravascular eosinophils, and (6) peripheral eosinophilia on CBC. The histology is that of both a necrotizing small-vessel vasculitis and eosinophilic inflammatory infiltrate (which accounts for the new naming convention).

The most common radiographic findings are of transient bilateral areas of consolidation. There is a predilection of the lung periphery and some evidence of a slightly upper lung predominance (as opposed to organizing pneumonia with a lower lung predominance). Bronchial wall thickening and small centrilobular nodules are also common features, especially given the association with asthma. Upward of 70% of patients will be p-ANCA positive.

Wegener does not have any specific association with asthma although other features of vasculitis and sinus disease can be present. It has a much stronger association with cANCA. Organizing pneumonia also has no specific association with the clinical picture shown but can be due to a variety of connective tissue disease or drug toxicities. Microscopic polyangiitis is a nongranulomatous necrotizing systemic vasculitis and the most common cause of pulmonary renal syndrome (concurrent pulmonary hemorrhage and glomerulonephritis); however, the manifestations are much more commonly renal with 90% of patients having rapidly progressive glomerulonephritis but pulmonary hemorrhage in only up to 30%.

Reference: Castañer E, Alguersuari A, Gallardo X, et al. When to suspect pulmonary vasculitis: radiologic and clinical clues. *Radiographics* 2010;30(1):33–53.

42 Answer A.   The CT images demonstrate lower lung predominant peribronchovascular and perilobular consolidation with a mild degree of resulting fibrosis. Of the choices listed, the pattern is most consistent with organizing pneumonia. The history of chronic UTI should specifically draw to mind the possibility of drug toxicity. This was a case of nitrofurantoin-related organizing pneumonia. Cessation of the drug resulted in significant improvement.

Septic emboli would be expected to be more nodular and cavitary (although peripheral opacities are common). Pulmonary hemorrhage would be more diffuse without a specific peripheral predominance. The features of UIP including subpleural reticular abnormality and honeycomb cyst formation are not seen here. Nonspecific interstitial pneumonia (NSIP) would be a consideration for this appearance, but the degree of consolidative abnormality is much more than typically seen without concurrent organizing pneumonia.

A good website to evaluate if a drug has potential pulmonary toxicity and how it might manifest is www.pneumotox.com.

Other manifestations of drug toxicity include eosinophilic pneumonia, diffuse alveolar damage, pulmonary edema, pulmonary hemorrhage, fibrosing interstitial pneumonias, lupus, vasculitis, hypersensitivity pneumonitis, and constrictive bronchiolitis.

References: Rossi SE, Erasmus JJ, McAdams HP, et al. Pulmonary drug toxicity: radiologic and pathologic manifestations. *Radiographics* 2000;20(5):1245–1259.

Webb WR, Higgins CB. *Thoracic imaging*. Philadelphia, PA: Lippincott Williams & Wilkins, 2010.

43a Answer A.

43b Answer A.   The head cheese sign reflects adjacent low, normal, and high attenuation in adjacent secondary pulmonary lobules. It reflects a combination of airspace disease (high attenuation) and obstructive disease (low attenuation). The low attenuation small airway disease component reflects mosaic attenuation, and the high attenuation component reflects ground-glass opacity.

The disease is most highly associated with subacute hypersensitivity pneumonitis and was initially considered pathognomonic. However, other diseases including sarcoidosis, atypical infections (such as *Mycoplasma*), respiratory bronchiolitis, and DIP have demonstrated this feature. Additionally, in patients with multiple pathologic processes, this sign can manifest, such as constrictive bronchiolitis and pulmonary hemorrhage.

Reference: Chong BJ, Kanne JP, Chung JH, et al. Headcheese sign. *J Thorac Imaging* 2014;29(1):W13.

44 **Answer B.** The radiograph demonstrates asymmetric, right greater than left airspace disease in an alveolar pattern. The airspace disease is greatest in the central lungs, and there are no identifiable effusions. Also, the heart is not enlarged. Given patient age and the lack of cardiac findings and effusions, cardiogenic edema is less likely. The other three considerations are possible; however, the history of recent high-altitude travel should make one strongly suspicious of high-altitude pulmonary edema (HAPE), a non-cardiogenic pulmonary edema.

HAPE is a potentially fatal condition that occurs after traveling to a low oxygen and low atmospheric pressure environment (generally found at high altitudes). Most frequently, it occurs in young male patients 1 to 2 days after rapid ascent to elevations above 3,000 m. The mechanism is not well understood but likely is related to vasoconstriction and acute-onset pulmonary hypertension with resulting capillary leak. Treatment is supportive with return to normal altitude being critical.

Reference: Gluecker T, Capasso P, Schnyder P, et al. Clinical and radiologic features of pulmonary edema. *Radiographics* 1999;19(6):1507–1531.

45 **Answer B.** The reverse halo sign is characterized by a peripheral rim of consolidation with central ground-glass opacity (not central necrosis, cavitation, or pseudocavitation). Originally thought to be specific for organizing pneumonia, it is now recognized to occur in other pathologies such as some infections (paracoccidioidomycosis—South American blastomycosis, mucormycosis, tuberculosis), pulmonary infarct, vasculitis, or sarcoidosis. Alternative names for the reverse halo sign include the atoll sign and fairy ring sign.

Reference: Walker CM, Mohammed TL, Chung JH. Reversed halo sign. *J Thorac Imaging* 2011;26(3):W80.

46 **Answer A.** The pattern of disease is almost identical on inspiration and expiration. There is diffuse ground glass with some areas of geographic sparing and mosaic attenuation (air trapping) as well as peripheral reticular abnormality and fibrosis. One common cause of upper lung predominant fibrosis with this degree of mosaic air trapping is chronic hypersensitivity pneumonitis (findings of subacute HP with superimposed fibrosis). Although sarcoidosis does cause upper lung fibrosis and can have air trapping, the pattern is generally more bronchovascular, radiating from the hilar with bronchiectasis being a significant feature. Progressive massive fibrosis can also cause upper lung fibrosis but is more similar to sarcoid-related fibrosis with the addition of mass-like perihilar consolidation. Idiopathic pulmonary fibrosis is the idiopathic form of usual interstitial pneumonitis generally producing lower lung predominant, subpleural, and reticular fibrosis, with or without honeycomb cyst formation.

Reference: Silva CI, Churg A, Müller NL. Hypersensitivity pneumonitis: spectrum of high-resolution CT and pathologic findings. *AJR Am J Roentgenol* 2007;188(2):334–344.

Section 4: Airway Disease

47a **Answer A.**

47b **Answer D.**

47c **Answer B.** Tree-in-bud nodularity represents dilated and impacted lobular bronchioles. On CT images, these appear as centrilobular branching structures that resemble a budding tree. Multiple causes have been described such as infectious (mycobacteria, fungal, viral, parasitic), congenital (cystic fibrosis,

Kartagener syndrome), idiopathic (obliterative bronchiolitis, panbronchiolitis), aspiration, immunologic (allergic bronchopulmonary aspergillosis), connective tissue disorders, and neoplastic pulmonary embolic phenomenon.

The constellation of imaging findings (tree-in-bud nodularity, bronchiectasis with mucous plugging, and air trapping) predominantly in the right middle lobe and lingula are highly suggestive of MAI infection. This is frequently referred to as Lady Windermere syndrome, which reflects one of the demographic groups frequently affected by NTM infection. The other group is the "classic" form and occurs in older men with emphysema and COPD with an imaging appearance identical to that of postprimary tuberculosis.

Organism diagnosis by culture is important for these cases as it guides antibiotic therapy (which often lasts for years). Culture can be difficult even with appropriate steps, so the suggest of NTM infection by imaging can be important to alert the bronchoscopist prior to the procedure.

Reference: Martinez S, et al. The many faces of pulmonary nontuberculous mycobacterial infection. *AJR Am J Roentgenol* 2007;189(1):177–186.

48a Answer C.

48b Answer B. Tracheobronchial anatomic variants can be divided into minor variants in lobar and segmental subdivisions (common) and major variants that include abnormal origin or supernumerary bronchus (rare). The major bronchial abnormalities include accessory cardiac bronchus (ACB) and tracheal bronchus. The ACB is a supernumerary bronchus that arises from the inner wall of the right mainstem bronchus or the intermediate bronchus opposite to the origin of the right upper lobe bronchus.

A tracheal bronchus is an anatomic variant characterized by an abnormal origin of a segmental or lobar bronchus arising within 2 cm of the carina and supplying a portion or the entire upper lobe. This term can also be used to describe an accessory bronchus that arises from the mainstem bronchus and serves the right upper lobe. When it serves the entire right upper lobe, as in this case, it is also known as "pig bronchus" or "bronchus suis." One in 400 normal persons has a tracheal bronchus.

Most of the time this anatomic variant is asymptomatic, however can become symptomatic in the setting of intubation, given the predisposition to develop atelectasis and/or pneumonia.

Reference: Ghaye B, et al. Congenital bronchial abnormalities revisited. *Radiographics* 2001;21(1):105–119.

49a Answer: D.

49b Answer: B. Tracheomalacia or tracheobronchomalacia (TBM) is defined as diffuse or segmental tracheal weakness with luminal area narrowing of 70% as criteria on dynamic expiratory CT. Correlation of CT findings with pulmonary functional evidence of airway obstruction is important as the degree of normal can vary. TBM can be divided into primary (congenital) and secondary (acquired) depending on the etiology. Congenital associations include numerous cardiovascular abnormalities, gastroesophageal reflux, and tracheoesophageal fistulas. Acquired conditions are more common and include prolonged intubation, chronic tracheal infections, extrinsic compressions (such as aortic aneurysms), or chronic tracheal inflammation such as relapsing polychondritis. It can be classified as severe if the anterior and posterior walls touch. A lunate configuration of the trachea on inspiratory CT images is highly specific for tracheomalacia, but low in sensitivity. Tracheomalacia "frown sign" describes the characteristic anterior bowing of the posterior membranous trachea on expiratory CT images resulting in a reversed U-shaped air column. Saber sheath trachea and tracheal wall thickening can be seen the setting of tracheomalacia, but are not specific.

References: Chung J, Kanne J, Gilman M. CT of diffuse tracheal diseases. *AJR Am J Roentgenol* 2011;196:w240–w246.

Ridge CA, O'Donnell CR, Lee, et al. Tracheobronchomalacia: current concepts and controversies. *J Thorac Imaging* 2011;26:278–289.

50a **Answer: A.**

50b **Answer: D.**   Aspiration-related lung disease is an underrecognized clinicopathologic entity that is estimated to account for at least 5% to 15% of community-acquired pneumonias. It is also considered the most common cause of death in patients with dysphagia due to neurologic insult. The most common imaging findings of acute aspiration-related lung disease include filling defects in the airway, lobar airway thickening, tree-in-bud nodularity, ground-glass centrilobular nodularity, and air–space disease. Chronic changes of aspiration-related lung disease include bronchiectasis, parenchymal granulomas, reticulation, and honeycombing.

Reference: Prather AD, et al. Aspiration related lung diseases. *J Thorac Imaging* 2014;29(5):304–309.

51 **Answer: A.**   Granulomatosis with polyangiitis (GPA) is a systemic granulomatous process with necrotizing vasculitis involving the lung, upper respiratory tract, and kidneys. This disease was formerly referred to as Wegener granulomatosis but has now been renamed. Characteristic imaging findings in the chest include pulmonary nodules and ground-glass opacities. Central cavitation occurs in up to 50% of nodules larger than 2 cm. Involvement of the trachea and bronchi is present in 16% to 23% of cases. Circumferential wall thickening is characteristic and helps differentiate from other common tracheal pathologic entities such as tracheobronchopathia osteochondroplastica (TBPO or TO) and relapsing polychondritis, which characteristically spare the posterior membrane.

Reference: Chung J, Kanne J, Gilman M. CT of diffuse tracheal diseases. *AJR Am J Roentgenol* 2011;196:w240–w246.

52 **Answer: A.**   Postintubation tracheal stenosis is the most common case of focal tracheal stenosis. It can present as a weblike stenosis (<1 cm), membranous concentric stenosis without damage of the cartilage, and the "A"-shaped stenosis, which happens secondary to lateral impacted fracture of the cartilage in patients with prior tracheostomy (as seen in this case). These are referred to as "pseudoglotic stenosis" during bronchoscopy due to their appearance. Critical tracheal narrowing is generally defined as <10 mm by imaging.

Long segment tracheal wall thickening and/or narrowing may be secondary to saber sheath trachea, relapsing polychondritis, or tracheobronchopathia osteochondroplastica. Less common causes include amyloidosis, granulomatosis with polyangiitis (Wegner granulomatosis), tumors, inflammatory bowel disease, or thermal injury. Saber sheath trachea is characterized by a tracheal index <0.6 (transverse dimension of the trachea divided by the anteroposterior dimension). Note that some abnormalities such as relapsing polychondritis and tracheobronchopathia osteochondroplastica tend to spare the posterior membrane (which lacks cartilage), which can help limit the differential diagnosis.

Differential considerations for more short segment narrowing in the trachea includes granulomatosis with polyangiitis, squamous papillomatosis, rhinoscleroma (Klebsiella rhinoscleromatis), cicatricial pemphigoid, sarcoidosis, and amyloidosis.

References: Chung J, Kanne J, Gilman M. CT of diffuse tracheal diseases. *AJR Am J Roentgenol* 2011;196:w240–w246.

Grenier PA, Beigelman-Aubry C, Brillet PY. Nonneoplastic tracheal and bronchial stenoses. *Radiol Clin North Am* 2009;47(2):243–260

53a Answer: A.

53b Answer: C.   The images demonstrate lower lung predominant findings of cylindrical and varicoid bronchiectasis with significant mosaic attenuation that is likely related to small airway disease. Cysts would not connect with the bronchi as shown, and there is no significant nodularity. Of the diseases listed, asthma can present with significant small airway disease, especially in acute exacerbation, but air trapping predominates in asthma as opposed to mosaic attenuation as seen here. Additionally, the degree of bronchiectasis would be atypical in asthma alone. Both cystic fibrosis and ABPA would be expected to be upper lung predominant and generally exhibit more nodules and mucoid impaction. The mucoid impaction in ABPA can be characteristically high density, which is nearly pathognomonic. Atypical mycobacterial disease has a classic predilection for the right middle lobe and lingular (Lady Windermere syndrome) but can present with the distribution shown. However, there should be evidence of nodules (possibly cavitary or tree-in-bud) to suggest active disease that is not seen. Bronchiolitis obliterans (constrictive bronchiolitis) is the best choice given the images seen. Careful clinical history should be obtained to evaluate for potential causes such as prior infection, inhalational exposures, connective tissue disease (especially rheumatoid arthritis), or drug toxicity.

Reference: Hansell DM, Lynch DA, McAdams HP, et al. *Imaging of diseases of the chest*. 5th ed. Mosby, 2009.

54a Answer: D.

54b Answer: A.   The chest x-ray demonstrates severe deviation of the trachea to the right due to a superior mediastinal mass. Subsequent CT confirms the presence of a mass at the thoracic inlet and the extrinsic compression of the trachea. The mass itself is intermediate to low density, but well circumscribed and despite its large size, does not seem to invade any adjacent structures as would be seen in carcinomas. The location is atypical for a foregut duplication cyst, and there is no contrast enhancement to suggest an aneurysm. However, there does appear to be a claw sign involving the thyroid (noted at the superior margin of the mass) consistent with thyroid etiology.

Reference: Hansell DM, Lynch DA, McAdams HP, et al. *Imaging of diseases of the chest*. 5th ed. Mosby, 2009.

55a Answer: A.

55b Answer: D.   The most common primary malignant neoplasm of the trachea is squamous cell carcinoma, followed by adenoid cystic cell carcinoma and mucoepidermoid, respectively. The most common metastatic lesion to the trachea is secondary to local extension from thyroid cancer, esophageal cancer, and lung cancer. Hematogenous spread of tumor to the trachea is rare but can be seen in melanoma and breast cancer.

Reference: Hansell DM, Lynch DA, McAdams HP, et al. *Imaging of diseases of the chest*. 5th ed. Mosby, 2009.

56a **Answer: B.**

56b **Answer: C.**   There is significant lower lung predominant bronchial wall thickening and varicoid bronchiectasis with areas of consolidation and tree-in-bud opacity. Considerations for only those findings would include immunodeficiency (such as CVID), ciliary dyskinesia, or diffuse panbronchiolitis. However, this patient also has situs inversus totalis (note the right aortic arch and dextrocardia). This combination is characteristic of Kartagener syndrome, a subtype of primary ciliary dyskinesia, which also features infertility and chronic sinus disease. Fifty percent of patients with immotile cilia syndrome will have situs inversus totalis as the determination of situs during embryologic development requires normal ciliary beating. Nonfunctioning cilia result in situ being determined randomly with half being normal and half inverted.

Other common associations for the other answer choices include splenomegaly with CVID and East Asian heritage with diffuse panbronchiolitis. Sarcoid can present with central bronchiectasis related to fibrosis, but the distribution is typically upper lobe predominant.

Reference: Hansell DM, Lynch DA, McAdams HP, et al. *Imaging of Diseases of the Chest*. 5th ed. Mosby, 2009.

57 **Answer: A.**   The National Emphysema Treatment Trial (NETT) demonstrated important information about treatment of hyperinflation in the setting of emphysema. One of the most important findings was that LVRS offers a focused group of patients' clinically significant improvements over medical therapy. Specifically, those patients with upper lung predominant emphysema and low exercise capacity demonstrated improved survival compared to medical therapy alone. As such, preoperative assessment of the distribution of emphysema by CT or ventilation–perfusion scan is critical for those considering undergoing LVRS.

Reference: Criner GJ, Cordova FSternberg AL, et al. The National Emphysema Treatment Trial (NETT) Part II: lessons learned about lung volume reduction surgery. *Am J Respi Crit Care Med* 2011;184(8):881–893.

58a **Answer: B.**

58b **Answer: A.**   In the setting of bronchiectasis (including cystic fibrosis), hypertrophied bronchial arteries are formed with sometimes significant collateralization (>90% of cases). These hypertrophied arteries are prone to recurrently bleed with sometimes catastrophic consequences. Bronchial artery anatomy is highly variable but typically arises from the descending thoracic aorta at the T5 or T6 level. The pulmonary arteries would be an atypical source of bleeding due to the lower pressure system unless a mycotic aneurysm has formed. The internal thoracic arteries and intercostal arteries form parenchymal collaterals much less frequently.

Surgical resection is a possible therapy, but bronchial artery particle embolization is preferred as a less invasive treatment. Although useful for controlling the underlying parenchymal disease, antimicrobial therapy and steroids do not play a primary role in treating the hemoptysis itself.

References: Bruzzi JF, Rémy-Jardin M, Delhaye D, et al. Multi-detector row CT of hemoptysis. *Radiographics* 2006;26(1):3–22.

Flume PA, Mogayzel PJ Jr, Robinson KA, et al. Cystic fibrosis pulmonary guidelines: pulmonary complications: hemoptysis and pneumothorax. *Am J Respir Crit Care Med* 2010;182(3):298–306.

Yoon W, Kim JK, Kim YH, et al. Bronchial and nonbronchial systemic artery embolization for life-threatening hemoptysis: a comprehensive review. *Radiographics* 2002;22(6):1395–1409.

59a **Answer: D.**

59b **Answer: B.** Chest radiograph demonstrates upper lobe predominant tram tracking, bronchiectasis, and nodularity consistent with an airway pattern. CT of the chest in another patient with the same disease process reveals airway disease with bronchiectasis, bronchial wall thickening, mucous plugging, and nodularity. Mediastinal kernel through the upper abdomen shows near complete fatty replacement of the pancreas in this 27-year-old female. The constellation of findings are most consistent with cystic fibrosis. Allergic bronchopulmonary aspergillosis (ABPA) would be a consideration for the pulmonary findings alone, but is not associated with pancreatic atrophy. Likewise, Kartagener syndrome and common variable immunodeficiency can cause bronchiectasis and airway disease, but airway disease generally has a lower lobe predominance. Also, these diseases have other characteristic-associated imaging findings.

Cystic fibrosis is increasingly seen in adults due to improvements in disease treatment and recognition of cases of adult-onset cystic fibrosis. It is the "most common life-limiting inherited disease" of Caucasians and results from a genetic mutation on chromosome 7 at the CF transmembrane conductance regulator (CFTR) causing impaired transport of chloride ions across membranes. This results in increased thickening of airway secretions leading to repetitive infections and inflammation followed by progressive bronchiectasis, further perpetuating the cycle. In the abdomen, cystic fibrosis often first manifests in intestinal dysfunction as meconium ileus. Adult manifestations of cystic fibrosis still include intestinal disease but also hepatobiliary, pancreatic, and less commonly renal disease. In the pancreas, proximal duct obstruction from inspissated secretions in cystic fibrosis causes fibrotic and fatty replacement of the pancreas as seen in this case.

References: Helbich TH, Heinz-Peer G, Eichler I, et al. Cystic fibrosis: CT assessment of lung involvement in children and adults. *Radiology* 1999;213:537–544.

Robertson MB, Choe KA, Joseph PM. Review of the abdominal manifestations of cystic fibrosis in the adult patient. *Radiographics* 2006;26:679–690.

60a **Answer: C.**

60b **Answer: A.** 60c Answer: C. The pattern of emphysema in alpha-1 antitrypsin deficiency is that of panlobular (panacinar) emphysema, which is typically lower lung predominant (shown). The other forms of emphysema are associated with smoking (centrilobular and paraseptal) or a result of scarring and fibrosis (cicatricial). Interestingly, IV methylphenidate abuse is associated with the development of panlobular emphysema similar to that seen in antitrypsin deficiency. Other rare causes of panlobular emphysema include hypocomplementemic urticarial vasculitis syndrome or Ehlers-Danlos. HIV and Marfan are also rare causes of emphysema but tend to produce apical bullae as the emphysema pattern.

References: Hansell DM, Lynch DA, McAdams HP, et al. *Imaging of diseases of the chest.* 5th ed. Mosby, 2009.

Lee P, Gildea TR, Stoller JK. Emphysema in nonsmokers: alpha 1-antitrypsin deficiency and other causes. *Cleve Clin J Med* 2002;69(12):928–929.

Stern EJ, Frank MS, Schmutz JF, et al. Panlobular pulmonary emphysema caused by i.v. injection of methylphenidate (Ritalin): findings on chest radiographs and CT scans. *AJR Am J Roentgenol* 1994;162(3):555–560.

61a **Answer: A.**

61b **Answer: C.**   The CT demonstrates normal-appearing main bronchi but markedly dilated and bronchiectatic parahilar bronchi bilaterally (cystic bronchiectasis). The process is relatively diffuse involving both the upper lobes and the lower lobes and spars the periphery. There is a component of mosaic attenuation related to airway disease noted as well. These findings are most consistent with Williams-Campbell syndrome. This is a rare congenital cause of bronchiectasis due to abnormal cartilage in the fourth to sixth generations of bronchi. This limited bronchial involvement results in a characteristic appearance of central cystic bronchiectasis. The other choices demonstrate tracheal and main bronchi involvement. Additionally, cystic fibrosis is upper lung predominant, and ciliary dyskinesia demonstrates a lower lung predominance.

Reference: Hansell DM, Lynch DA, McAdams HP, et al. *Imaging of diseases of the chest.* 5th ed. Mosby, 2009.

62 **Answer: B.**   Although there is perihilar and central bronchiectasis, there is also dilation of the main bronchi and the trachea. The trachea here is almost as large as the vertebral body. Additionally, there are focal outpouchings and early diverticula formation along the main bronchi. These features are consistent with Mounier-Kuhn disease. The tracheal and main bronchi involvement help distinguish this case from what would otherwise be very similar to Williams-Campbell. Tracheobronchomegaly is most frequently found in 20- to 40-year-old men, and patients frequently have a history of recurrent respiratory infections and chronic cough. The defect is related to a deficiency of smooth muscle and elastic fibers and has an association with other disorders such as Marfan, Ehlers-Danlos, and cutis laxa. A tracheal diameter on frontal radiograph exceeding 25 mm (transverse diameter) should suggest the diagnosis in men, 21 mm in women. Add 2 mm each for the lateral projections (AP diameter). The diameter used on CT is 3 cm, measured 2 cm above the aortic arch. Tracheomalacia is frequently seen in conjunction.

Reference: Webb WR, Higgins CB. *Thoracic imaging.* Philadelphia, PA: Lippincott Williams & Wilkins, 2010.

63 **Answer: A.**   On the frontal projection, the round foreign body overlaps the right hilum. Rounded objects such as this are almost always related to aspiration rather than embolization (more commonly thin wires or vascular sheaths). As such, from the frontal projection only, both esophageal and airway placement are possible. However, on the lateral projection, the foreign body is identified as a thin coin overlapping the airway just distal to the carina at the level of the right mainstem bronchus. The item is too far anterior on this projection to be esophageal.

Right bronchial positioning of an aspirated foreign body occurs in approximately 70% of cases. The proximal or distal location within the bronchial tree appears to be predominantly determined by foreign body size. When removing the foreign body, special attention should be paid to complete removal as some foreign bodies such as tablets, teeth, and organics (i.e., peanuts) can fragment requiring repeat procedures if unrecognized.

It is important to remember that not all aspirated foreign bodies are radiodense and the only sign of an obstructing lesion could be the secondary findings of atelectasis or hyperinflation. Clinical history and a low threshold for bronchoscopic evaluation are important in these cases.

Reference: Baharloo F, Veyckemans F, Francis C, et al.Tracheobronchial foreign bodies: presentation and management in children and adults. *Chest* 1999;115(5):1357–1362.

Section 5: Thoracic Manifestations of Systemic Disease

64a **Answer: C.**

64b **Answer: A.** Several systemic diseases may develop cystic lung disease, to include but not limited to tuberous sclerosis, neurofibromatosis, Sögren syndrome, amyloidosis, and Langerhans cell histiocytosis. Of these, tuberous sclerosis will cause a diffuse random distribution of lung cysts, fat containing renal lesions (AMLs), and cerebral cortical tubers as seen in this patient. Neurofibromatosis, while also a neurocutaneous disorder and able to cause scattered cysts, causes neurofibromas often seen on chest imaging as intercostal nodular soft tissue cords or as cutaneous nodules. Pulmonary Langerhans cell histiocytosis is most commonly a disease localized to the lung in smokers, but the systemic form of Langerhans cell histiocytosis can cause lung disease and lytic bone lesions in a younger population. Lastly, lymphocytic interstitial pneumonia (LIP) is a lymphoproliferative disorder that can result in cystic lung disease commonly in the setting of Sögren syndrome.

Major and minor criteria have been established for the diagnosis of tuberous sclerosis given the highly variable manifestations of the disease both within and between families. Lymphangioleiomyomatosis, renal angiomyolipomas, and cardiac rhabdomyomas are all common major criteria, while only the subependymal giant-cell tumors are uncommon although classic manifestation of tuberous sclerosis.

References: Adriaensen ME, et al. Radiological evidence of lymphangioleiomyomatosis in female and male patients with tuberous sclerosis complex. *Clin Radiol* 2011;66:625–628.

Umeoka S, et al. Pictorial review of tuberous sclerosis in various organs. *RadioGraphics* 2008;28(7):e32.

65a **Answer: D.**

65b **Answer: C.**

65c **Answer: A.** The CT images provided demonstrate focal nodular opacities that are partially calcified and centered on the secondary pulmonary lobule. Of the options provided, metastatic pulmonary calcification would be the most likely cause in this patient with chronic renal failure. Pulmonary edema would not account for the focal nature, nodularity, nor calcification of the opacities. Similarly, pulmonary fibrosis would not cause these findings, but generally result in architectural distortion with reticular opacities. Finally, calcified pulmonary metastases in the setting of osteosarcoma or adenocarcinoma can cause calcified nodules, but the focal cluster and uniform centering on the pulmonary lobule would be very atypical.

While not 95% to 100%, metastatic pulmonary calcification is seen in the majority of patients who have required hemodialysis (60% to 75%). The remaining options incorrectly indicate that metastatic pulmonary calcification occurs in the minority of this patient population.

Starting dialysis, parathyroidectomy, and new renal transplantation have all been associated with CT imaging improvement in metastatic pulmonary calcification. Of these choices, only failed renal transplantation correlates with described cases of accelerated metastatic pulmonary calcification.

Reference: Belem LC, et al. Metastatic pulmonary calcification: State-of-the-art review focused on imaging findings. *Respir Med* 2014;108:668–676.

66a **Answer: C.**

66b **Answer: D.** The contrast CT of the chest in soft tissue kernel demonstrates a paraspinal soft tissue mass-like density with associate extension into the neural foramen resulting in foraminal widening. None of the other options would be expected to widen the adjacent foramen. Additionally, an intercostal arterial aneurysm would enhance similar to aorta (unless clotted), and a pulmonary nodule would be centered in the lung.

Diffuse lung disease is an uncommon manifestation in neurofibromatosis. A case series of 55 patients with neurofibromatosis revealed only 3 with diffuse lung disease. When combined with a literature review, a total of 64 cases of neurofibromatosis-associated diffuse lung disease were compared. Ground-glass opacities, basilar reticular opacities, and bullae were the most common CT findings, but cystic lung disease was found in 25% of patients. In the setting of cystic or interstitial lung disease, CT evidence of paraspinal tumors, intercostal nodular cords, and cutaneous nodules raises the possibility for neurofibromatosis.

Reference: Zamora AC, et al. Neurofibromatosis-associated lung disease: a case series and literature review. *Eur Respir J* 2007;29:210–214.

67 **Answer: B.** In a study of 973 patients diagnosed with polymyositis–dermatomyositis, 58 demonstrated associated lung disease, and of those, 18 out of 22 patients with lung biopsies were diagnosed with nonspecific interstitial pneumonia (NSIP). Other less common pulmonary manifestations included usual interstitial pneumonia, diffuse alveolar damage, and organizing pneumonia. More recent medical literature will include antisynthetase syndrome with PM-DM as myositis syndromes that cause interstitial lung disease. Also, more recent experience suggests that a combined NSIP–OP pattern is the most common pulmonary manifestation of the myositis syndromes.

Reference: Douglas WW, et al. Polymyositis-dermatomyositis-associated interstitial lung disease. *Am J Respir Crit Care Med* 2001;164:1182–1185.

68a **Answer: A.**

68b **Answer: B.**

68c **Answer: B.** The chest radiographs provided demonstrate reticular basilar opacities typical of fibrosing interstitial pneumonias and characterized by the fine netlike radio-opaque lines over the lower lung fields. The corresponding CT through the lung bases reveals peripheral predominant, basal predominant reticular abnormality with honeycombing, a finding that defines the CT pattern of usual interstitial pneumonia and differentiates it from nonspecific interstitial pneumonia, bronchiolitis, and organizing pneumonia.

When studying 63 patients with rheumatoid arthritis-related lung disease, Tanaka et al. found that the most common pulmonary CT findings are ground-glass opacities and reticulation and the most common pattern was usual interstitial pneumonia.

Reference: Tanaka N, et al. Rheumatoid arthritis-related lung diseases: CT findings. *Radiology* 2004;232:81–91.

69a **Answer: B.**

69b **Answer: D.** Obscuration of the pulmonary vascular marking by hazy poorly defined opacities with associated air bronchograms is consistent with consolidation. Some component of interstitial thickening may be present in this patient with pulmonary hemorrhage, but the other choices of reticular, cystic, or nodular are not the predominant pattern. Additionally, diffuse pulmonary hemorrhage generally spares the lung apices.

With the placement of a dialysis catheter, the radiograph raises concern for a renopulmonary disease. Any one of the options provided can cause consolidation on chest radiograph. Only pulmonary hemorrhage, as demonstrated by hemoptysis or present on bronchoscopy, specifically favors Goodpasture syndrome. Caused by antiglomerular basement membrane antibodies, Goodpasture syndrome classically results in glomerulonephritis and diffuse pulmonary hemorrhage (DPH). Once diffuse pulmonary hemorrhage has been identified, the differential etiologies are commonly categorized as (1) Goodpasture syndrome/antiglomerular basement membrane disease, (2) other immunologically mediated diseases such as systemic lupus erythematosus or granulomatosis with polyangiitis, (3) nonimmunologically mediated causes such as medications or idiopathic pulmonary hemosiderosis, or (4) immunocompromised conditions with infection such as leukemia, HIV, or transplant.

Reference: Primack SL, Miller RR, Muller NL. Diffuse pulmonary hemorrhage: clinical, pathologic and imaging features. *AJR Am J Roentgenol* 1995;164:295–300.

70a **Answer: B.**

70b **Answer: B.**

70c **Answer: C.**   The CT image provided demonstrates a focal pulmonary artery filling defect consistent with pulmonary embolism in a patient also diagnosed with systemic lupus erythematosus (SLE). Approximately one-third of patients with SLE also have antiphospholipid antibody syndrome, placing them at significant risk for recurrent pulmonary embolism and venoocclusive disease, but even SLE patients without antiphospholipid antibody syndrome are at increased risk of pulmonary embolism. In a study of over 500,000 patients hospitalized with autoimmune disorder in Sweden over 44 years, subjects with autoimmune disease had an overall relative risk of 6.38 for subsequent pulmonary embolism within 1 year relative to with those without autoimmune disease. The autoimmune conditions with highest risk for pulmonary embolism in this study were polymyositis–dermatomyositis (relative risk 16.44), polyarteritis nodosa (relative risk 13.26), immune thrombocytopenic purpura (relative risk 10.79), and systemic lupus erythematosus (relative risk 10.23). Still, the most common thoracic manifestation of SLE is pleural effusion, followed by pulmonary parenchymal disease, diaphragmatic dysfunction, and pulmonary arterial hypertension.

References: Lalani TA, et al. Imaging findings in systemic lupus erythematosus. *Radiographics* 2004;24:1069–1086.

Zoller B, et al. Risk of pulmonary embolism in patients with autoimmune disorders: a nationwide follow-up study from Sweden. *Lancet* 2012;379:244–249.

71a **Answer: D.**

71b **Answer: A.**   Acute chest syndrome is the most common "circumstance" associated with death in adults with sickle cell anemia in a study of 209 patients older than 20 years who died after study enrollment, followed by stroke, infection, and perioperative complications. Chronic organ failure was a common additional associated condition, but rarely found in the study as the primary cause of death.

By definition, acute chest syndrome patients must exhibit fever or chest pain, pulmonary symptoms such as wheezing, and pulmonary opacities on chest imaging in the setting of sickle cell anemia. Often seen following vasoocclusive crisis, acute chest syndrome may be complicated by infection, fluid overload, splinting from chest wall bone pain, and fat emboli. Recommended treatments for acute chest syndrome include antibiotics, supplemental oxygen, monitoring for bronchospasm, and potential transfusions for anemia.

References: Platt OS, et al. Mortality in sickle cell disease: life expectancy and risk factors for early death. *New Engl J Med* 1994;330(23):1639–1644.

Minter KR, Gladwin MT. Pulmonary complications of sickle cell anemia: a need for increased recognition, treatment and research. *Am J Respir Crit Care Med* 2001;164:2016–2019.

Yawn BP, et al. Management of sickle cell disease: summary of the 2014 evidence-based report by Expert Panel Members. *JAMA* 2014;312(10):1033–1048.

72a Answer: D.

72b Answer: A.   Lower lung predominant, perilymphatic cysts are seen in approximately 70% of patients with lymphocytic interstitial pneumonia. Other common CT findings are bilateral ground-glass and centrilobular opacities. Lymphocytic interstitial pneumonia results from bronchus-associated lymphoid tissue (BALT) hyperplasia and is most commonly seen in Sögren syndrome and other autoimmune diseases. Other diseases associated with LIP can be categorized as immunodeficiencies such as HIV and miscellaneous/idiopathic.

  The differential diagnosis for chronic consolidations on chest CT includes chronic infection, sarcoidosis, and lipoid pneumonia, but in the setting of Sögren syndrome (SS)–associated lung disease, lymphoma becomes a primary concern. Patients with Sögren syndrome have 44 times the incidence of lymphoma compared to the equivalent general population. The most common subtype of lymphoma in Sögren syndrome is MALT lymphoma, an extranodal marginal zone B-cell (non-Hodgkin) lymphoma.

References: Egashira R, et al. CT findings of thoracic manifestations of primary Sögren syndrome: radiologic-pathologic correlation. *Radiographics* 2013;33:1933–1949.

Johkoh T, et al. Lymphocytic interstitial pneumonia: thin-section CT findings in 22 patients. *Radiology* 1999;212:567–572.

Swigris JJ, et al. Lymphoid interstitial pneumonia: a narrative review. *Chest* 2002;122:2150–2164.

Tonami H, et al. Clinical and imaging findings of lymphoma in patients with Sögren syndrome. *J Comput Assist Tomogr* 2003;27(4):517–524.

73a Answer: B.

73b Answer: C.

73c Answer: A.   Each finding is present on the provided chest radiograph, but of the provided choices, only pulmonary cavitation suggests granulomatosis with polyangiitis (GPA), formerly known as Wegener granulomatosis. A granulomatous vasculitis, GPA most commonly presents in the lungs as pulmonary nodules or masses. Pulmonary cavitation is seen in 50% of patient with granulomatosis with polyangiitis. Other manifestations on chest CT of GPA include halo nodules, reverse halo nodules, pulmonary hemorrhage with consolidation and ground-glass opacities, and tracheobronchial thickening. The lungs and kidneys are involved in the majority of cases, but the upper respiratory tract is the most common.

References: Comarmond C, Cacoub P. Granulomatosis with polyangiitis (Wegener): clinical aspects and treatment. *Autoimmun Rev* 2014;13(11):1121–1125.

Martinez F, et al. Common and uncommon manifestations of Wegener granulomatosis at chest CT: radiologic-pathologic correlation. *Radiographics* 2012;32:51–69.

74a **Answer: C.**

74b **Answer: B.** Necrobiotic nodules are an uncommon manifestation of rheumatoid-associated pulmonary disease, occurring in <1% of patients with rheumatoid arthritis. Other findings in this case more common in RA include pleural and pericardial effusions. When rheumatoid nodules occur, they can cavitate in 50% of cases and generally predominate in the upper and midlungs. Tissue diagnosis of rheumatoid nodules reveals that "a central zone of eosinophilic fibrinoid necrosis is surrounded by palisading fibroblasts."

In the setting of an occupational exposure such as silicosis, coal workers' pneumoconiosis (CWP), or asbestosis, rheumatoid arthritis may manifest with scattered pulmonary nodules known as rheumatoid pneumoconiosis or Caplan syndrome. Pulmonary nodules are a central component of this disease with CT presence of pneumoconiosis being variable. In this patient, eggshell calcified mediastinal lymph nodes are characteristic for silicosis or CWP and raise concern for the disease in this patient with known rheumatoid arthritis and rheumatoid nodules. Sarcoidosis and granulomatous infections are in the differential and have been reported to be associated with RA treatments, although Heerfordt syndrome refers to uveoparotid sarcoidosis. Carney triad and Sögren syndrome do not produce these findings.

References: Ozkaya S, Bilgin S, Hamsici S, et al. The pulmonary radiologic findings of rheumatoid arthritis. *Resp Med* 2011;4:187–192.

Schreiber J, Koschel D, Kekow J, et al. Rheumatoid pneumoconiosis (Caplan's syndrome). *Eur J Intern Med* 2010;21:168–172.

Tanaka N, Kim JS, Newell JD, et al. Rheumatoid arthritis-related lung diseases: CT findings. *Radiology* 2004;232(81):91.

75 **Answer: D.** The dilated peripheral vessels seen in hepatopulmonary syndrome directly demonstrate intrapulmonary arteriovenous shunting. Together with an increased A-a gradient and cirrhosis, intrapulmonary shunting defines hepatopulmonary syndrome. Shunting can be confirmed by contrast echocardiography, pulmonary perfusion scintigraphy, or pulmonary angiography.

Main pulmonary artery enlargement suggests pulmonary artery hypertension, which can occur in the setting of chronic liver disease, but is not a defining component of hepatopulmonary syndrome. Likewise, pulmonary fibrosis and mixed pulmonary interstitial and ground-glass opacities are not findings of hepatopulmonary syndrome.

Reference: McAdams HP, et al. The hepatopulmonary syndrome: radiologic findings in 10 patients. *AJR Am J Roentgenol* 1996;166:1379–1385.

76 **Answer: C.** Shrinking lungs syndrome occurs in the setting of systemic lupus erythematosus with progressive weakening in the diaphragms and/or restricted chest wall expansion. In this patient, no significant reticular opacity is present to suggest volume loss associated with fibrosing interstitial pneumonia as can be seen with systemic sclerosis/scleroderma. Sögren syndrome classically causes lymphocytic interstitial pneumonia (LIP), and only isolated cases of combined SLE and Sögren syndrome have been associated with shrinking lungs syndrome. Granulomatosis with polyangiitis generally causes pulmonary hemorrhage or cavitating pulmonary lesions without known association with shrinking lungs syndrome.

Reference: Warrington KJ, Moder KG, Brutinel WM. The shrinking lungs syndrome in systemic lupus erythematosus. *Mayo Clin Proc* 2000;75:467–472.

77a **Answer: C.**

77b **Answer: A.** Obliterative bronchiolitis, also known as bronchiolitis obliterans and constrictive bronchiolitis, most commonly demonstrates mosaic attenuation on inspiratory CT images and air trapping on expiratory CT images, as seen in the case provided. In a series comparing obliterative bronchiolitis and severe asthma, mosaic attenuation in obliterative bronchiolitis proved to be the best differentiator between the two.

Airway disease can occur in multiple autoimmune diseases, but obliterative bronchiolitis is most characteristic of rheumatoid arthritis. Systemic lupus erythematosus is an alternative, but less common, cause in the setting of collagen vascular disease.

References: Jensen SP, et al. High-resolution CT features of severe asthma and bronchiolitis obliterans. *Clin Radiol* 2002;57:1078–1085.

Lynch DA. Lung disease related to collagen vascular disease. *J Thorac Imaging* 2009;24:299–309.

78a **Answer: B.**

78b **Answer: A.** The normal diameter of the main pulmonary artery is approximately 25 mm. The 90th percentile cutoff value is 29 mm in men and 27 mm in women. A measurement of 37 mm, as found in this case, is highly likely to be associated with pulmonary arterial hypertension. A recent meta-analysis showed that pulmonary arterial hypertension was found in about 13% of subjects with scleroderma, compared with 3% of patients with lupus. The prevalence of pulmonary hypertension in subjects with Sögren syndrome and polymyositis–dermatomyositis is low. In patients with scleroderma, the NSIP pattern of lung fibrosis is found in 78% of surgical lung biopsies, substantially more common than other pathologies including UIP.

References: Bouros D, Wells AU, Nicholson AG, et al. Histopathologic subsets of fibrosing alveolitis in patients with systemic sclerosis and their relationship to outcome. *Am J Respir Crit Care Med* 2002;165(12):1581–1586.

Truong QA, Massaro JM, Rogers IS, et al. Reference values for normal pulmonary artery dimensions by noncontrast cardiac computed tomography: the Framingham Heart Study. *Circ Cardiovasc Imaging* 2012;5(1):147–154.

Yang X, Mardekian J, Sanders KN, et al. Prevalence of pulmonary arterial hypertension in patients with connective tissue diseases: a systematic review of the literature. *Clin Rheumatol* 2013;32(10):1519–1531.

Section 6: Atelectasis and Collapse

79a **Answer: B.**

79b **Answer: A.**

79c **Answer: B.**

79d **Answer: D.** The posteroanterior chest radiograph shows a large left hilar mass with left upper lobe collapse. There are several indirect signs of volume loss including leftward tracheal shift, a juxtaphrenic peak, and left hilar elevation as evidenced by outward and upward rotation of the left interlobar pulmonary artery, which is obscured laterally by the hilar mass (silhouette sign).

The Luftsichel or air crescent sign is classically seen in patients with left upper lobe collapse. The sign is produced by a hyperexpanded superior segment of the left lower lobe, which interposes between the collapsed left upper lobe and aortic arch. The flat waist sign is seen with left lower lobe collapse, and the S sign of Golden is most commonly seen with right upper lobe collapse. The comet tail sign is seen on CT and represents a swirling of vessels and is used in the diagnosis of rounded atelectasis.

Lobar collapse in an adult outpatient is malignancy until proven otherwise, usually from a primary lung cancer. Other causes of lobar collapse include endobronchial tumors such as carcinoid, hamartoma, and metastatic disease. The most common cause of lobar collapse in an intubated or sedated patient is a mucus plug, which is optimally treated with aggressive suctioning or bronchoscopy. Foreign body is a frequent cause of lobar collapse in pediatric patients.

References: Molina PL, Hiken JN, Glazer HS. Imaging evaluation of obstructive atelectasis. *J Thorac Imaging* 1996;11:176–186.

Woodring JH, Reed JC. Radiographic manifestations of lobar atelectasis. *J Thorac Imaging* 1996;11:109–144.

80a **Answer: D.**

80b **Answer: A.**

80c **Answer: C.** The anteroposterior chest radiograph shows right upper lobe atelectasis, pulmonary edema, and small pleural effusions. Radiograph obtained hours later shows near complete resolution of right upper lobe atelectasis following bronchoscopy. There are a few direct and several indirect signs of volume loss. The direct signs include fissural displacement and crowding of the bronchovascular structures, the latter is optimally assessed on CT. In this case, there is upward and medial displacement of the minor fissure, a direct sign of volume loss. Indirect signs of volume loss that are present include right hemidiaphragm elevation, rightward tracheal shift, and increased pulmonary opacity.

The most common cause of lobar collapse in an intubated or sedated patient is a mucus plug, which is optimally treated with aggressive suctioning or bronchoscopy. Lobar collapse in an adult outpatient is malignancy until proven otherwise, usually from a primary lung cancer. Other causes of lobar collapse include endobronchial tumors such as carcinoid, hamartoma, and metastatic disease. Foreign body is a frequent cause of lobar collapse in pediatric patients.

Woodring JH, Reed JC. Radiographic manifestations of lobar atelectasis. *J Thorac Imaging* 1996;11:109–144.

81 **Answer: A.** Originally described in the case of a calcified granuloma, the shifting granuloma sign reflects a change in the degree of atelectasis with the associated change in position of a visible lesion on radiograph. This "movement" of an internal marker is an easily recognizable sign of significant atelectasis or collapse.

Reference: Rohlfing B. The shifting granuloma: an internal marker of atelectasis. *Radiology* 1977;123:283–285.

82a **Answer: A.**

82b **Answer: A.**

82c **Answer: D.** The frontal and lateral chest radiographs show a right lower lobe rounded mass (>3 cm) with associated volume loss evidenced by ipsilateral shift of the heart. The mass abuts an area of pleural effusion or pleural thickening. This raises the possibility of rounded atelectasis, which is confirmed on CT. There are four features that are needed to confidently diagnose rounded atelectasis on CT:

1. Volume loss in the affected lobe (usually identified by fissural displacement)
2. Comet tail sign (i.e., curving of ipsilateral bronchovascular structures toward the mass)
3. Adjacent pleural abnormality (e.g., pleural thickening or pleural effusion)
4. Rounded opacity must have significant contact with pleural abnormality.

Rounded atelectasis is frequently metabolically inactive with FDG activity equal to or less than mediastinal blood pool. CT follow-up of rounded atelectasis is controversial with some thoracic radiologists advising no follow-up and some suggesting follow-up at intervals (3 to 6 months) to ensure stability.

References: Batra P, Brown K, Hayashi K, et al. Rounded atelectasis. *J Thorac Imaging* 1996;11:187–197.

Gurney JW. Atypical manifestations of pulmonary atelectasis. *J Thorac Imaging* 1996;11:165–175.

McAdams HP, Erasums JJ, Patz EF, et al. Evaluation of patients with round atelectasis using 2-[18F]-fluoro-2-deoxy-D-glucose PET. *J Comput Assist Tomogr* 1998;22:601–604.

83a **Answer: A.**

83b **Answer: D.**

83c **Answer: C.**   The initial chest radiograph shows life support devices in expected locations. There are perihilar and basal lung opacities with vascular indistinctness, which is most consistent with pulmonary edema. The absence of fever and a normal white blood cell count argues against the diagnosis of pneumonia. While there are likely small bilateral pleural effusions, the majority of the opacities are related to pulmonary edema.

A radiograph obtained at the time of hypoxia shows new left lung collapse. There is ipsilateral mediastinal shift with displacement of the gastric tube, endotracheal tube, and right internal jugular central venous catheter. In an intubated or sedated patient, sudden lung collapse is frequently from an obstructing mucus plug. Tumor is more common in outpatients presenting with lobar collapse. There are only a few conditions that change rapidly over a few hours on chest radiography and include atelectasis, pulmonary edema, and aspiration.

References: Woodring JH, Reed JC. Radiographic manifestations of lobar atelectasis. *J Thorac Imaging* 1996;11:109–144.

Woodring JH, Reed JC. Types and mechanisms of pulmonary atelectasis. *J Thorac Imaging* 1996;11:92–108.

84a **Answer: C.**

84b **Answer: A.**   The axial contrast-enhanced chest CT shows densely enhancing left lower lobe surrounded by a left pleural effusion. This is most characteristic of relaxation atelectasis. While pneumonia is not entirely excluded, it is less likely given lack of hypodense enhancement within the collapsed lung.

There are four types of atelectasis related to etiology. **Relaxation or passive atelectasis** occurs when a pleural effusion, pneumothorax, or mass allows the lung to collapse to its normal lower volume. **Adhesive atelectasis** is seen primarily in premature infants with surfactant deficiency or adults following smoke inhalation and is caused by alveolar collapse secondary to insufficient surfactant production or surfactant dysfunction. **Cicatricial atelectasis** occurs in patients with lung fibrosis, which leads to adjacent lung atelectasis. **Resorption atelectasis** results from proximal bronchial obstruction and may be seen with tumor, mucus plug, or foreign body aspiration.

Reference: Woodring JH, Reed JC. Types and mechanisms of pulmonary atelectasis. *J Thorac Imaging* 1996;11:92–108.

85 **Answer: B.** Prone imaging is generally part of a standard initial HRCT evaluation for patients suspected to have interstitial lung disease. Prone imaging enhances evaluation of the subpleural dependent lower lungs. Since the peripheral lower lung is frequently the initial site of abnormality for many interstitial pneumonias, the presence of atelectasis can obscure subtle, early ILD. Thus, prone imaging is performed to eliminate any dependent atelectasis and confirm the presence of absence of any mild underlying lung disease.

Reference: Lynch DA, Newell JD, Lee JS. *Imaging of diffuse lung disease.* Hamilton, ON: B.C. Decker, Inc., 2000.

86a **Answer: D.**

86b **Answer: D.**

86c **Answer: D.**

86d **Answer: A.** The posteroanterior chest radiograph shows combined right middle and right lower lobe collapse. The vertically oriented major fissure intersects the inferiorly displaced minor fissure, and the right interlobar pulmonary artery is invisible. There is rightward mediastinal shift and compensatory hyperinflation of the right upper lobe. A mediastinal mass with paratracheal and subcarinal lymphadenopathy is also noted. The lateral radiograph shows a band of opacity extending from anterior to posterior in the expected location of the right middle and right lower lobes.

The coronal contrast-enhanced chest CT confirms collapse caused by a large mediastinal mass, likely lymphadenopathy. In the absence of a primary tumor elsewhere in the lung or body, the leading considerations would include small cell lung cancer or lymphoma. Carcinoid typically is an endobronchial mass, which is often well defined and may contain calcium in about 25% of cases.

Reference: Woodring JH, Reed JC. Radiographic manifestations of lobar atelectasis. *J Thorac Imaging* 1996;11:109–144.

87a **Answer: D.**

87b **Answer: B.**

87c **Answer: A.**

87d **Answer: A.** The posteroanterior chest radiograph shows complete left lower lobe collapse manifesting as a triangular-shaped opacity in the retrocardiac region. The flat waist sign represents a flattening of the left heart border and mediastinum with loss of the normal left-sided moguls or contours including the aortic arch, pulmonary trunk, left atrial appendage, and left ventricular border. It occurs from posterior rotation and leftward shift of the heart. The lateral radiograph shows increased opacity posteriorly over the spine resulting in the spine sign. Normally, the spine should become more lucent inferiorly. Other radiographic signs associated with left lower lobe collapse include the "top-of-the-knob" and "Nordenström" signs. The top-of-the-knob sign results in obscuration of the superomedial aspect of the aortic arch due to leftward mediastinal shift and rotation. The Nordenström sign represents lingular subsegmental atelectasis from kinking and reorientation of the lingular bronchi.

The S sign of Golden is classically associated with right upper lobe collapse from a centrally obstructing tumor, usually lung cancer. The central lung cancer causes a convex inferior bulge with the adjacent elevated minor fissure resulting in a reverse S configuration. The Luftsichel or air crescent sign is classically seen in patients with left upper lobe collapse. The sign is produced by a hyperexpanded superior segment of the left lower lobe, which interposes between the collapsed left upper lobe and aortic arch. The comet tail sign is a CT finding that helps diagnose rounded atelectasis and represents a swirling of vessels into the mass-like opacity.

Lobar collapse in an adult outpatient is malignant until proven otherwise, usually from a primary lung cancer. Other causes of lobar collapse include endobronchial tumors such as carcinoid, hamartoma, and metastatic disease. Foreign body is the most common cause of lobar collapse in pediatric patients. Mucus plug and aspiration are common causes of collapse in intubated or sedated patients.

References: Kattan KR, Wlot JF. Cardiac rotation in left lower lobe collapse. "The flat waist sign." *Radiology* 1976;118(2):275–279.

Woodring JH, Reed JC. Radiographic manifestations of lobar atelectasis. *J Thorac Imaging* 1996;11:109–144.

88a **Answer: B.**

88b **Answer: A.**

88c **Answer: D.**

88d **Answer: B.**   The frontal chest radiograph shows subtle obscuration of the right heart border. The lateral radiograph confirms right middle lobe collapse. There is inferior displacement of the minor fissure and anterior and superior displacement of the right major fissure, both direct radiographic signs of volume loss. The intermediate stem line is composed of the posterior wall of the bronchus intermedius and right main bronchus and is not responsible for the radiographic abnormality.

The axial chest CT confirms complete right middle lobe collapse. CT is necessary to exclude a centrally obstructing lung mass or endobronchial tumor. Bronchoscopy is often necessary in addition to CT to exclude small endobronchial nodules. The middle lobe syndrome is a condition, which describes chronic right middle lobe collapse and may be seen with both obstructive and nonobstructive etiologies. It is more common in middle or elderly adults, usually women. The most common cause of the middle lobe syndrome in adults is nonobstructive inflammatory conditions including tuberculosis infection. When it occurs in children, it is usually associated with asthma or repeated infection.

References: Gudbjartsson T, Gudmundsson G. Middle lobe syndrome: a review of clinicopathological features, diagnosis and treatment. *Respiration* 2012;84:80–86.

Sekerel BE, Nakipoglu F. Middle lobe syndrome in children with asthma: review of 56 cases. *J Asthma* 2004;41:411–417.

Wagner RB, Johnston MR. Middle lobe syndrome. *Ann Thorac Surg* 1983;35:679–686.

89a **Answer: D.**

89b **Answer: A.**

89c **Answer: A.**

89d **Answer: B.** The posteroanterior chest radiograph shows right upper lobe atelectasis and the S sign of Golden. The S sign of Golden is classically associated with right upper lobe collapse from a centrally obstructing tumor, usually lung cancer. The central lung cancer causes a convex inferior bulge with the adjacent elevated minor fissure resulting in a reverse S configuration.

The Luftsichel or air crescent sign is classically seen in patients with left upper lobe collapse. The sign is produced by a hyperexpanded superior segment of the left lower lobe, which interposes between the collapsed left upper lobe and aortic arch. The flat waist sign is seen with left lower lobe collapse. The comet tail sign is a CT finding, which helps diagnose rounded atelectasis and represents a swirling of vessels into the mass-like opacity.

Lobar collapse in an adult outpatient is malignancy until proven otherwise, usually from a primary lung cancer. Other causes of lobar collapse include endobronchial tumors such as carcinoid, hamartoma, and metastatic disease. The tumor may be differentiated from atelectatic lung by looking at density on postcontrast CT. Atelectatic lung enhances homogeneously and intensely following contrast as the bronchovascular structures are closely opposed, whereas tumor will typically have heterogeneous and hypodense enhancement.

Reference: Woodring JH, Reed JC. Radiographic manifestations of lobar atelectasis. *J Thorac Imaging* 1996;11:109–144.

90a **Answer: A.**

90b **Answer: B.** The initial chest radiograph shows diffuse fine granular airspace opacities typical of surfactant deficiency. The follow-up radiograph obtained for desaturation shows low lung volumes with complete white out of both lungs, most compatible with adhesive atelectasis.

As stated before, but for review, there are four types of atelectasis. **Adhesive atelectasis** is seen primarily in premature infants with surfactant deficiency or in adults following smoke inhalation and is caused by alveolar collapse secondary to insufficient surfactant production or surfactant dysfunction. **Relaxation or passive atelectasis** occurs when a pleural effusion, pneumothorax, or mass allows the lung to collapse "relax" to its normal lower volume. **Cicatricial atelectasis** occurs in patients with lung fibrosis, which leads to adjacent lung atelectasis. **Resorption atelectasis** results from proximal bronchial obstruction and may be seen with tumor, mucus plugging, or foreign body aspiration. With proximal bronchial obstruction, the air within alveoli is progressively absorbed by circulating blood in the pulmonary arterial system. In a nonintubated patient, complete air absorption occurs in 24 hours. In an intubated patient receiving a high concentration of oxygen, the air may be absorbed from the alveoli in as little as an hour.

Reference: Woodring JH, Reed JC. Types and mechanisms of pulmonary atelectasis. *J Thorac Imaging* 1996;11:92–108.

Section 7: Pulmonary Physiology

91a **Answer: A.**

91b **Answer: C.** The low FEV_1/FVC ratio (<70%) represents obstruction. The FEV_1 at 60% of predicted indicates moderate obstruction ($50\% \le FEV_1 < 80\%$ predicted). When evaluating a spirogram, the interpreter must interpret the values and the flow–volume loops. Understanding the flow–volume loops is very important as it can provide valuable information about different abnormalities in the airway physiology. The arm under the x axis corresponds to the inspiratory part whereas the arm above the axis corresponds to the expiratory phase of the test.

In this case, the flow–volume loop shows the classic scooped-out appearance in the expiratory phase characteristic of obstructive lung diseases. Variable intrathoracic obstruction would cause a flattening of the expiratory arm of the flow–volume loop. Since the FVC is normal, there is no evidence of a restrictive pattern. However, restriction can only be diagnosed in the presence of a low total lung capacity (TLC). Hyperinflation can be diagnosed when the TLC exceeds 120% of predicted.

The patient presented in this case has a significant smoking history, and the spirogram shows moderate airflow obstruction with scooped-out pattern. Therefore, the disease that would most likely cause this pattern is chronic obstructive pulmonary disease. Vocal cord dysfunction would cause a variable extrathoracic obstruction pattern on flow–volume loops, affecting the inspiratory phase. Tracheal stenosis would cause a fixed airway obstruction, characterized by an abnormality in both inspiratory and expiratory arms of the flow–volume loops. Idiopathic pulmonary fibrosis would cause a restrictive pattern.

References: Barreiro TJ, Perillo I. An approach to interpreting spirometry. *Am Fam Physician* 2004;69(5):1107–1114. http://www.attud.org/docs/interpretingspirometry.pdf.

Davies LK. Intrathoracic vs extrathoracic obstructive lesions. http://anest.ufl.edu/files/2011/08/Intrathoracic-vs-Extrathoracic-Airway-Obstruction.pdf

Pocket Guide. The global initiative for chronic obstructive disease. http://www.goldcopd.org/uploads/users/files/GOLD_Pocket_2010Mar31.pdf

92a **Answer: C.**

92b **Answer: C.**   The FEV_1/FVC ratio is normal (>70%); therefore, there is no obstruction. There is a marked reduction in FVC, which suggests a restrictive lung process. However, this must be confirmed by evaluating the total lung capacity (TLC). In this case, the TLC is reduced (<80%) confirming the presence of a restrictive process. The flow–volume loop shows the classic narrowing as a result of decreased volumes.

Variable intrathoracic obstruction presents a flattening in the expiratory phase in the flow–volume loop. Airway obstruction causes a scooped-out pattern in the flow–volume loop.

The patient presented in this case has significant asbestos exposure and restriction on pulmonary function tests. The disease that will most likely cause this presentation is asbestosis (chronic lung disease resulting from the inhalation of asbestos particles marked by severe fibrosis).

Chronic obstructive pulmonary disease would cause an obstructive pattern with a scooped-out flow–volume loop. Bronchiolitis obliterans would typically cause an obstructive defect that is poorly responsive to bronchodilators. Tracheal stenosis would cause a fixed airway obstruction abnormality in the flow–volume loop.

References: Barreiro TJ, Perillo I. An approach to interpreting spirometry. *Am Fam Physician* 2004;69(5):1107–1114. http://www.attud.org/docs/interpretingspirometry.pdf.

Davies LK. Intrathoracic vs extrathoracic obstructive lesions. http://anest.ufl.edu/files/2011/08/Intrathoracic-vs-Extrathoracic-Airway-Obstruction.pdf

Pocket Guide. The global initiative for chronic obstructive disease. http://www.goldcopd.org/uploads/users/files/GOLD_Pocket_2010Mar31.pdf

93 **Answer: B.**   The FEV_1/FVC ratio is normal (>70%); therefore, there is no obstruction. The FVC and FEV_1 are normal and the flow–volume loop does not show significant abnormalities. Total lung capacity (TLC) and residual volume

(RV) are normal. A decreased TLC (<80%) indicates a restrictive process, whereas an increased TLC (>120%) indicates hyperinflation. An increased RV (>120%), typically seen in obstructive lung diseases, indicates air trapping. Given the normal FEV1/FVC, FEV_1, FVC, and lung volumes, this is a normal spirogram.

Pulmonary vascular disease typically produces a low diffusion capacity of carbon monoxide (DLCO). Chronic obstructive pulmonary disease causes obstruction pattern with a scooped-out flow–volume loop. Pulmonary fibrosis causes restriction, characterized by a low TLC.

References: Barreiro TJ, Perillo I. An approach to interpreting spirometry. *Am Fam Physician* 2004;69(5):1107–1114. http://www.attud.org/docs/interpretingspirometry.pdf.

Davies LK. Intrathoracic vs extrathoracic obstructive lesions. http://anest.ufl.edu/files/2011/08/Intrathoracic-vs-Extrathoracic-Airway-Obstruction.pdf

Pocket Guide. The global initiative for chronic obstructive disease. http://www.goldcopd.org/uploads/users/files/GOLD_Pocket_2010Mar31.pdf

94a Answer: D.

94b Answer: D. This patient has airway obstruction as the FEV_1/FVC ratio is <70%. The FEV_1 at 38% of predicted indicates severe obstruction (30% $\leq FEV_1$ < 50% predicted). Moderate obstruction is defined as an FEV_1 50% to 79% of predicted. Following the administration of bronchodilators, there was an increase of 160 ml in FEV_1 and an absolute change of 10% of the baseline FEV_1. However, this change is not enough to be considered significant (>200 ml and 12% of baseline FEV_1).

The disease presented demonstrates obstruction that is not reversible to bronchodilators, which is seen in chronic obstructive pulmonary disease, either tobacco related or secondary to alpha-1 antitrypsin deficiency. The early onset, lack of history of smoking, and severe obstruction support this diagnosis.

Asthma typically gives significant response to bronchodilators. Pulmonary fibrosis is a restrictive disease and is not consistent with the case presented. Primary pulmonary hypertension typically presents with a normal spirogram and an isolated decrease in DLCO (not presented in this case).

References: Barreiro TJ, Perillo I. An approach to interpreting spirometry. *Am Fam Physician* 2004;69(5):1107–1114. http://www.attud.org/docs/interpretingspirometry.pdf.

Davies LK. Intrathoracic vs extrathoracic obstructive lesions. http://anest.ufl.edu/files/2011/08/Intrathoracic-vs-Extrathoracic-Airway-Obstruction.pdf

Pocket Guide. The global initiative for chronic obstructive disease. http://www.goldcopd.org/uploads/users/files/GOLD_Pocket_2010Mar31.pdf

95 Answer: C. This patient has airway obstruction as the FEV_1/FVC ratio is <70%. The FEV_1 at 75% of predicted indicates moderate obstruction (50% $\leq FEV_1$ < 80% predicted). Significant reversibility is present given that following the administration of bronchodilators, there was an increase of 360 ml (>200 ml) in FEV_1 and an absolute change of 13% (>12%) of the baseline FEV_1. This study does not show a restrictive pattern.

References: Barreiro TJ, Perillo I. An approach to interpreting spirometry. *Am Fam Physician* 2004;69(5):1107–1114. http://www.attud.org/docs/interpretingspirometry.pdf.

Davies LK. Intrathoracic vs extrathoracic obstructive lesions. http://anest.ufl.edu/files/2011/08/Intrathoracic-vs-Extrathoracic-Airway-Obstruction.pdf

Pocket Guide. The global initiative for chronic obstructive disease. http://www.goldcopd.org/uploads/users/files/GOLD_Pocket_2010Mar31.pdf

96 Answer: B. This patient has airway obstruction as the FEV_1/FVC ratio is <70%. The FEV_1 at 45% of predicted indicates severe obstruction (30% $\leq FEV_1$ < 50%

predicted). The flow–volume loop shows flattening in both the inspiratory and expiratory phases. This is characteristic of fixed airway obstruction given the lack of changes in the obstructed airway caliber during inspiration or expiration producing a constant degree of airflow limitation during the entire respiratory cycle. A fixed lesion may be extrathoracic or intrathoracic, but the changes in the flow–volume loop are similar. Given this patient's history, it is likely secondary to tracheal stenosis. Other possible causes include goiter and tracheal tumors.

Variable intrathoracic obstruction is characterized by a flattening of the expiratory phase, whereas variable extrathoracic obstruction presents with a flattening in the inspiratory phase of the flow–volume loop. Although there is a low FVC, a low TLC is required to diagnose restriction. The flow–volume loop does not support a restrictive process.

References: Barreiro TJ, Perillo I. An approach to interpreting spirometry. *Am Fam Physician* 2004;69(5):1107–1114. http://www.attud.org/docs/interpretingspirometry.pdf.

Davies LK. Intrathoracic vs extrathoracic obstructive lesions. http://anest.ufl.edu/files/2011/08/Intrathoracic-vs-Extrathoracic-Airway-Obstruction.pdf

Pocket Guide. The global initiative for chronic obstructive disease. http://www.goldcopd.org/uploads/users/files/GOLD_Pocket_2010Mar31.pdf

97 **Answer: A.**   This patient has airway obstruction as the FEV_1/FVC ratio is <70%. The FEV_1 at 83% of predicted indicates mild obstruction (FEV1 ≥ 80% predicted). The flow–volume loop shows flattening in the inspiratory phase with a preserved expiratory phase, a characteristic of variable extrathoracic obstruction.

Variable lesions are characterized by changes in airway lesion caliber during breathing. Depending on their location (intrathoracic or extrathoracic), they tend to behave differently during inspiration and expiration. Airway abnormalities located above the thoracic inlet (extrathoracic) are affected during inspiration because there is an increased flow of air from the atmosphere toward the lungs, resulting in a decreased intraluminal pressure respective to the atmosphere. The decrease in intraluminal pressure during inspiration causes a limitation of inspiratory flow seen as a flattening in the inspiratory limb of the flow-volume loop. During expiration, the positive pressure generated to force the air out expands the narrowed extrathoracic airway. Therefore, the maximal expiratory flow–volume curve is usually normal. Causes of variable extrathoracic lesions include vocal cord paralysis, vocal cord adhesions, vocal cord constriction, laryngeal edema, glottic strictures, and tumors.

Tracheomalacia is an intrathoracic problem, and tracheal stenosis is a fixed defect that would not produce the described change in the flow–volume loop. Emphysema would produce obstruction and a scooped-out configuration in the flow–volume loop.

References: Barreiro TJ, Perillo I. An approach to interpreting spirometry. *Am Fam Physician* 2004;69(5):1107–1114. http://www.attud.org/docs/interpretingspirometry.pdf.

Davies LK. Intrathoracic vs extrathoracic obstructive lesions. http://anest.ufl.edu/files/2011/08/Intrathoracic-vs-Extrathoracic-Airway-Obstruction.pdf

Pocket Guide. The global initiative for chronic obstructive disease. http://www.goldcopd.org/uploads/users/files/GOLD_Pocket_2010Mar31.pdf

98 **Answer: B.**   The flow–volume loop shows flattening in the expiratory phase with a preserved inspiratory phase, a characteristic of variable intrathoracic obstruction. Variable lesions are characterized by changes in airway lesion caliber during breathing. Depending on their location (intrathoracic or extrathoracic), they tend to behave differently during inhalation and exhalation.

Variable intrathoracic constrictions expand during inspiration, causing an increase in airway lumen and resulting in a normal inspiratory limb of the flow–volume loop. During expiration, compression by increasing pleural pressures leads to a decrease in the size of the airway lumen at the site of intrathoracic obstruction, producing a flattening of the expiratory limb of the flow–volume loop. Causes of variable intrathoracic lesions include tumors of the lower trachea or mainstem bronchus, tracheomalacia, and airway changes associated with polychondritis.

Vocal cord dysfunction would cause an extrathoracic abnormality, whereas tracheal stenosis would cause a fixed defect. Emphysema would produce obstruction and a scooped-out configuration in the flow–volume loop.

References: Barreiro TJ, Perillo I. An approach to interpreting spirometry. *Am Fam Physician* 2004;69(5):1107–1114. http://www.attud.org/docs/interpretingspirometry.pdf.

Davies LK. Intrathoracic vs extrathoracic obstructive lesions. http://anest.ufl.edu/files/2011/08/Intrathoracic-vs-Extrathoracic-Airway-Obstruction.pdf

Pocket Guide. The global initiative for chronic obstructive disease. http://www.goldcopd.org/uploads/users/files/GOLD_Pocket_2010Mar31.pdf

99a **Answer: C.**

99b **Answer: C.** This patient has obstruction as the FEV_1/FVC ratio is <70%. The FEV_1 at 42% of predicted indicates severe obstruction ($30\% \leq FEV_1 < 50\%$ predicted). The total lung capacity is reduced (<80%), evidencing restriction. Hyperinflation is defined as a TLC > 120%. The diffusion capacity is decreased.

The combined obstruction and restriction associated with an upper lobe predominant reticulonodular pattern on chest-x-ray are compatible with pulmonary Langerhans cell histiocytosis. Chronic obstructive pulmonary disease and obliterative bronchiolitis produce obstruction and may cause hyperinflation but would not cause restriction. Idiopathic pulmonary fibrosis produces a restrictive defect but would not typically produce obstruction unless associated with a concomitant obstructive disease. Moreover, the radiologic findings are not compatible with any other of the presented alternatives. Other diseases that can produce concurrent obstruction and restriction are sarcoidosis, lymphangioleiomyomatosis, and hypersensitivity pneumonitis.

References: Barreiro TJ, Perillo I. An approach to interpreting spirometry. *Am Fam Physician* 2004;69(5):1107–1114. http://www.attud.org/docs/interpretingspirometry.pdf.

Davies LK. Intrathoracic vs extrathoracic obstructive lesions. http://anest.ufl.edu/files/2011/08/Intrathoracic-vs-Extrathoracic-Airway-Obstruction.pdf

Pocket Guide. The global initiative for chronic obstructive disease. http://www.goldcopd.org/uploads/users/files/GOLD_Pocket_2010Mar31.pdf

100a **Answer: B.**

100b **Answer: A.** This patient has obstruction as the FEV_1/FVC ratio is <70%. The FEV_1 at 42% of predicted indicates very severe obstruction ($FEV_1 < 30\%$ predicted). The total lung capacity is markedly increased (>120%), evidencing hyperinflation. The residual volume (RV) is also significantly increased (>120%) showing air trapping. The diffusion capacity is decreased.

The combined very severe obstruction, hyperinflation, and air trapping is compatible with chronic obstructive pulmonary disease. Idiopathic pulmonary fibrosis produces a restrictive defect, but it does not produce obstruction unless associated with a concomitant obstructive disease. Sarcoidosis can produce obstruction and can also be associated with restriction, but it is not commonly associated with hyperinflation. Primary pulmonary hypertension is a cause of low diffusion capacity but is not typically a cause obstruction, hyperinflation, and air trapping.

References: Barreiro TJ, Perillo I. An approach to interpreting spirometry. *Am Fam Physician* 2004;69(5):1107–1114. http://www.attud.org/docs/interpretingspirometry.pdf.

Davies LK. Intrathoracic vs extrathoracic obstructive lesions. http://anest.ufl.edu/files/2011/08/Intrathoracic-vs-Extrathoracic-Airway-Obstruction.pdf

Pocket Guide. The global initiative for chronic obstructive disease. http://www.goldcopd.org/uploads/users/files/GOLD_Pocket_2010Mar31.pdf

6 Diseases of the Pleura, Chest Wall, and Diaphragm

QUESTIONS

1a A 63-year-old female presents with shortness of breath. What is the predominant imaging finding?

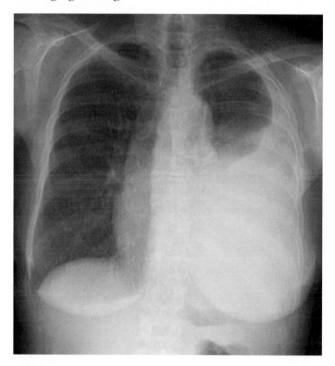

    A. Pneumonia
    B. Pleural effusion
    C. Atelectasis
    D. Cardiomegaly

1b What underlying etiology should be excluded with a massive pleural effusion?
    A. Heart failure
    B. Protein deficiency
    C. Malignancy
    D. Hemorrhage

1c What subtype of pleural effusion would you expect most often with malignancy?

    A. Transudative
    B. Chylous
    C. Hemorrhagic
    D. Exudative

1d What is the most common cause of transudative pleural effusion?

    A. Heart failure
    B. Renal failure
    C. Malignancy
    D. Pneumonia

2 What subtype of pleural effusion would you expect with this diagnosis?

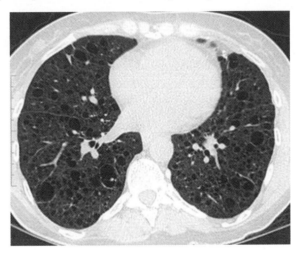

    A. Chylous
    B. Exudative
    C. Transudative
    D. Hemorrhagic

3 The patient is asymptomatic and afebrile. What is the most likely diagnosis?

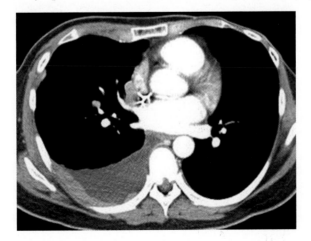

    A. Empyema
    B. Metastases
    C. Fibrous tumor
    D. Lymphoma

4a A 54-year-old male presents with fever and chest pain. What abnormality would most likely account for the radiographic findings?

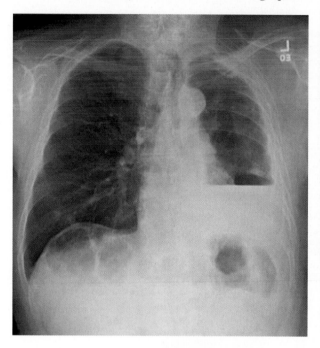 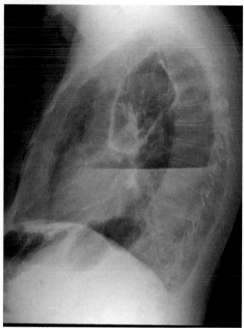

A. Bronchopleural fistula
B. Cardiogenic pulmonary edema
C. Chest wall abscess
D. Interrupted pulmonary artery

4b Which imaging feature is most suggestive of bronchopleural fistula?

A. Volume loss
B. Exudative effusion
C. Persistent air fluid level
D. Pleural thickening

4c A chest CT was obtained. What is the most likely diagnosis?

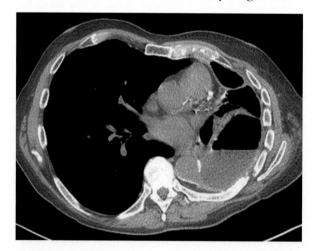

A. Simple effusion
B. Empyema
C. Hemothorax
D. Consolidation

4d What sign is demonstrated?

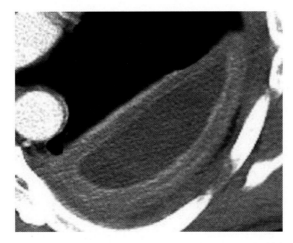

    A. Luftsichel
    B. Split pleura
    C. Bulging fissure
    D. Doughnut

4e What is the preferred management of empyema?

    A. Antibiotics and close follow-up
    B. Aspiration of pleural fluid
    C. Antibiotics and drainage
    D. Pneumonectomy

5a A 72-year-old male presents for routine evaluation. What are the radiographic findings?

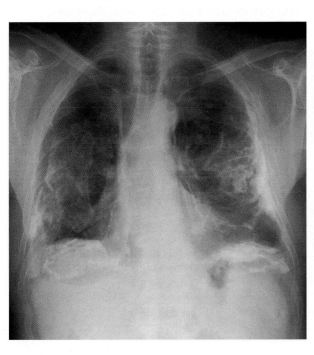
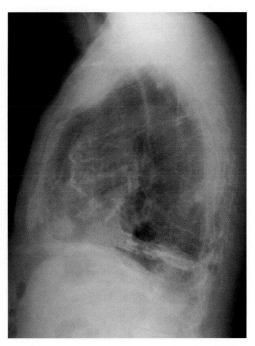

    A. Metastatic disease
    B. Calcified pleural plaques
    C. Multifocal pneumonia
    D. Calcified granulomas

5b A chest CT was obtained. What is the most likely diagnosis?

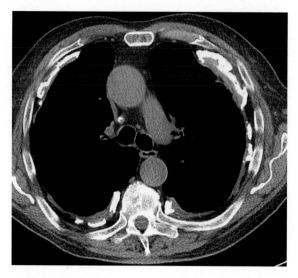

    A. Tuberculous empyema
    B. Asbestos-related pleural disease
    C. Posttraumatic pleural thickening
    D. Metastatic mesothelioma

5c Approximately when do pleural plaques occur after asbestos exposure?

    A. 1 year
    B. 5 years
    C. 20 years
    D. 40 years

6a Another patient with asbestos exposure presents to your clinic with chest pain and hemoptysis. What imaging finding is present?

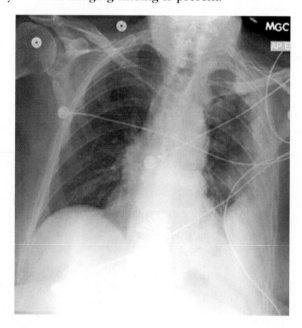

    A. Pneumothorax
    B. Dependent pleural effusion
    C. Peripheral consolidation
    D. Pleural thickening

6b A chest CT was obtained. What is the diagnosis until proven otherwise?

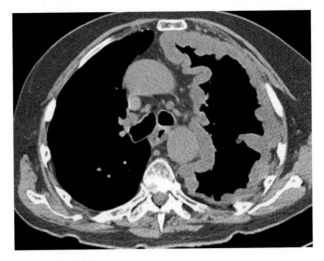

A. Empyema
B. Mesothelioma
C. Hemothorax
D. Amyloidosis

7a A 45-year-old male presents for routine physical. Where is the primary abnormality located?

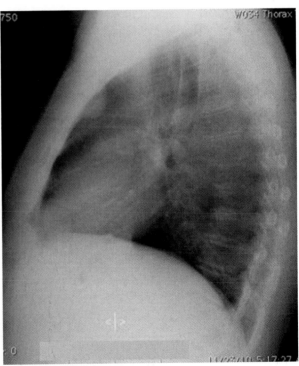

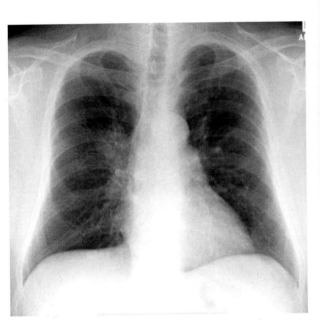

A. Pulmonary parenchyma
B. Chest wall or pleura
C. Mediastinal soft tissues
D. Osseous structures

7b   What sign indicates this abnormality does not originate within the lung?

A. Hilum overlay
B. Comet tail
C. Incomplete border
D. Air crescent

7c   A chest CT was obtained. What is the diagnosis?

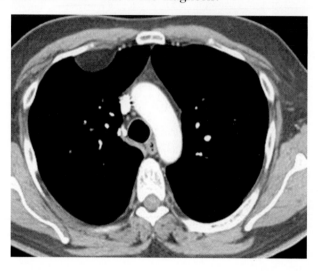

A. Lipoma
B. Desmoid tumor
C. Solitary fibrous tumor
D. Metastasis

8a   A 37-year-old male presents to the emergency room with chest pain. What diagnosis would you consider most likely?

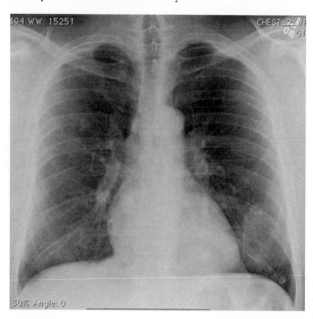

A. Round pneumonia
B. Pleural mass
C. Primary bone neoplasm
D. Loculated pleural fluid

8b A chest CT was obtained. The patient discloses a remote history of gunshot to the left upper quadrant requiring surgical intervention. What is the most likely diagnosis?

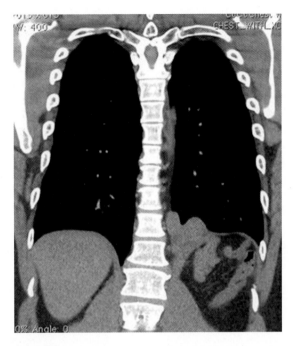

A. Metastatic disease
B. Thoracic splenosis
C. Solitary fibrous tumor
D. Extramedullary hematopoiesis

9a What is the radiographic finding?

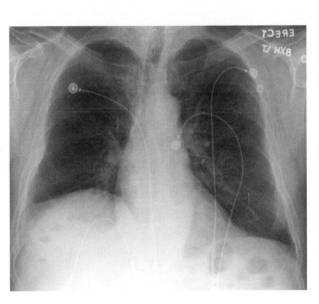
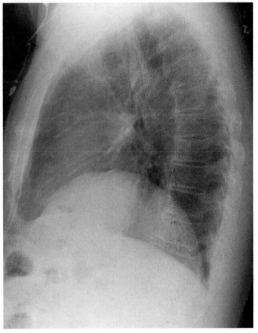

A. Elevated hemidiaphragm
B. Deep sulcus sign
C. Pleural mass
D. "V" sign of Naclerio

9b What cause of the imaging findings would be your primary consideration if this patient had a history of cardiac surgery with subsequent increased shortness of breath?

A. Direct injury of the diaphragm
B. Phrenic nerve injury
C. Ischemic heart disease
D. Esophageal rupture

9c What would be the next test of choice to confirm suspected diaphragmatic paralysis?

A. Ventilation–perfusion scintigraphy
B. Inspiratory–expiratory chest CT
C. Nerve conduction studies
D. Fluoroscopic sniff test

10a A 19-year-old female presented with chest pain. What is the diagnosis?

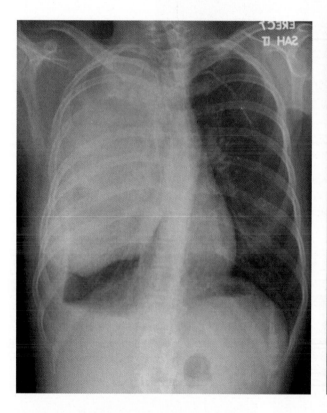 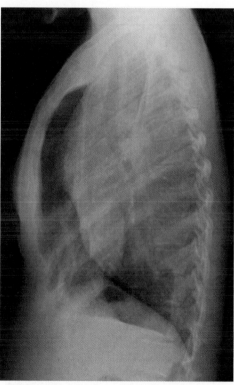

A. Chest wall mass
B. Anterior mediastinal mass
C. Large congenital cyst
D. Unilateral pulmonary edema

10b What is the best diagnosis?

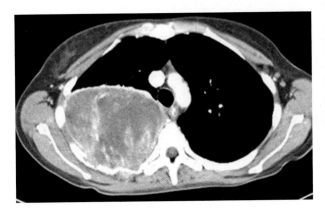
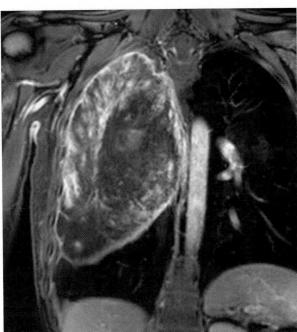

    A. Lipoma
    B. Loculated effusion
    C. Aneurysm
    D. Chest wall sarcoma

11a A 73-year-old female presents with shortness of breath. What is the abnormality?

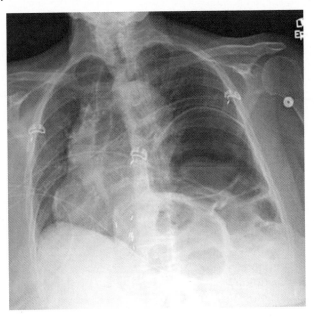

    A. Cystic mass
    B. Bullous emphysema
    C. Intrathoracic bowel
    D. Pneumothorax

11b A CT was obtained. What is the diagnosis?

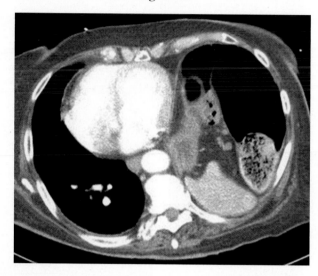

   A. Elevated hemidiaphragm
   B. Abdominal mass
   C. Diaphragmatic hernia
   D. Pneumonectomy

12a Having the opacity longer in length in one projection versus the orthogonal view suggests:

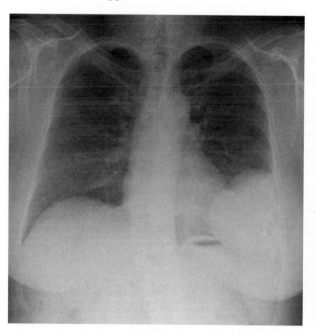
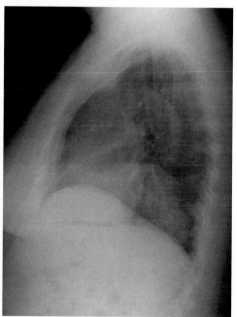

   A. Lower lobe pulmonary process
   B. Posttraumatic etiology
   C. Extrapulmonary location
   D. Subdiaphragmatic location

12b A chest CT was obtained. What imaging findings would be exclusive to solitary fibrous tumor of the pleura?

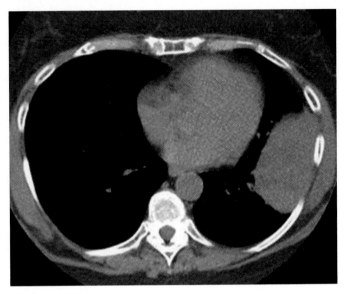

A. Fat
B. None
C. Calcification
D. Fluid

13a A 55-year-old male presents for pulmonary nodule follow-up. What is the diagnosis?

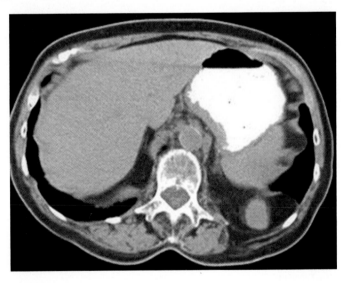

A. Hiatus hernia
B. Spigelian hernia
C. Morgagni hernia
D. Bochdalek hernia

13b A different 52-year-old male presents for routine checkup. What is the finding?

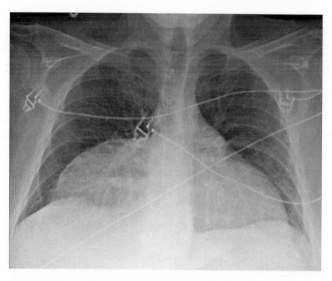

   A. Elevated hemidiaphragm
   B. Pericardial effusion
   C. Lymphadenopathy
   D. Cardiophrenic angle mass

13c A chest CT was obtained. What is the best diagnosis?

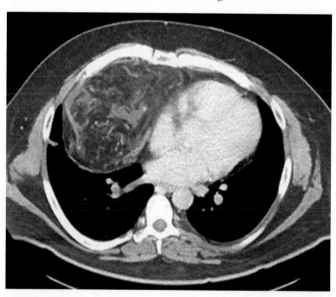

   A. Morgagni hernia
   B. Bochdalek hernia
   C. Hiatal hernia
   D. Hematoma

14a What is the primary abnormality?

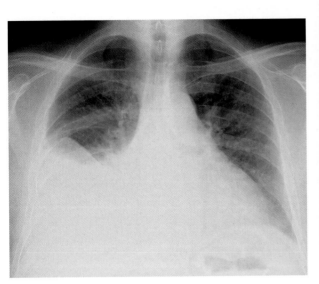
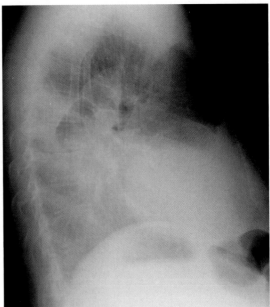

    A. Right lung consolidation
    B. Right pleural effusion
    C. Right pneumothorax
    D. Right hydropneumothorax

14b Given this CT image of the same patient, what is the cause of the right pleural effusion?

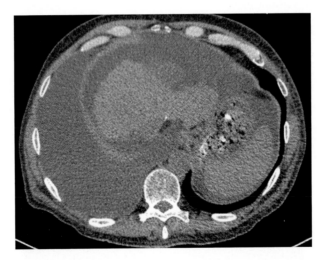

    A. Hepatic cirrhosis
    B. Heart failure
    C. Malignancy
    D. Parapneumonic

14c What percentage of hepatic hydrothoraces are bilateral?
    A. 1% to 2%
    B. 10% to 15%
    C. 50%
    D. >80%

15 The patient has a history of Eloesser flap. What is the most likely cause of his pleural findings?

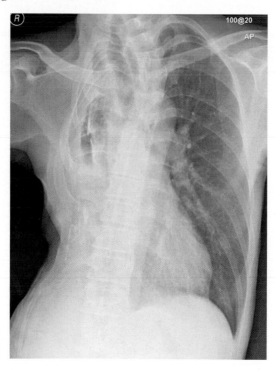

    A. Remote hemothorax
    B. Asbestos-related pleural disease
    C. Remote tuberculous empyema
    D. Pleural mesothelioma

16a What is the most likely cause of the right rib deformities?

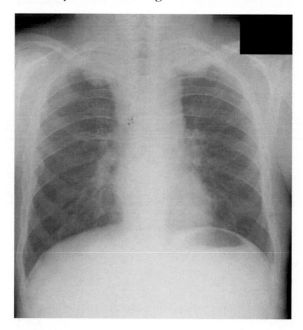

    A. Neurofibromatosis
    B. Aortic coarctation
    C. Posttraumatic fractures
    D. Metastases

16b What abnormality is associated with neurofibromatosis type 1?

    A. Cardiac rhabdomyomas

    B. Lateral meningoceles

    C. Hemiplegia

    D. Choroid plexus papillomas

17 What stage of thymoma is demonstrated?

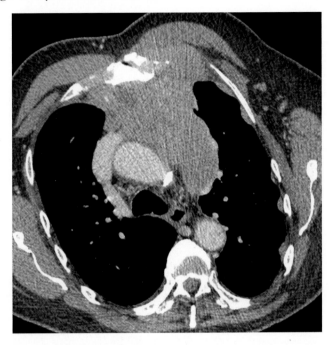

    A. Stage I

    B. Stage II

    C. Stage III

    D. Stage IV

18a What does the soft tissue focus represent?

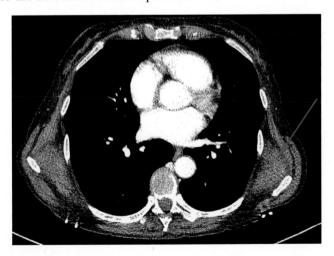

    A. Normal muscle

    B. Vascular malformation

    C. Benign tumor

    D. Malignant tumor

18b This was an incidental finding. What is the best recommendation?

    A. No follow-up

    B. Follow-up CT in 6 months

    C. Needle biopsy

    D. Surgical resection

19 Chest wall desmoid tumor is most commonly associated with which condition?

    A. Carney triad

    B. Gardner syndrome

    C. Lofgren syndrome

    D. Osler-Weber-Rendu syndrome

20 CT pulmonary angiography in a 32-year-old female with shortness of breath and 5 days after oocyte retrieval following HCG administration for infertility. What is the most likely cause of the CT findings?

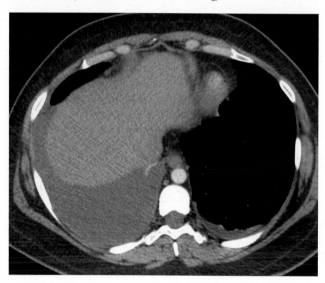

    A. Meadow syndrome

    B. Hepatic failure

    C. Ovarian hyperstimulation syndrome

    D. Meigs syndrome

ANSWERS AND EXPLANATIONS

1a **Answer B.**

1b **Answer C.**

1c **Answer D.**

1d **Answer A.**   The pleural space is composed of inner visceral and outer parietal layers. The pleural space normally holds 10 to 15 mL of fluid and is a potential space. An effusion as small as 50 mL on the lateral and 200 mL on the frontal radiograph can be detected. The most common effusion subtypes are transudative and exudative. Transudative effusions are more common, caused by increased hydrostatic or decreased oncotic pressures. Examples include heart, liver, and renal failure. Exudative effusions result from increased pleural permeability and can be seen with infection or neoplasm.

Of importance, malignancy should be excluded in the presence of a massive pleural effusion. Although only a small number of malignant effusions are massive, most massive effusions are of malignant etiology.

References: Evans AL, Gleeson FV. Radiology in pleural disease: state of the art. *Respirology* 2004;9:300–312.

Kuhlman JE, Singha NK. Complex disease of the pleural space: radiographic and CT evaluation. *Radiographics* 1997;17:63–79.

Maskell NA, Butland RJ. BTS guidelines for the investigation of a unilateral pleural effusion in adults. *Thorax* 2003;58:8–17.

2 **Answer A.**   Chylous effusions are a rare subtype of pleural effusion caused by thoracic duct (or its tributaries) disruption or lymphatic obstruction resulting in leakage of chyle into the pleural space. Causes include lymphangioleiomyomatosis (LAM), lymphangiomatosis, and lymphoma, among others. This case demonstrates the typical appearance of LAM with diffuse cystic lung disease.

References: Evans AL, Gleeson FV. Radiology in pleural disease: state of the art. *Respirology* 2004;9:300–312.

Kuhlman JE, Singha NK. Complex disease of the pleural space: radiographic and CT evaluation. *Radiographics* 1997;17:63–79.

Maskell NA, Butland RJ. BTS guidelines for the investigation of a unilateral pleural effusion in adults. *Thorax* 2003;58:8–17.

3 **Answer B.**   This case demonstrates enhancing pleural nodules and pleural thickening in association with the moderate-sized effusion. This is a case of metastatic pleural disease from a breast malignancy. Metastatic disease to the pleura may manifest as effusion, thickening, or nodularity. While pleural soft tissue nodularity may suggest the diagnosis, pleural effusion without nodules does NOT exclude the diagnosis of metastatic pleural involvement. Lung and breast are the two most common origins of metastatic malignancies to the pleura.

Top differentials for pleural nodularity include metastases (most common), lymphoma, fibrous tumor, mesothelioma, and invasive thymoma.

References: Dynes MC, White EM, Fry WA, et al. Imaging manifestations of pleural tumors. *Radiographics* 1992;12:1191–1201.

Hussein-Jelen T, Bankier AA, Eisenberg RL. Solid pleural lesions. *AJR Am J Roentgenol* 2012;198:W512–W520.

4a **Answer A.**

4b **Answer C.**

4c **Answer B.**

4d **Answer B.**

4e **Answer C.** Empyema refers to an infected, purulent collection within the pleural space, which can be life threatening. Empyema often develops secondary to pneumonia with parapneumonic effusion, which later becomes infected. As discussed, infection causes increased pleural permeability, which may result in pleural fluid accumulation.

Over the split pleura sign is associated with empyema. This sign results from separation of the visceral and parietal pleura, which become thickened and inflamed. Contrast-enhanced imaging often shows pleural enhancement.

Preferred treatment consists of appropriate medical therapy and drainage. This typically consists of antibiotics and thoracostomy tube placement. Complicated empyemas (i.e., internal septation or loculation) may need multiple chest tubes or surgical debridement.

Bronchopleural fistula refers to abnormal communication between the bronchial tree and pleural space. This can be seen with many causes, including infection or empyema as in this case. This abnormality accounts for the air fluid level seen on imaging and is suspected when attempted drainage fails to clear the pneumothorax component. Another potential complication of empyema is extrathoracic extension, referred to as empyema necessitans.

References: Kraus GJ. The split pleura sign. *Radiographics* 2007;243:297–298.

Kuhlman JE, Singha NK. Complex disease of the pleural space: radiographic and CT evaluation. *Radiographics* 1997;17:63–79.

Stark DD, Federle MP. Differentiating lung abscess and empyema: radiography and computed tomography. *AJR Am J Roentgenol* 1983;141:163–137.

5a **Answer B.**

5b **Answer B.**

5c **Answer C.** Asbestos-related disease of the lung and pleura may be neoplastic and nonneoplastic. Findings generally take years to manifest, although recent data from asbestos exposures in Libby Montana have demonstrated pleural disease in shorter time periods and younger patients. Pleural effusion is one of the earliest findings and may present within 10 years of exposure (effusion may be hemorrhagic). Pleural plaques (with or without calcification) are the most common manifestation, generally occurring 20 to 30 years postexposure. Common distribution sites include the chest wall underlying the ribs and diaphragm.

Important ancillary findings associated with asbestos-related lung disease include rounded atelectasis, asbestosis (parenchymal manifestations of exposure), mesothelioma, and bronchogenic carcinoma. Individuals who smoke have significantly increased risk (50 times or more) of developing primary lung neoplasm.

References: Larson TC, Meyer CA, Kapil V, et al. Workers with libby amphibole exposure: retrospective identification and progression of radiographic changes. *Radiology* 2010;255(3):924–933.

Roach HD, Davies GJ. Asbestos: when the dust settles—an imaging review of asbestos-related disease. *Radiographics* 2002;22:167–184.

6a **Answer D.**

6b **Answer B.** Mesothelioma is the most common primary pleural malignancy and has a delayed presentation, often 35 to 40 years after asbestos exposure. Characteristic imaging shows extensive, circumferential pleural thickening, usually several centimeters thick. Note the extension along the mediastinal pleura as well as the fissural extension, much more common in malignant pleural thickening than benign pleural thickening. Pleural effusion may also be seen, and delayed development (more than 20 years after exposure) of a pleural effusion in the setting of asbestos exposure should raise concern for the diagnosis. Mesothelioma is not thought to arise from preexisting plaques.

Reference: Wang ZJ, Reddy GP. Malignant pleural mesothelioma: evaluation with CT, MR imaging, and PET. *Radiographics* 2004;24:105–119.

7a **Answer B.**

7b **Answer C.**

7c **Answer A.** Pleural or chest wall lipomas are benign fatty lesions. Radiographs show an abnormality along the anterior chest wall demonstrating the incomplete border sign, indicating this lesion cannot originate with the lung. The lesion creates obtuse margins on the lateral radiograph, also suggesting extraparenchymal origin. Additionally, this case demonstrates a positive hilum overlay sign indicating that the opacity on frontal view does not reside in the hilum, but does not necessarily indicate pleural or chest wall location. CT characterizes this lesion as fat, confirming the diagnosis of lipoma.

Reference: Mullan CP, Rachna M. Radiology of chest wall masses. *AJR Am J Roentgenol* 2011;197:460–470.

8a **Answer B.**

8b **Answer B.** Thoracic splenosis refers to autotransplantation of splenic tissue within the thorax, typically after trauma and disruption of the diaphragm. Ectopic locations include both the abdomen and chest. Thoracic splenosis may be asymptomatic or present with hemoptysis and pleurisy. Imaging findings include multiple, enhancing (if IV contrast given) pleural implants of varying sizes within the left hemithorax. CT imaging in this case shows nodularity extending along the hemidiaphragm into the chest with abnormal configuration of the spleen secondary to remote trauma. Additional tests to help confirm the diagnosis include technetium 99m (^{99m}Tc) sulfur colloid, indium 111–labeled platelet, ^{99m}Tc heat–damaged erythrocyte, or ^{99m}Tc white blood cell scans.

References: Huang AH, Shaffer K. Thoracic splenosis. *Radiographics* 2006;239:293–296.

Malik UF, Martin MR. Parenchymal thoracic splenosis: history and nuclear imaging without invasive procedures may provide diagnosis. *J Clin Med Res* 2010;2(4):180–184.

9a **Answer A.**

9b **Answer B.**

9c **Answer D.** Radiographic images show elevation of the right hemidiaphragm (which is normally slightly higher than the left). The diaphragm separates the chest from the abdomen and is the primary muscle of respiration. An elevated hemidiaphragm may have many causes. Phrenic nerve (which innervates the diaphragm) injury is a common etiology, often resulting from surgery, trauma, or tumor invasion. Diaphragmatic eventration refers to asymmetric thinning of diaphragm muscle, typically involving only a segment, producing a focal bulge.

Diaphragmatic paralysis can be confirmed using the fluoroscopic sniff test. A positive exam demonstrates a normal functioning contralateral hemidiaphragm with paradoxical motion of the affected hemidiaphragm as the patient sniffs, which results from negative intrathoracic pressure during rapid inspiration. CT of the chest may be warranted to exclude an underlying process such as malignancy, but does not directly evaluate the hemidiaphragm for paralysis.

Differentials for an apparent elevated hemidiaphragm include normal expiration, congenital hypoplastic lung, decreased lung volume from atelectasis or lung resection, subpulmonic effusion, and mass effect from abdominal neoplasm or organomegaly.

References: Nason LK, Walker CM. Imaging of the diaphragm: anatomy and function. *Radiographics* 2012;32:E51–E70.

Verhey PT, Gosselin MV. Differentiating diaphragmatic paralysis and eventration. *Acad Radiol* 2007;4:420–425.

10a Answer A.

10b Answer D. When lesions become large, it can be difficult to distinguish point of origin, and cross-sectional imaging is usually performed. The provided radiographs demonstrate a well-defined large opacity involving the right upper and midthorax, but it is the erosion and partial absence of the posterior fifth rib that confirms chest wall involvement. The lateral chest radiograph demonstrates an open retrosternal window with a posterior localization of the process. Unilateral pulmonary edema and congenital cysts would not create the chest wall changes.

CT and MR imaging show a heterogeneously enhancing mass with chest wall, pleural, and bony involvement. This particular diagnosis was Ewing sarcoma, also known as Askin tumor. Ewing sarcoma is seen in children and young adults and may be associated with 11;22 chromosomal translocation. Imaging features include small to large heterogeneous mass, which may be associated with pleural effusion and lymphadenopathy. Calcifications are less common, but can occur. Large sarcomas generally show internal necrosis and sometimes hemorrhage. Avid enhancement is common, which becomes more heterogeneous as lesions become larger and necrotic.

References: Murphy MD, Senchak LT, Mambalam PK. From the radiologic pathology archives: Ewing sarcoma family of tumors: radiologic-pathologic correlation. *Radiographics* 2013;33:803–813.

Tateishi U, Gladish GW, Kusumoto M. Chest wall tumors: radiologic findings and pathologic correlation. Part 2: malignant tumors. *Radiographics* 2003;23:1491–1508.

11a Answer C.

11b Answer C. Radiographs from question 11a demonstrate abdominal contents within the left hemithorax. Bowel has a characteristic radiographic signature, often allowing for exclusion of pneumothorax or cystic lesion. CT confirms the diagnosis of diaphragmatic hernia with a classic "dependent viscera sign" where the intra-abdominal contents come in direct contact with the posterior ribs indicating an absence of an intact diaphragm.

A diaphragmatic hernia is a congenital or acquired defect, which may allow abdominal contents to herniate into the thorax. Common causes of acquired defects include trauma and surgery. Hiatal hernias are the most common diaphragmatic hernia overall. Other forms include Morgagni and Bochdalek.

Reference: Sandstrom CK, Stern EJ. Diaphragmatic hernias: a spectrum of radiographic appearances. *Curr Probl Diagn Radiol* 2011;3:95–115.

12a **Answer C.**

12b **Answer B.** Radiographs show a peripheral, defined mass with an incomplete border and dimension that are much greater in the anterior–posterior diameter versus the lateral width on frontal view. The incomplete border sign suggests extrapulmonary origin (obtuse margins also suggest extraparenchymal origin, and acute margins suggest parenchymal origin). The asymmetric dimensions on frontal and lateral are more characteristic of a pleural lesion, and using the same logic with air fluid levels assists in differentiating pulmonary abscess from empyema. CT demonstrates a well-defined, homogeneous pleural mass. The pathologic diagnosis of fibrous tumor of the pleura was obtained (also known as solitary or localized fibrous tumor).

Fibrous tumor of the pleura is a rare diagnosis most common in adults (fourth through sixth decades). Imaging features depend on size and tumor aggression. Benign and malignant forms exist, benign being more common. Small nonaggressive tumors tend to be homogeneous with obtuse margins and lack chest wall extension. Larger lesions can become heterogeneous and show more acute margins, mimicking pulmonary mass. Malignant forms may have chest wall or bony involvement. Enhancement is typical, and calcifications are rare. Pedunculated forms with fibrovascular stalk can be seen. No imaging finding of the primary lesion is specific for solitary fibrous tumor of the pleura, and no finding differentiates benign versus malignant short of metastatic lesions. Some may demonstrate systemic symptoms in relation to fibrous tumors including hypertrophic osteoarthropathy and in some cases hypoglycemia. Treatment of localized fibrous tumors of the pleura is surgical resection, with a recurrence rate of up to 15%.

PET/CT may demonstrate low-grade FDG uptake in benign forms and more avid uptake in malignant forms. Malignant lesions may be multiple and show a recurrence rate up to 63%. Differentials include metastasis, mesothelioma, and lymphoma.

References: Ginat DT, Bokhari A, Bhatt S, et al. Imaging features of solitary fibrous tumors. *AJR Am J Roentgenol* 2011;196:487–495.

Luciano C, Francesco A, Giovanni V. CT signs, patterns and differential diagnosis of solitary fibrous tumors of the pleura. *J Thorac Dis* 2010;2:21–25.

Rosado-de-Christenson ML, Abbott GF, McAdams HP, et al. From the Archives of the AFIP: localized fibrous tumor of the pleura. *Radiographics* 2003;23:759–783.

13a **Answer D.**

13b **Answer D.**

13c **Answer A.** These cases demonstrate both congenital diaphragmatic hernias, Bochdalek and Morgagni. The first case shows a small Bochdalek hernia containing fat and a small portion of bowel. The second case demonstrates a large cardiophrenic opacity on chest radiograph with subsequent CT revealing a large Morgagni hernia containing fat and engorged vasculature, likely from omentum.

Bochdalek hernias are far more common, occurring through the foramen of Bochdalek. These are typically unilateral and occur posteriorly on the left. They can also be seen on the right, or may be bilateral. Morgagni hernias occur along the anteromedial right hemidiaphragm. Differentials for right cardiophrenic angle mass on chest radiography include Morgagni hernia, pericardial cyst, lymphadenopathy, and pericardial/mediastinal fat.

References: Mullins ME, Stein J, Saini CC, et al. Prevalence of incidental bochdalek's hernia in a large adult population. *AJR Am J Roentgenol* 2001;177:363–366.

Sandstrom CK, Stern EJ. Diaphragmatic hernias: a spectrum of radiographic appearances. *Curr Probl Diagn Radiol* 2011;3:95–115.

14a **Answer B.**

14b **Answer A.**

14c **Answer A.** The chest x-ray demonstrates a large layering right effusion. There is no air fluid level or pleural line to suggest a pleural air component. The associated CT demonstrates significant liver cirrhosis and ascites confirming the likely etiology as hepatic hydrothorax.

Hepatic hydrothorax is defined as a significant effusion in the setting of cirrhosis without other identifiable cause. Overall, it is uncommon (5% to 10% of cirrhotic patients) although centers that treat a large number of liver disease patients may see this frequently. The most accepted etiology is leakage of ascitic fluid through small defects in the diaphragm. The majority of hepatic hydrothorax cases are right sided (85%). Only 10% to 15% of causes are left sided with <2% being bilateral. Note that the absence of ascites does not exclude this disease as the normal intra-abdominal and intrathoracic pressure gradient can preferentially fill the pleural space in some cases.

Reference: Kim YK, Kim Y, Shim SS. Thoracic complications of liver cirrhosis: radiologic findings. *Radiographics* 2009;29(3):825–837.

15 **Answer C.** Chest radiograph demonstrates a unilateral process with severe volume loss, pleural thickening, and pleural calcifications. While remote hemothorax and asbestos-related pleural disease can both produce a fibrothorax with pleural calcifications, tuberculous empyema would be the most characteristic, and the history of Eloesser flap used for treatment of chronic empyema confirms the diagnosis.

Chronic tuberculous empyema arises from tuberculous pleurisy as a complication of primary pulmonary tuberculosis. The chronic pleural mycobacterial infection causes a calcified pleural thickening around the empyema, which may progress to volume loss in the setting of fibrothorax. Significant extrapleural fat proliferation has been described in the setting of tuberculous empyema as seen in the following CT from the same patient:

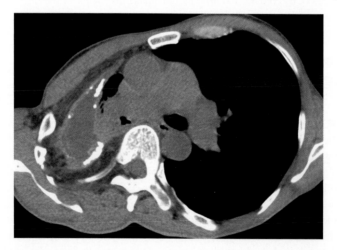

Chylous-like fluid in the empyema may also be seen manifesting as a fluid fat level.

References: Kim HY, Song K, Goo JM, et al. Thoracic sequelae and complications of tuberculosis. *Radiographics* 2001;21:839–860.

Thourani VH, Lancaster RT, Mansour KA, et al. Twenty-six years of experience with the modified eloesser flap. *Ann Thorac Surg* 2003;76:401–406.

16a **Answer A.**

16b **Answer B.**   While many indolent conditions can cause resorptive changes of the ribs, few cause multilevel erosions. Neither traumatic fractures nor metastases would result in the rib changes seen. Aortic coarctation can cause "rib notching" similar to the findings here, but the chest radiograph also reveals biapical mass lesions as well as subpleural lesions along the inner aspects of the lateral ribs. These findings are consistent with "ribbon ribs" of neurofibromatosis.

Neurofibromatosis type 1 (NF1 or von Recklinghausen disease) is the most common phakomatosis, commonly manifesting with cutaneous neurofibromas, café au lait spots, freckling, optic nerve gliomas, sphenoid wing dysplasia, and other characteristic bony changes. Accompanying NF1, the inactivation of tumor suppression results in multiple different potential tumors although the potential tumors provided as alternative answers are associated with other phakomatoses (cardiac rhabdomyomas–tuberous sclerosis and choroid plexus papillomas–von Hippel-Lindau disease). Hemiplegia is associated with Sturge-Weber syndrome. Finally, dural ectasia and lateral meningoceles are associated with neurofibromatosis type 1, commonly seen with associated scoliosis.

Reference: Rossi SE, Erasmus JJ, McAdams HP, et al. Thoracic manifestations of neurofibromatosis-I. *AJR Am J Roentgenol* 1999;173:1631–1638.

17 **Answer D.**   A large anterior mediastinal mass at the root of the aorta and projecting to one side is demonstrated on CT with multiple associated left pleural lesions representing "drop metastases." The combination is most consistent with thymoma with direct invasion into the left pleural space. By the Masaoka-Koga staging of thymoma, pleural and pericardial dissemination indicate stage IVa disease with hematogenous metastases representing stage IVb disease. The distinction between stage IVa and IVb diseases is the difference between neoadjuvant chemotherapy and surgical resection (with or without radiation therapy) and palliative chemotherapy, respectively.

Reference: Benveniste MFK, Rosado-de-Christensen ML, Sabloff BS, et al. Role of imaging in the diagnosis, staging, and treatment of thymoma. *Radiographics* 2011;31:1847–1861.

18a **Answer C.**

18b **Answer A.**   Elastofibroma dorsi is a benign tumor of the chest wall that occurs in the infrascapular region deep to the adjacent musculature. In this case, the lesions are relatively symmetric, although they can be asymmetric or unilateral. Elastofibroma dorsi is most common in elderly women, and some have postulated that mechanical friction is the cause of the right side predominance of unilateral lesions. The characteristic location and CT appearance is sufficient for diagnosis, particularly in bilateral cases such as this, and requires no further follow-up in the asymptomatic patient. Some cases of elastofibroma dorsi do cause symptoms of shoulder pain or "snapping" scapula, for which resection may be considered.

References: Naylor MF, Nascimento AG, Sherrick AD, et al. Elastofibroma dorsi: radiologic findings in 12 patients. *AJR Am J Roentgenol* 1996;167:683–687.

Ochsner JE, Sewall SA, Brooks GN, et al. Best cases from the AFIP: elastofibroma dorsi. *Radiographics* 2006;26:1873–1876.

19 **Answer B.**   Chest wall desmoid tumor, also called aggressive fibromatosis, is the most common low-grade sarcoma of the chest wall. While this lesion does not metastasize, it is infiltrative and can even invade the intrathoracic cavity.

Desmoid tumors have several associations, the most common being Gardner syndrome and trauma. On imaging, desmoid tumors can have variable density on CT, signal lower than muscle on T1, and intermediate signal on T2.

The alternative options have associate thoracic lesions. Carney triad is pulmonary chondromas, extra-adrenal paragangliomas, and gastrointestinal stromal tumors. Lofgren syndrome is sarcoidosis with thoracic adenopathy, erythema nodosum, and arthralgia. Finally, Osler-Weber-Rendu syndrome manifests with multiple arteriovenous malformations and mucocutaneous telangiectasias.

Reference: Tateishi U, Gladish GW, Kusumoto M, et al. Chest wall tumors: radiologic findings and pathologic correlation. *Radiographics* 2003;23:1491–1508.

20 **Answer C.** Right greater than left pleural effusions are shown on CT pulmonary angiogram. With the clinical history and patient symptoms, the constellation is consistent with ovarian hyperstimulation syndrome (OHSS). The syndrome occurs around 6 days following oocyte retrieval and manifests with enlargement of the ovaries with third spacing of fluid. Severity is classified as mild (ovarian enlargement with abdominal symptoms), moderate (evidence of ascites on imaging), and severe (ascites or hydrothorax with respiratory symptoms, hemoconcentration, or coagulopathy). Most cases are uncomplicated with supportive measures provided until resolution around 12 days after HCG administration. More common complications include pulmonary embolism, ARDS, and pulmonary infection.

Reference: McNeary M, Stark P. Radiographic findings in ovarian hyperstimulation syndrome. *J Thorac Imaging* 2002;17:230–232.

Mediastinal Disease

QUESTIONS

1a What best explains the radiographic appearance below?

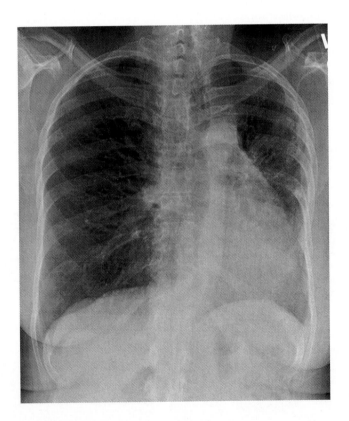

A. Consolidation
B. Cardiomegaly
C. Pulmonary volume loss
D. Pneumothorax

1b Pre- and post-IV contrast CT images provided are oblique MPR contrast image through the right and left pulmonary arteries. What diagnosis best explains the findings?

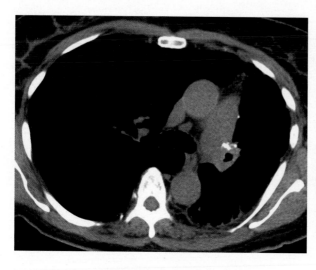 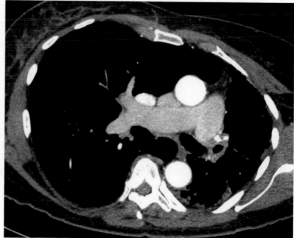

A. Chronic pulmonary embolism
B. Fibrosing mediastinitis
C. Untreated lymphoma
D. Takayasu arteritis

1c What is the most common cause of fibrosing mediastinitis in the United States?

A. Histoplasmosis
B. Idiopathic
C. Tuberculosis
D. Radiation

2a Given the CT findings, what is the patient's most likely presenting symptom?

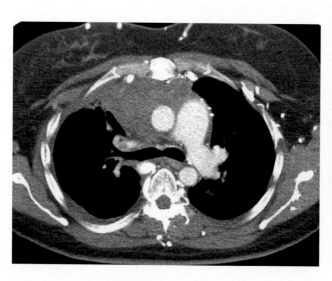 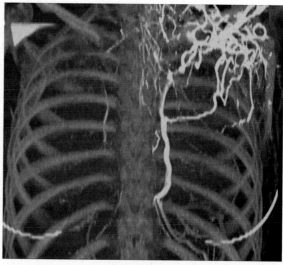

A. Stridor
B. Facial swelling
C. Mental status changes
D. Nausea

2b Additional CT image from the same study. What is the salient finding?

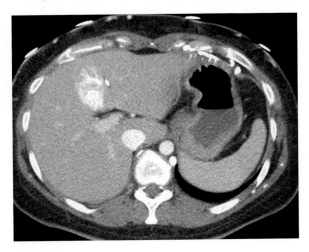

A. Porcelain gallbladder
B. Splenic enlargement
C. Focal hepatic enhancement
D. Gastric wall thickening

2c What is the most common cause of superior vena cava syndrome?

A. Cancer
B. Iatrogenic
C. Fibrosing mediastinitis
D. Behcet disease

3a What mediastinal compartment is abnormal?

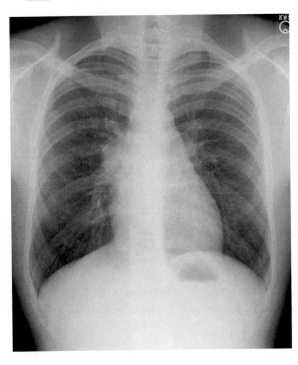
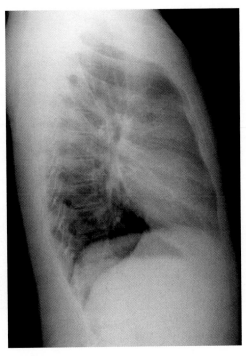

A. Superior
B. Anterior
C. Middle
D. Posterior

3b   Which CT imaging characteristic in this case is typical for thymoma?

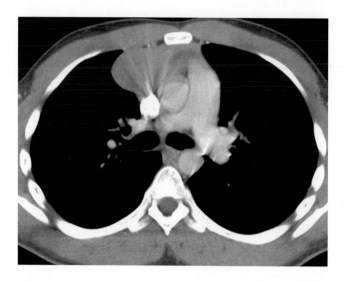

A. Partial fat attenuation
B. Pleural metastasis
C. Projects to one side of the mediastinum
D. Calcification

3c   Excision of the lesion reveals thymoma. Which of the following would be the most common associated condition?

A. Ischemic heart disease
B. Hypogammaglobulinemia
C. Pure red cell aplasia
D. Myasthenia gravis

4   These two contrast-enhanced CTs were separated in time by 2 weeks (earlier on the left). What is the most likely diagnosis?

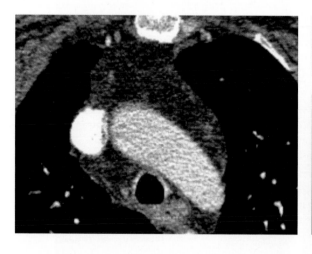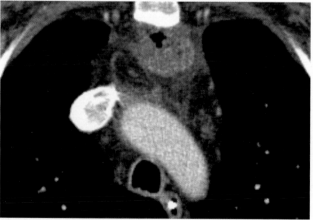

A. Thymoma
B. Thymic carcinoma
C. Mediastinal abscess
D. Normal thymus

5 What is the most common source of pneumomediastinum in the setting of ARDS?

A. Alveolar rupture
B. Extension from pneumothorax
C. Tracheal rupture from endotracheal tube cuff overinflation
D. Esophageal rupture

6a In what mediastinal compartment is the abnormality most likely located based on the chest radiographs?

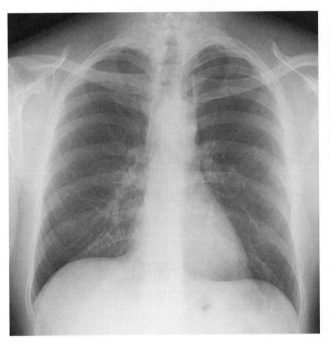
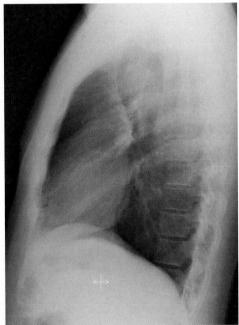

A. Anterior
B. Middle
C. Posterior
D. Superior

6b On evaluation of that patient's CT, what is the likely cause of the abnormality?

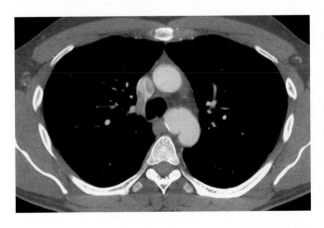
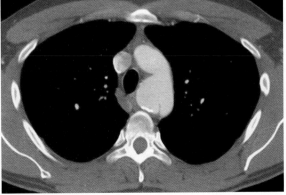

A. Acute traumatic pseudoaneurysm
B. Chronic traumatic pseudoaneurysm
C. Acute mycotic pseudoaneurysm
D. Chronic mycotic pseudoaneurysm

7 An esophageal mass is identified in this patient with a known retroperitoneal liposarcoma. What is the likely etiology of the esophageal mass?

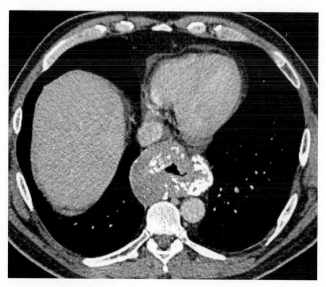

A. Liposarcoma metastasis
B. Primary esophageal carcinoma
C. Esophageal leiomyoma
D. Esophageal lymphoma

8a In what mediastinal space is the abnormality based on these chest x-rays?

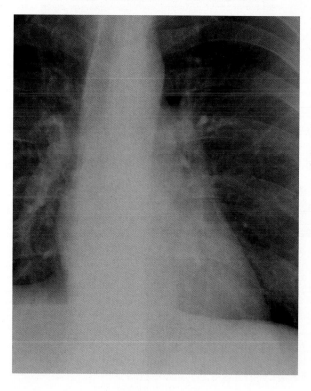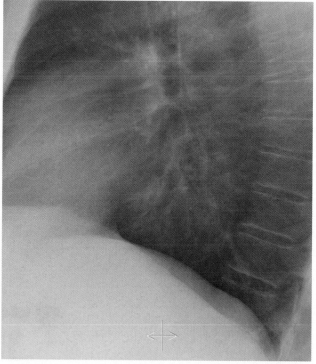

A. Anterior
B. Middle
C. Posterior
D. Superior

8b Based on the corresponding CT, what is the cause of the middle mediastinal opacity on chest x-ray?

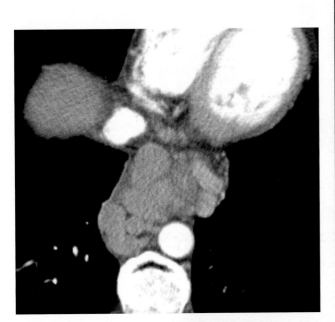 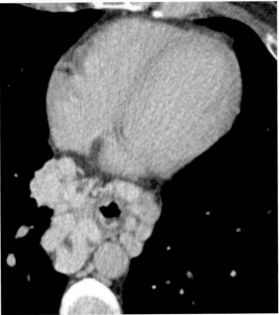

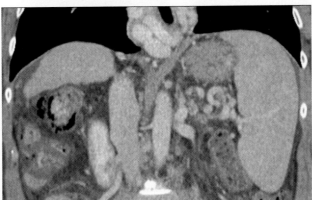

A. Esophageal cancer
B. Esophageal varices
C. Lymphadenopathy
D. Mediastinitis

9a Which of these complications is most common in the setting of a proximal esophageal rupture?

A. Right pleural effusion
B. Left pleural effusion
C. Pneumopericardium
D. Left hydropneumothorax

9b What is the most common feature identified on initial radiograph after esophageal perforation?

A. Mediastinal widening
B. Pneumomediastinum
C. Left pleural effusion
D. Right pleural effusion

10a   Based on this CT, what is the most likely diagnosis?

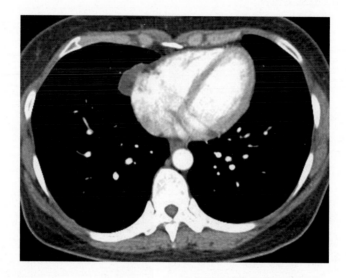

    A. Pericardial nodule
    B. Pericardial cyst
    C. Loculated pleural effusion
    D. Pleural implant

10b   If clinical scenario warrants, what is the next best imaging modality for confirmation?

    A. MRI
    B. PET/CT
    C. Radiographs
    D. Echocardiography

10c   An MRI was performed, based on this. What is the likely diagnosis?

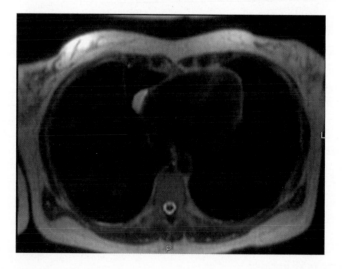

    A. Pericardial nodule
    B. Pericardial cyst
    C. Loculated pleural effusion
    D. Pleural implant

11a On evaluation of these radiographs, what is the best diagnosis?

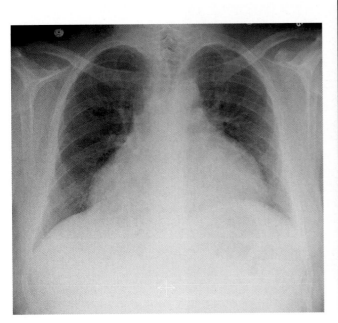
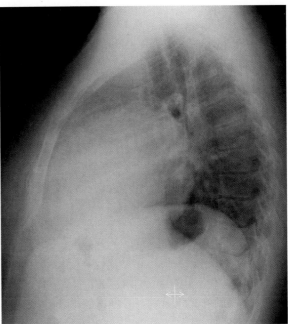

    A. Cardiomegaly
    B. Anterior mediastinal mass
    C. Pneumomediastinum
    D. Pericardial effusion

11b What is the upper limit of normal for volume of pericardial fluid?

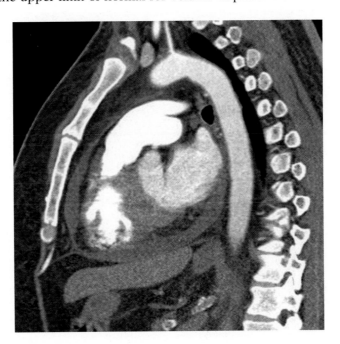

    A. 5 mL
    B. 50 mL
    C. 100 mL
    D. 200 mL

12 Which would be the most likely precipitating event for this spontaneous presentation?

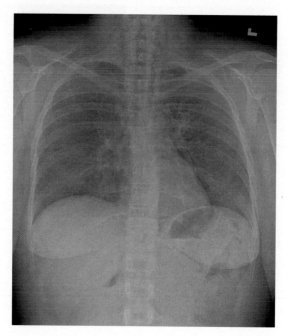

    A. Apical blebs
    B. Intense screaming
    C. Recent long plane flight
    D. Chemotherapy

13a Given the salient abnormality on this axial CT, what is the next best step?

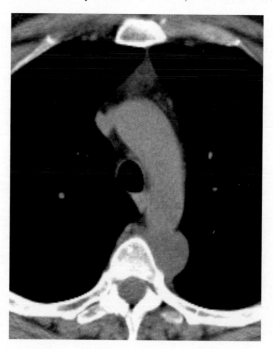

    A. PET/CT
    B. MRI
    C. Follow-up CT in 1 year
    D. CT-guided biopsy

13b An MRI was performed with T1-weighted imaging (left), T2-weighted imaging (middle), and T1 postcontrast imaging (right). What is the likely diagnosis?

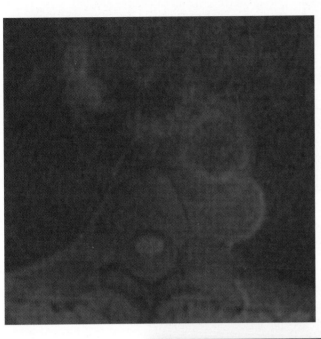
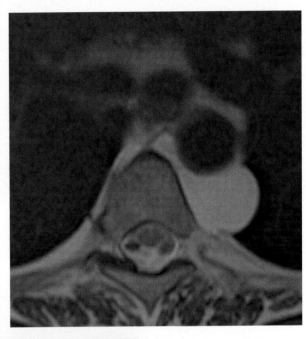
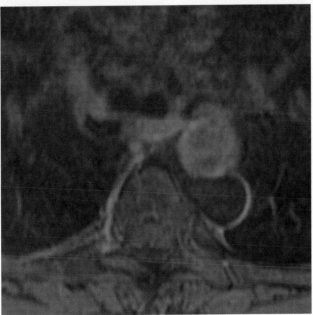

A. Schwannoma
B. Pleural metastasis
C. Foregut duplication cyst
D. Descending aortic pseudoaneurysm

14a What is the most likely diagnosis?

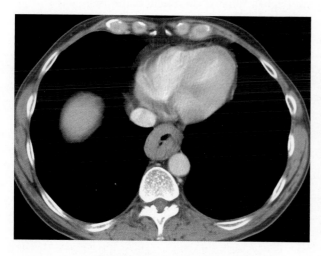
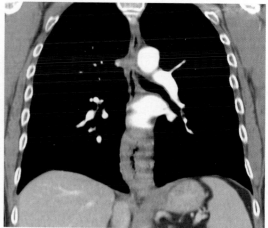

   A. Esophageal duplication cyst
   B. Esophageal varices
   C. Esophageal carcinoma
   D. Barrett esophagus

14b Endoscopy with biopsy confirms esophageal carcinoma. If the CT demonstrates direct invasion of the adjacent lung, what tumor category would it be?

   A. T1
   B. T2
   C. T3
   D. T4

15a In which mediastinal compartment is the lesion?

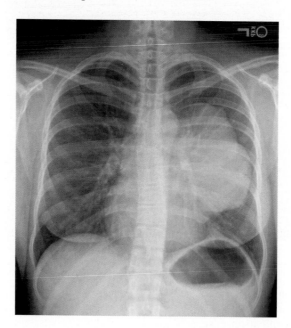

   A. Anterior
   B. Superior
   C. Posterior
   D. Middle

15b What is the most likely diagnosis?

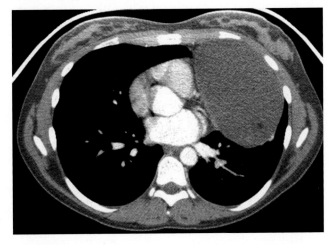

- A. Thymoma
- B. Teratoma
- C. Pericardial cyst
- D. Lymphoma

15c What is the most common extragonadal location of germ cell tumors?

- A. Retroperitoneum
- B. Mediastinum
- C. Intraperitoneum
- D. Head and neck

16a What shadow is abnormal?

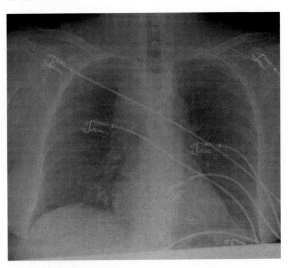

- A. Azygoesophageal border
- B. Right paratracheal stripe
- C. Aortopulmonary window
- D. Interlobar artery

16b The patient presents with recent development of chest pain and history of prior pulmonary embolism currently on oral anticoagulation. A CT pulmonary angiogram was obtained. Localize the abnormality.

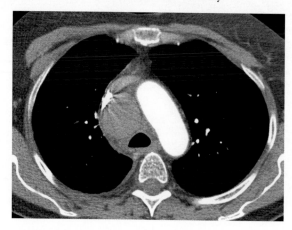

    A. Anterior mediastinum
    B. Intrapulmonary
    C. Middle mediastinum
    D. Endotracheal

16c T1 noncontrast (A), T1 contrast, and T2 (C) were obtained. The patient's INR is supratherapeutic. Which would be the best recommendation after correcting the INR in this hemodynamically stable patient?

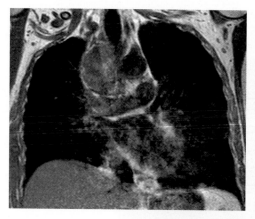 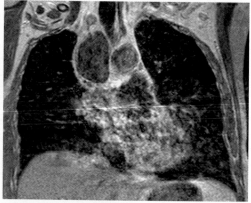

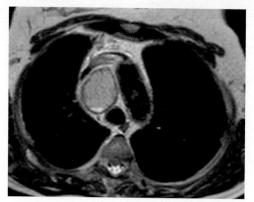

    A. Observation
    B. Bronchoscopy with biopsy
    C. Surgical resection
    D. PET/CT

17a What is the best recommendation based on the image alone?

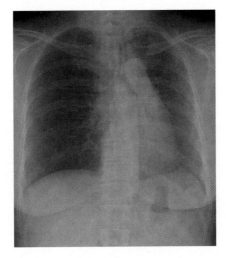

    A. No follow-up
    B. Surveillance radiograph in 6 to 8 weeks
    C. Chest CT
    D. Chest tube placement

17b Which diagnosis best matches the CT findings?

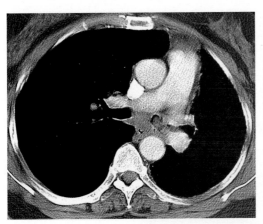
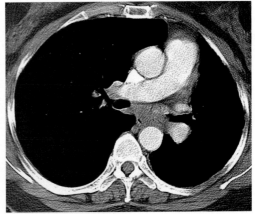

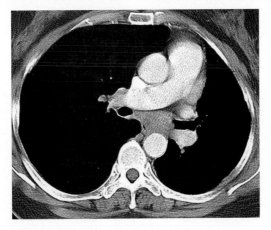

    A. Pulmonary embolism
    B. Endobronchial mass
    C. Aortic aneurysm
    D. Duplication cyst

17c What is the most common tracheal tumor?

    A. Bronchial carcinoid

    B. Adenoid cystic carcinoma

    C. Mucoepidermoid carcinoma

    D. Squamous cell carcinoma

18a This patient presents after recent pneumonia followed by progressive back pain then abrupt loss of feeling and use of lower extremities. What is the most likely diagnosis?

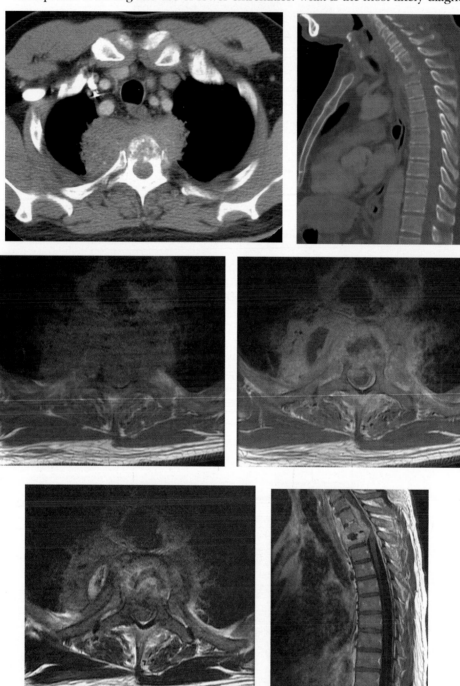

    A. Lymphoma

    B. Extramedullary hematopoiesis

    C. Bronchogenic carcinoma with spinal invasion

    D. Paraspinal abscess with discitis

18b What is the most common infectious cause of discitis?

    A. Staphylococcus

    B. Streptococcus

    C. Salmonella

    D. Tuberculosis

19a The cervicothoracic sign dictates that the abnormality is in the:

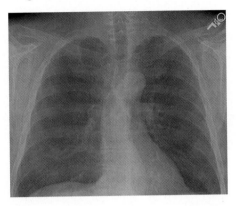

    A. Posterior mediastinum

    B. Anterior mediastinum

    C. Upper lobe lung

    D. Intrathoracic trachea

19b CT (B), T1 without contrast (C), and T1 with contrast (D) are provided. What is the most likely diagnosis?

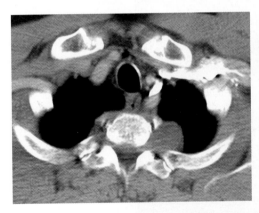
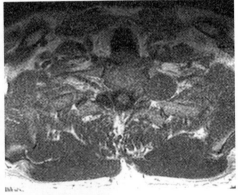
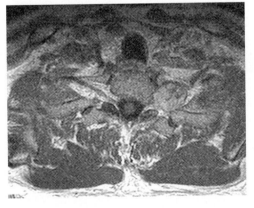

    A. Lung cancer

    B. Apical scarring

    C. Neurogenic tumor

    D. Neurenteric cyst

19c What is the most common neurogenic tumor of the mediastinum?

    A. Neurofibroma

    B. Ganglioneuroma

    C. Paraganglioma

    D. Schwannoma

20a What diagnosis is most likely?

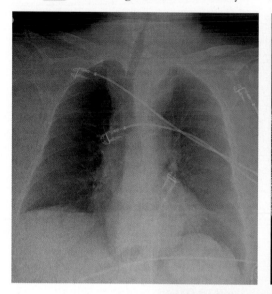
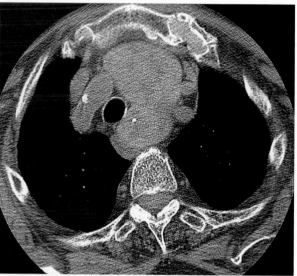
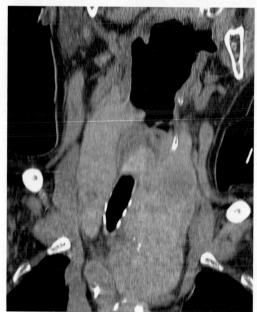

    A. Multinodular goiter

    B. Thymoma

    C. Teratoma

    D. Lymphoma

20b What percentage of intrathoracic goiter lesions are posterior?

    A. 0% to 5%

    B. 20% to 25%

    C. 35% to 40%

    D. 50% to 55%

ANSWERS AND EXPLANATIONS

1a **Answer C.**

1b **Answer B.**

1c **Answer A.** The chest radiograph demonstrates leftward shift of the mediastinum to include the heart and trachea. Lung markings are seen to the periphery bilaterally, excluding pneumothorax as a potential cause of mediastinal shift. Cardiomegaly cannot explain the findings as the heart is not enlarged and would not explain tracheal displacement. Consolidation is absent with diaphragm and mediastinal borders well maintained. Therefore, pulmonary volume loss is the only provided explanation for the radiographic appearance.

CT images reveal left parahilar masslike calcification in addition to an obstructed left pulmonary artery. Chronic pulmonary embolism could cause calcification associated with narrowing of the pulmonary artery, but not extrinsic calcification with occlusion. Also, chronic pulmonary embolism will not cause unilateral volume loss of the lung. Untreated lymphoma is a mediastinal process, which can engulf and obstruct vessels within the mediastinum, but will not cause calcification. Takayasu arteritis can occlude pulmonary vessels and cause calcification, but will not create masslike lesions within the mediastinum or hilum. By elimination, fibrosing mediastinitis can cause each of the findings of hilar masslike calcification, vascular obstruction, and unilateral pulmonary volume loss.

The most common cause of fibrosing mediastinitis in the United States is chronic histoplasma capsulatum infection with alternative infections such as Mycobacterium tuberculosis and Aspergillus being less common. Radiation-caused mediastinitis is less common and requires a history of prior radiation exposure. Idiopathic fibrosing mediastinitis is a less common cause but should be considered in the setting of mediastinal fibrosis without calcification or with associated alternative sites of fibrosis such as Riedel thyroiditis or retroperitoneal fibrosis.

References: Gurney JW, Conces DJ. Pulmonary histoplasmosis. *Radiology* 1996;199:297–306.

McNeeley MF, Chung JH, Bhalla S, et al. Imaging of granulomatous fibrosing mediastinitis. *AJR Am J Roentgenol* 2012;199:319–327.

2a **Answer B.**

2b **Answer C.**

2c **Answer A.** Imaging demonstrates a right anterior mediastinal mass, which is infiltrating around the aorta and pulmonary arteries. The superior vena cava is not visualized secondary to complete obstruction. Maximum intensity projection (MIP) and axial CT image both demonstrate contrast filling of large collateral vessels predominantly in the chest wall. While each of these symptoms have been described in the setting of SVC syndrome, head and neck swelling is one of the most common presenting symptoms. Other common presenting symptoms include headache and dyspnea. Stridor and altered mental status can be seen with severe cases of SVC syndrome but are not as common. Nausea has been described with SVC syndrome but is neither characteristic nor specific.

With obstruction of the SVC, multiple collateral venous pathways develop, generally tracking to the abdomen to reach the IVC. In this case, the collaterals are transiting the liver and creating a classic hot quadrate lobe or "hot spot sign." Multiple dense collateral pathways are also seen. While the region of liver is near the gallbladder fossa, it does not demonstrate the expected eggshell calcification of a porcelain gallbladder. Likewise, the stomach wall and spleen are within normal limits on this exam.

Collectively, cancers are by far the most common cause of SVC syndrome, with common cancers including bronchogenic carcinoma, lymphoma (as in this case), and metastatic disease. Iatrogenic causes, fibrosing mediastinitis, and Behcet disease all are potential benign causes of SVC syndrome but are less common etiologies than cancer.

Reference: Sheth S, Ebert MD, Fishman EK. Superior vena cava obstruction evaluation with MDCT. *AJR Am J Roentgenol* 2010;194:336–346.

3a **Answer B.**

3b **Answer C.**

3c **Answer D.** Dividing up the mediastinum into specific compartments (anterior, middle, posterior, and occasionally superior) allows for a narrowing of the differential diagnosis to a manageable number. Here, the lateral chest radiograph best demonstrates an opacity in the retrosternal window. The frontal chest radiograph exhibits the hilum overlay sign, with a rounded border overlying the right hilum but not obscuring the hilar vessels, further confirming the anterior location of the lesion.

Location and internal characteristics on CT can occasionally narrow the differential for an anterior mediastinal mass. Unfortunately, the lesion on the CT provided does not help differentiate the lesion. Its location at the junction of the heart and great vessels, homogeneous density, and projecting to one side of the mediastinum are all characteristic of thymoma, but they are not specific.

Multiple conditions are seen associated with thymoma, the most common being myasthenia gravis with 15% of patients with thymoma having myasthenia gravis and 35% of patients with myasthenia gravis having thymoma. Other common conditions have been grouped into "parathymic syndromes" and include pure red cell aplasia, hypogammaglobulinemia, and disorders of the endocrine system, skin, or connective tissue. Relationships with cardiac disease and renal disease have been published, but the specific conditions listed have not shown any significant association.

References: Rosado-de-Christenson ML, Galobardes J, Moran CA. From the archives of the AFIP Thymoma: radiologic-pathologic correlation. *Radiographics* 1992;12:151–168.

Whitten CR, Khan S, Munneke GJ, et al. A diagnostic approach to mediastinal abnormalities. *Radiographics* 2007;27:657–671.

4 **Answer C.** There has been rapid development of a focal rim-enhancing lesion in the anterior mediastinum. Note the new surrounding inflammatory changes as well. Thymoma would be expected to be better defined and homogeneous. Necrosis and internal gas such as in this case would be unusual. Thymic carcinoma and invasive thymoma can have a more aggressive appearance but still would not develop over such a short interval. Normal thymus should not be space occupying such as the lesion demonstrated and would be triangular or bilobed in shape.

Acute mediastinitis is uncommon but most frequently occurs after recent surgery, esophageal perforation, or direct spread from neck infections. Of note, diffuse mediastinitis has a very high mortality (upwards of 80% at 30 days). Gas bubbles, such as those seen, can be identified in up to 50% of cases and are an important differentiator for infection versus neoplasm.

Of note, differentiation of normal postmedian sternotomy changes from mediastinal infection or hemorrhage can be difficult in the immediate postoperative period. The normal postoperative appearance can include variable degrees of retrosternal fluid, air, and hematoma but should largely resolve by 2 to 3 weeks.

Reference: Webb WR, Higgins CB. *Thoracic imaging*. Philadelphia: Lippincott Williams & Wilkins, 2010.

5 **Answer A.** Alveolar rupture is the most common cause of pneumomediastinum in this setting. This is referred to as the Macklin effect and is characterized by (1) alveolar rupture, (2) air dissection along the bronchovascular bundles (resulting in pulmonary interstitial emphysema), and (3) spread into the mediastinum. This can also occur in other settings such as blunt force trauma, although excluding a direct bronchial or tracheal laceration in that case would be critical. Extension from pneumothorax would be unusual as the parietal pleura would normally prevent gas from entering the mediastinum unless there is a preexisting violation of the pleura such as in the setting of recent thoracic surgery. Tracheal rupture from cuff overinflation is an unusual iatrogenic cause of pneumomediastinum that should be avoidable in most cases due to early identification of the overinflated cuff on chest x-ray and new endotracheal tubes that limit cuff volume and pressure. Esophageal rupture would be unusual without an underlying esophageal abnormality such as esophageal cancer, trauma, foreign body ingestion, or corrosive ingestion. Improper Blakemore tube placement for varices can result in esophageal rupture if the gastric balloon is inflated in the esophagus.

References: Webb WR, Higgins CB. *Thoracic imaging*. Philadelphia: Lippincott Williams & Wilkins, 2010.

Wintermark M, Schnyder P. The Macklin effect: a frequent etiology for pneumomediastinum in severe blunt chest trauma. *Chest* 2001;120(2):543–547.

6a **Answer B.**

6b **Answer B.** The aortic knob demonstrates an unexpected contour abnormality that mildly displaces the trachea. This identifies the abnormality as middle mediastinal in location based on the frontal projection alone. The lateral radiograph confirms an abnormality immediately posterior to the trachea resulting in anterior displacement of the normal tracheal air column.

On CT, the abnormality is identified as focal saccular dilatation of the distal aortic arch and proximal descending aorta at the level of the aortic isthmus. Note there is a degree of calcified peripheral thrombus adherent to the wall of the pseudoaneurysm (or false aneurysm) consistent with a chronic time course. Acutely presenting aneurysms of either cause would be likely associated with a degree of periaortic inflammatory change, aortic wall thickening, or mediastinal hemorrhage. Based on location, this is likely posttraumatic. Mycotic aneurysms are very unusual with current antibiotic regimens with the classic example being related to syphilis (more frequently involving the ascending aorta and aortic root). The most common cause of a true aneurysm is aortic atherosclerosis, but those aneurysms tend to be more fusiform in the thoracic aorta.

Reference: Marcu CB, Nijveldt R, Van Rossum AC. Unsuspected chronic traumatic aortic pseudoaneurysm-what to do about it. Late post-traumatic aortic pseudoaneurysm. *Can J Cardiol* 2008;24(2):143–144.

7 **Answer C.** Although this mass appears large and circumferential, the likely diagnosis is that of leiomyoma given the dystrophic areas of calcification (biopsy proven in this case). Metastases only rarely calcify with possible calcification in osteogenic or cartilaginous tumors and some mucinous GI tumors. Liposarcoma metastases are very unlikely to calcify (although they could potentially contain fat elements). Similarly, primary esophageal malignancies, either squamous cell carcinoma or adenocarcinoma, are unlikely to calcify. Untreated lymphoma almost never calcifies.

Leiomyomas are the most common benign tumor of the esophagus. The majority are asymptomatic and smaller than 3 cm in size although some can grow larger. They are most frequently round or mildly lobulated although some grow circumferentially (~10%) as this example demonstrates. They are more frequently seen in men than women (2:1) and less frequently in children. They are generally found in the mid and lower esophagus, and the vast majority are intramural arising from esophageal smooth muscle cells. Unlike the remainder of the gastrointestinal tract, gastrointestinal stromal tumors (GISTs) are less common in the esophagus. GISTs can calcify but have a higher predilection for necrosis or cyst formation within the mass than leiomyoma, which is generally more homogeneous. Duplication cysts and granular cell tumors are less frequent benign esophageal masses. There is a rare pattern of esophageal leiomyomatosis, which is a more diffuse smooth muscle proliferation giving rise to multiple leiomyomas. This is associated with genetic abnormalities such as Alport syndrome with an increased risk of leiomyomas elsewhere in the body such as the airways.

Reference: Lewis RB, Mehrotra AK, Rodriguez P, et al. From the radiologic pathology archives: esophageal neoplasms: radiologic-pathologic correlation. *Radiographics* 2013;33(4):1083–1108.

8a Answer B.

8b Answer B.   The initial chest radiographs demonstrate a rounded opacity overlying the heart that is difficult to see on the lateral but is localized to the middle mediastinum as a subtle opacity anterior to the spine. The corresponding CT demonstrates tubular structures that enhance more on venous phase imaging than arterial (note the difference in aortic enhancement to distinguish arterial from venous phase imaging). These are large esophageal varices in the setting of cirrhosis. Note, esophageal cancer and lymphadenopathy would not be expected to be tubular as seen here. The esophageal wall is thickened in this case, but that is related to esophagopathy rather than malignancy. Secondary features include splenomegaly and a small nodular liver with a small amount of perihepatic ascites in this case.

Esophageal varices develop as a collateral drainage pathway in the setting of portal hypertension. The collateral pathway is from the portal system into the azygos system. These are the classic "uphill" varices seen in the setting of cirrhosis and portal hypertension. "Downhill" varices can also be seen due to SVC obstruction but are typically noted more superiorly in the upper third of the esophagus. Typical causes of downhill varices include lung cancer, lymphoma, and mediastinal fibrosis.

Reference: Gore RM, Livine MS, eds. *Textbook of gastrointestinal radiology*, 2nd ed. Philadelphia, PA: WB Saunders Co, 2000:454–463, 2082.

9a Answer A.

9b Answer B.   Although distal esophageal ruptures are more common (classically the distal left posterior wall for spontaneous rupture), proximal esophageal ruptures do occur. In the setting of a proximal esophageal rupture, a right effusion is the most common feature of those listed. For distal esophageal rupture, left effusion or hydropneumothorax is more common. On initial radiograph, pneumomediastinum is the most common feature and generally takes at least 1 hour to manifest after initial injury. Pleural effusion and mediastinal widening may take several hours. Etiologies to consider for esophageal perforation include esophagitis, foreign body impaction, trauma, and increasingly iatrogenic causes (such as related to balloon dilatation). Life-threatening mediastinitis, empyema, and lung abscess are complications to consider on follow-up imaging.

References: Wu JT, Mattox KL, Wall MJ Jr. Esophageal perforations: new perspectives and treatment paradigms. *J Trauma* 2007;63(5):1173–1184.

Young CA, Menias CO, Bhalla S, et al. CT features of esophageal emergencies. *Radiographics* 2008;28(6):1541–1553.

10a **Answer B.**

10b **Answer A.**

10c **Answer B.** The CT demonstrates a fluid attenuation lesion abutting the pericardium in the right chest. The location and imaging appearance are typical of a pericardial cyst, and in the majority of patients, no further imaging is warranted. However, in some patients, the appearance may be less typical or there may be a history of malignancy that warrants further evaluation. PET/CT of this area is sometimes difficult due to adjacent myocardial uptake. Additionally, a lack of uptake does not exclude malignancy. Radiographs would not demonstrate anything the CT has not already shown. Echocardiography is an option but can be of limited value due to available echo windows and body habitus. MRI is an excellent method for further evaluation and can demonstrate the fluid nature of the abnormality, even in cases with higher-density proteinaceous fluid. In this example, the high T2-weighted image (note the spinal fluid) confirms fluid within the lesion.

Reference: Jeung MY, Gasser B, Gangi A, et al. Imaging of cystic masses of the mediastinum. *Radiographics* 2002;22 Spec No:S79–S93.

11a **Answer D.**

11b **Answer B.** The cardiac silhouette is markedly enlarged on the frontal radiograph with a typical "water bottle" configuration. On the lateral, there is a vertically oriented density anterior to the heart and posterior to the sternum. This is visible because of vertically oriented low densities on either side. This is termed the "Oreo Cookie" or, less commonly, the sandwich sign, double-lucency sign, or epicardial fat pad sign and reflects pericardial effusion outlined by epicardial fat (anteriorly) and pericardial fat (posteriorly). This is a specific sign for pericardial effusion but is infrequently seen (low sensitivity). Note that there is no relationship with this sign and the double Oreo cookie sign of SLAP tears or the sandwich/hamburger sign of mesenteric lymphoma.

Classic clinical findings for significant effusion and tamponade are the Beck triad of hypotension, muffled heart sounds, and jugular venous distension. Symptomatology is variable and significantly related to acuity. As little as 80 mL of fluid may be symptomatic if acute, but more chronic effusions have been reported as large as 2 and even 3 L without symptoms. Up to 50 mL is considered physiologic in some patients with 15 to 50 mL generally considered the normal range (some quote a lesser volume of 25 mL as the upper limit of normal).

The causes of pericardial effusion are many, and understanding the clinical context of the patient is critical for determining the cause of effusion. Consider the general differential of infection (in the immunosuppressed, remember tuberculosis), malignancy (especially lung cancer, breast cancer, lymphoma, or melanoma), trauma, radiation therapy, collagen vascular disease (such as lupus), or metabolic disorders (such as uremia).

References: Bogaert J, Francone M. Pericardial disease: value of CT and MR imaging. *Radiology* 2013;267(2):340–356.

Rienmüller R, Gröll R, Lipton MJ. CT and MR imaging of pericardial disease. *Radiol Clin North Am* 2004;42(3):587–601.

Wang ZJ, Reddy GP, Gotway MB, et al. CT and MR imaging of pericardial disease. *Radiographics* 2003;23:S167–S180.

12 Answer B.   Spontaneous pneumomediastinum has been described associated with multiple precipitating events such as intense screaming, intense physical activity, and coughing. Associated histories include asthma, inhalational drug use, childbirth, and forceful emesis. Spontaneous pneumomediastinum occurs secondary to the "Macklin effect" where increased pressure ruptures an alveolus and air tracks along the axial interstitium to the mediastinum as describe above. On physical exam, the patient may exhibit the "Hamman sign" or "Hamman crunch" with crepitus on cardiac auscultation. Radiographically, lucency tracks along planes of the mediastinum, creating signs such as "ring around the artery" sign and continuous diaphragm sign. In practice, a significant portion of patients with spontaneous pneumomediastinum present without a clear precipitating event, typical history, or radiographic findings. In one study, 30% of spontaneous pneumomediastinum identified on CT was not evident on radiograph.

References: Caceres M, Ali SZ, Braud R, et al. Spontaneous pneumomediastinum: a comparative study and review of the literature. *Ann Thorac Surg* 2008;86:962–966.

Zylak CM, Standen JR, Barnes GR, et al. Pneumomediastinum revisited. *Radiographics* 2000;20:1043–1057.

13a Answer B.

13b Answer C.   On CT, there is a rounded left posterior mediastinal lesion that abuts the adjacent vertebral body as well as the proximal descending aorta. The lesion is homogeneous and slightly lower in attenuation than is the aortic blood pool suggesting that this could be fluid. Given the location, neurogenic tumors such as neuromas or paragangliomas are possible in addition to foregut duplication cysts or even a pseudoaneurysm. Further imaging is warranted, and MRI would be best suited to identify the exact relationship of the lesion to the adjacent structures and provide information as to its soft tissue or fluid nature.

On MRI, the lesion is homogeneous and of low intensity on T1-weighted sequence and high intensity on T2-weighted sequences. This is consistent with fluid content. Neurogenic tumors can have low T1 and high T2-weighted signal but would be expected to show vivid enhancement after contrast administration, which is not shown. Note that the thin rim of peripheral enhancement shown is typical of wall enhancement in foregut duplication cysts. Furthermore, the lesion does not invaginate into the neuroforamina, which is frequently found in schwannomas. There is no connection to the aorta to suggest pseudoaneurysm. There is a bilobed component more anteriorly to the vertebral body consistent with a middle mediastinal component. These findings are classic for a foregut duplication cyst.

Bronchogenic cysts, esophageal duplication cysts, and neurenteric cysts are all congenital foregut duplication cysts related to abnormality of the budding embryonic foregut. Mediastinal bronchogenic cysts are typically fluid attenuation and located in the middle mediastinum (80%) or less likely posterior mediastinum (17%). As many as 15% to 25% can be extramediastinal such as in the pleura, diaphragm, or lungs. MRI can be a very useful tool for confirmation of the cystic nature of the abnormality, especially for those cases that contain proteinaceous fluid or have had complications such as infection or internal hemorrhage. Treatment options favor surgical removal for larger lesions (especially if symptomatic or in a young patient). There is a theoretical risk of subsequent infection or hemorrhage. Some advise removal for all lesions, and some lesions have been treated percutaneously in high–surgical risk patients. The presence of any mural nodularity would be a reason to suggest removal as the lesion is more likely to be a cystic malignancy.

Reference: McAdams HP, Kirejczyk WM, Rosado-de-Christenson ML, et al. Bronchogenic cyst: imaging features with clinical and histopathologic correlation. *Radiology* 2000;217(2):441–446.

14a **Answer C.**

14b **Answer D.** While only massive circumferential esophageal thickening (>20 cm) can accurately differentiate esophageal carcinoma from other benign esophageal processes like esophagitis, significant thickening with additional imaging characteristics can help exclude certain conditions. The CT shown demonstrates circumferential thickening of the esophagus measuring up to 17 mm (measurement not given) that is soft tissue in density. Esophageal varices will generally contrast fill similar to the other vasculature with a serpentine appearance. A duplication cyst would not create circumferential thickening with central lumen. Barrett esophagus would not cause this degree of thickening.

CT is limited in its staging of esophageal cancer but can be useful in cases of identifying direct invasion, regional lymph node involvement, and distant metastases. If direct invasion of adjacent non-resectable structures is demonstrated, the lesion then meets criteria for a "T4" lesion in the TNM classification. A T4 lesion stages the cancer at III or IV dependent on the presence of distant metastases and excludes treatment with surgery alone.

References: Kim TJ, Kim HY, Lee KW, et al. Multimodality assessment of esophageal cancer: preoperative staging and monitoring of response to therapy. *Radiographics* 2009;29:403–421.

Reinig JW, Stanley JH, Schabel SI. CT Evaluation of thickened esophageal walls. *AJR Am J Roentgenol* 140:931–934.

15a **Answer A.**

15b **Answer B.**

15c **Answer B.** The hilum overlay sign indicates location of the lesion either anterior or posterior to the hilum as the hilar structures remain well visualized despite the overlying lesion. Therefore, this case cannot be in the middle mediastinum. The lesion also obscures the left heart border, meaning the large lesion is displacing the lingula, an anterior structure. The lesion is centered below the aortic arch. Altogether, these findings are consistent with an anterior mediastinal mass.

The subsequent CT redemonstrates the large anterior mediastinal mass, which is primarily cystic, but does contain a small portion of fat, making this lesion consistent with a mature teratoma. Approximately 15% of mediastinal mature teratomas do not exhibit fat or calcium on CT. The anterior mediastinum is the most common location of extragonadal germ cell tumors and represents about 1/7 of the total anterior mediastinal masses. Treatment for mediastinal teratoma is complete surgical resection.

References: Moeller KH, Rosado-de-Christenson ML, Templeton PA. Mediastinal mature teratoma: imaging features. *AJR Am J Roentgenol* 1997;169:985–990.

Rosado-de-Christenson ML, Templeton PA, Moran CA. Mediastinal germ cell tumors: radiologic and pathologic correlation. *Radiographics* 1992;12:1013–1030.

16a   Answer B.

16b   Answer C.

16c   Answer A.   Although rare, spontaneous mediastinal hematoma can present as a mediastinal mass. The main purpose of this case is localization to the middle mediastinum along the right paratracheal stripe with subsequent accurate analysis of the MR characteristics. T1 shows intermediate signal on noncontrast and no evidence of contrast enhancement. Axial T2 demonstrates a small, but present, fluid debris level, which makes this lesion cystic and happens to represent a hematocrit level. The patient's INR in this case was supratherapeutic. The combination of sudden-onset chest pain, plausible cause of spontaneous hemorrhage, and consistent imaging characteristics is sufficient for likely diagnosis with expected spontaneous resolution with removal of the underlying cause.

References: Kamiyoshihara M, Ibe T, Kakegawa S, et al. Spontaneous mediastinal hematoma presenting as a mass. *J Thorac Oncol* 2007;2(6):544–545.

Whitten CR, Khan S, Munneke GJ, et al. A diagnostic approach to mediastinal abnormalities. *Radiographics* 2007;27:657–671.

17a   Answer C.

17b   Answer B.

17c   Answer D.   Presenting chest radiograph demonstrates leftward shift of the mediastinum with some rotational change in the mediastinal contour. Some may be tempted to diagnose a pneumothorax and recommend chest tube placement, but no direct findings are present to suggest pneumothorax. Without a clear cause "pushing" the mediastinum, the shift is therefore due to left lung volume loss and without comparison needs further workup with CT or potentially bronchoscopy. Some may recognize an abrupt cutoff in the left mainstem bronchus, further supporting the need for timely workup.

The subsequent CT reveals an endobronchial mass obstructing the left mainstem bronchus and projecting beyond the expected bronchial borders. No additional findings are present, such as calcification, that may support a particular tumor type. Statistically, squamous cell carcinoma is the most common adult tracheal tumor, followed by adenoid cystic carcinoma. While this case is in the left mainstem bronchus, it is an adenoid cystic carcinoma (ACC), which is known to extend into or be centered in the mainstem bronchi. Regional adenopathy or distant disease is uncommon, with local recurrence being the primary concern following resection.

Reference: Ngo AH, Walker CM, Chung JH, et al. Tumors and tumorlike conditions of the Large Airways. *AJR Am J Roentgenol* 2013;201:301–313.

18a   Answer D.

18b   Answer A.   Pyogenic discitis/spondylitis most often affects the lumbar spine, although 35% of cases occur in the thoracic spine. This case displays the classic findings of pyogenic spondylitis generally involving at least one disc level and the adjacent vertebral bodies. Paraspinal soft tissues are thickened and enhancing with a focal fluid collection well demonstrated along the right spine. Destructive changes of the vertebral bodies are easily seen on CT with MR revealing vertebral enhancement. The patient's relatively rapid loss of lower extremity sensation and motor function is secondary to the epidural abscess along the anterior spinal canal and compressing the cord. Extramedullary hematopoiesis does not have this aggressive behavior, and neoplasms generally do not cause the pattern of disc and bilateral vertebral body involvement.

All of the listed organisms are known to cause infectious spondylitis, but *Staphylococcus aureus* is the most common and is the cause in this case. Spread of infection can be hematogenous, direct inoculation, or direct spread from adjacent soft tissue infection. While this case did have a history of recent pneumonia, it is unclear if the spinal involvement was hematogenous or by direct spread. The classic presentation for infectious spondylitis is progressive, "insidious" back pain with or without associated constitutional symptoms like fever or malaise.

Reference: Hong SH, Choi J, Lee JW, et al. MR imaging assessment of the spine: infection or an imitation? *Radiographics* 2009;29:599–612.

19a **Answer A.**

19b **Answer C.**

19c **Answer D.** Of the choices given, only neurogenic tumor would fit the imaging characteristics. While subtle, a smooth asymmetric lesion is present along the left lung apex with obtuse margins consistent with a pleural or extrapleural lesion. Following cervicothoracic sign, the borders of the lesion are well defined above the level of the clavicles, indicating that the lesion is posterior in location. Follow-up imaging with CT and MR demonstrates a lesion arising from the adjacent foramen (better shown on the single CT axial image) that intensely enhances on postcontrast MR imaging.

Some studies have demonstrated differentiation of neurogenic tumors based on the long axis of the lesion where a vertical long axis suggests ganglioneuroma and a horizontal axis suggests schwannoma. With only axial images provided, this distinction cannot be made on the provided images. This case represents a schwannoma, the most common mediastinal neurogenic tumor.

References: Marshall GB, Farnquist BA, MacGregor JH, et al. Signs in thoracic imaging. *J Thorac Imaging* 2006;21:76–90.

Nakazono T, White CS, Yamasaki F, et al. MRI findings of mediastinal neurogenic tumors. *AJR Am J Roentgenol* 2011;197:W643–W652.

20a **Answer A.**

20b **Answer B.** Extending through the thoracic inlet from the paratracheal thyroid bed, this lesion is consistent with a multinodular goiter with intrathoracic component. On radiograph, the lesion displaces the trachea to the right with widening of the superior mediastinum. Follow-up CT in axial and coronal planes reveals the mildly heterogeneous lesion with small calcifications directly connecting to the thyroid.

The goiter extends lateral and posterior to the trachea on axial image. Up to 25% of intrathoracic goiters are posterior in location and therefore should be included with the differential for a superior posterior mediastinal mass. This lesion is atypical for the fact that it extends along the left trachea, where the vast majority of thyroid goiter, which extends to the posterior mediastinum, descends along the right trachea.

References: Kawashima A, Fishman EK, Kuhlman JE, et al. CT of posterior mediastinal masses. *Radiographics* 1991;11:1045–1067.

Whitten CR, Khan S, Munneke GJ, et al. A diagnostic approach to mediastinal abnormalities. *Radiographics* 2007;27:657–671.

8 Vascular Disease

QUESTIONS

1a A chest radiograph demonstrated a lingular nodule for which a contrast-enhanced CT was performed. What is the likely cause of the nodule?

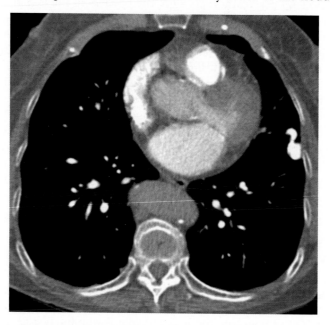

A. Bronchogenic carcinoma
B. Remote granulomatous infection
C. Pulmonary arteriovenous malformation (AVM)
D. Metastasis

1b In a patient with multiple pulmonary AVMs, what is the likely underlying diagnosis?

A. Osler-Weber-Rendu syndrome
B. Klippel-Trénaunay syndrome
C. Parkes Weber syndrome
D. Sturge-Weber syndrome

2a What is the salient abnormality on the chest radiograph of this patient?

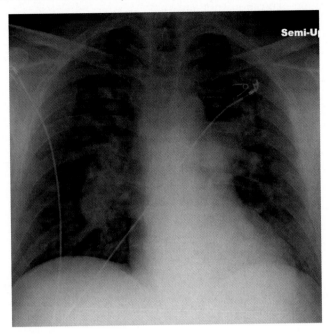

A. Pleural effusion
B. Hilar enlargement
C. Tracheal stenosis
D. Pneumothorax

2b What is the cause of pulmonary artery enlargement based on the corresponding CT?

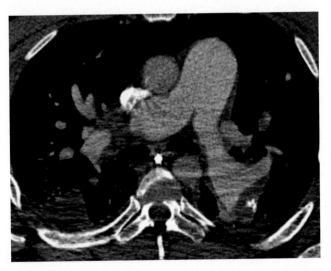

A. Acute pulmonary embolus
B. Chronic pulmonary embolus
C. Fat emboli
D. Septic emboli

3 What is the likely cause of mosaic attenuation on this CT given no evidence of air trapping on expiration (not shown)?

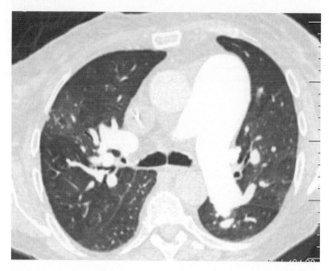

A. Obliterative bronchiolitis
B. Vascular abnormality
C. Emphysema
D. Asthma

4a What is the most likely diagnosis for this patient with new-onset fevers and neck pain with swelling?

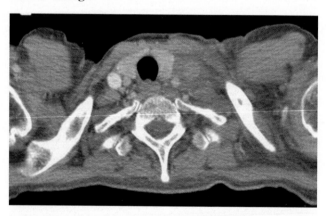

A. Leriche syndrome
B. Lhermitte-Duclos
C. Lemierre syndrome
D. Lambert-Eaton syndrome

4b What is the most frequent site of emboli in patients with internal jugular thrombophlebitis?

A. Brain
B. Lungs
C. Spleen
D. Bowel

5   In the setting of a young patient with pulmonary hypertension and these CT findings, what is the likely diagnosis?

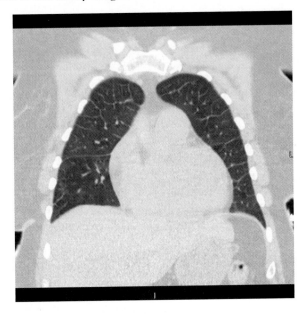

    A. Hepatopulmonary syndrome
    B. Scleroderma
    C. Lymphangitic carcinomatosis
    D. Pulmonary venoocclusive disease (PVOD)

6a   What is the salient abnormality on this upright PA chest x-ray?

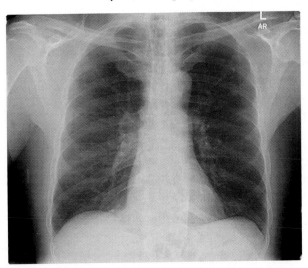

    A. Unilateral hyperlucency
    B. Unilateral hilar enlargement
    C. Unilateral pleural effusion
    D. Unilateral pneumothorax

6b   Unilateral hyperlucency due to oligemia is referred to as what eponym?

    A. Hampton hump
    B. Westermark sign
    C. Halo sign
    D. Reverse halo sign (atoll)

7a Which of the following radiographic signs are associated with pulmonary infarct?

A. Reversed halo (atoll) sign
B. Halo sign
C. Galaxy sign
D. Split pleura sign

7b The other leading differential diagnosis for a "reversed halo" sign is which of the following?

A. Eosinophilic pneumonia
B. Angioinvasive fungal infection
C. Minimally invasive adenocarcinoma
D. Organizing pneumonia

8a In the setting of suspected acute pulmonary embolism in pregnancy, which of the following exams is both appropriate AND results in the lowest radiation dose to the fetus?

A. CTA of the pulmonary arteries
B. V/Q scan
C. CT of the chest without contrast
D. MRA with contrast of the pulmonary arteries

8b In the setting of suspected acute pulmonary embolism in pregnancy, which of the following exams is both appropriate AND results in the lowest radiation dose to the mother?

A. CTA of the pulmonary arteries
B. V/Q scan
C. CT of the chest without contrast
D. MRA with contrast of the pulmonary arteries

9 Which of the following features is the most significant component of the Wells criteria for pulmonary embolism?

A. Clinical signs and symptoms of DVT
B. Tachycardia
C. Prior PE or DVT
D. Malignancy with recent treatment

10 Which of the following imaging findings would be most specific for pulmonary artery sarcoma instead of pulmonary artery embolism?

A. Multiple bilateral subsegmental filling defects
B. Unilateral central filling defect
C. PET/CT positivity
D. Local expansion of the involved pulmonary arteries

11 What is the most common pulmonary arterial manifestation of Behçet disease involving the lungs?

A. Pulmonary artery aneurysms
B. Pulmonary artery occlusion
C. Pulmonary embolism
D. Pulmonary hemorrhage

12 A patient suffers a high-speed motor vehicle collision, which included multiple long bone lower extremity fractures. He develops acute shortness of breath and new rash 24 hours later, which prompted a follow-up CT of the chest. What is the leading etiology for the lung abnormalities?

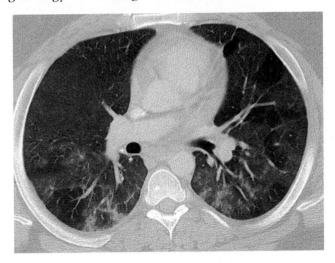

A. Aspiration
B. Contusion
C. Atypical infection
D. Fat embolism

13 What complication from pulmonary artery catheter placement is identified?

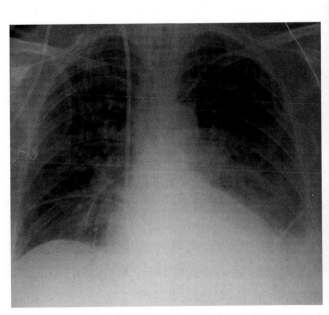

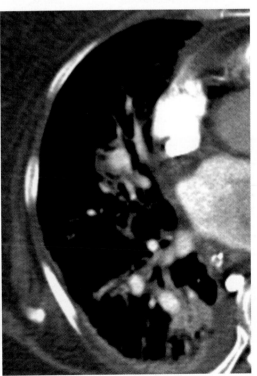

A. Pseudoaneurysm formation
B. Pulmonary artery dissection
C. Right heart rupture
D. Pulmonary artery occlusion

14 Which of the following vasculitides is most likely responsible for these imaging findings?

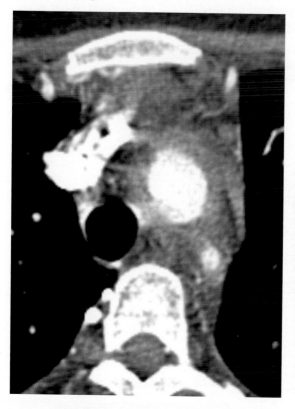
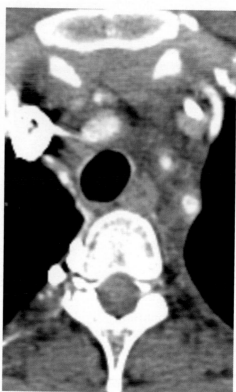

A. Behçet disease
B. Granulomatosis with polyangiitis
C. Takayasu's
D. Goodpasture syndrome

15 What is the cause of the linear high density in the right lower lobe pulmonary artery based on these CT images?

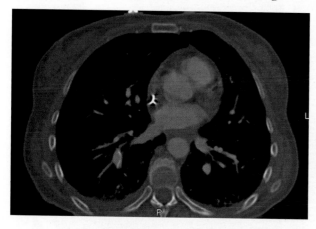
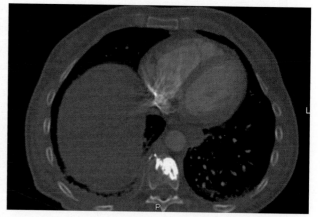

A. Dendriform pulmonary ossification
B. Methyl methacrylate embolization
C. Calcified chronic bland embolus
D. Embolized guidewire

16 Which clinical setting is associated with the highest percentage of amniotic fluid embolism?

   A. During spontaneous labor
   B. After spontaneous labor
   C. During cesarean section
   D. After cesarean section

17a What is the salient abnormality on these radiographs?

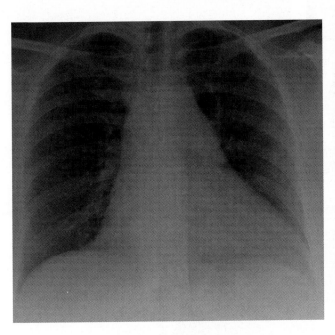
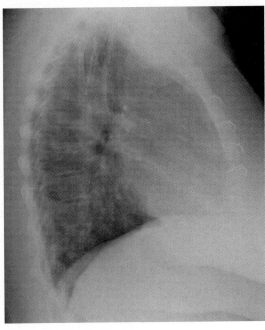

   A. Left hilar enlargement
   B. Aortic aneurysm
   C. Retrocardiac consolidation
   D. Pneumothorax

17b Based on CT, what is the likely underlying disease?

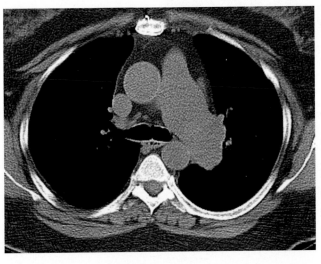
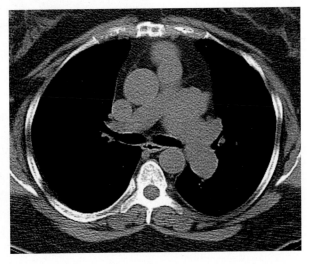

   A. Primary pulmonary hypertension
   B. Congenital absence of the right pulmonary artery
   C. Pulmonary valve stenosis
   D. Chronic thromboembolic disease

18 A Rasmussen aneurysm refers to what?

    A. A mycotic pulmonary artery aneurysm

    B. A mycotic aortic aneurysm

    C. A mycotic bronchial artery aneurysm

    D. A mycotic pulmonary vein aneurysm

19a What is the salient vascular abnormality?

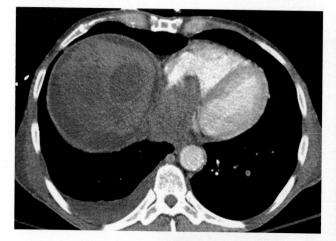 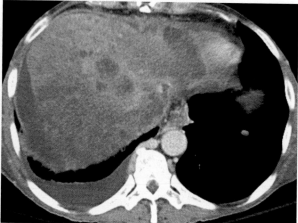

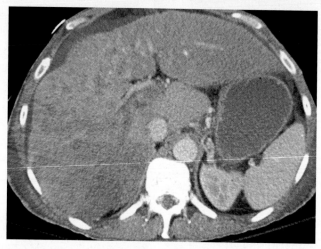

    A. IVC tumor thrombus extending into the right atrium

    B. Right atrial mixing artifact related to incomplete opacification of the hepatic veins and IVC

    C. Bland IVC thrombus

    D. Thrombus related to prior IVC filter placement

19b Which of the following tumors is most likely to present with inferior vena cava tumor thrombus?

    A. Renal cell carcinoma

    B. Hepatocellular carcinoma

    C. Adrenal carcinomas

    D. Bronchogenic carcinoma

20a What is the upper limit of normal for pulmonary artery size on chest CT in a male?

A. 20 mm

B. 25 mm

C. 30 mm

D. 35 mm

20b What is the upper limit of normal for size of the right interlobar pulmonary artery in women on chest x-ray?

A. 5 mm

B. 10 mm

C. 15 mm

D. 20 mm

ANSWERS AND EXPLANATIONS

1a **Answer C.**

1b **Answer A.** On contrast-enhanced CT, the "nodule" is identified as vividly enhancing. In fact, the nodule enhances identically to the pulmonary outflow tract with a large draining vein identified. As such, the "nodule" is actually a vascular lesion. Pulmonary AVMs can occasionally occur in isolation, and CT diagnosis requires the presence of a dilated artery and vein resulting in a right-to-left shunt as an AVM is a high-flow low-resistance fistulous connection. Treatment of pulmonary AVMs is generally advised for a nidus >3 mm.

Pulmonary AVMs (upwards of 60%) occur in the setting of Osler-Weber-Rendu (hereditary hemorrhagic telangiectasia or HHT). HHT is inherited in an autosomal dominant fashion with AVMs and telangiectasias. These are especially prone to develop on mucosal surfaces, the skin, and the lungs and can result in fatal hemorrhage. Diagnostic criteria for HHT include (1) epistaxis, (2) multiple vascular dilatations, (3) arteriovenous malformations in the internal organs, and (4) a first-degree relative with the conditions. Presence of three of these criteria is sufficient for a definitive diagnosis.

Klippel-Trénaunay syndrome is a syndrome of low-flow vascular malformations with (1) capillary malformations or port-wine stains on a limb, (2) congenital varicose veins or venous malformations, and (3) bone and soft tissue hypertrophy. Parkes Weber syndrome demonstrates overgrowth of the affected limb with small fistulas. The abnormality is similar to Klippel-Trénaunay except the vascular lesions are high flow instead of low flow. Sturge-Weber syndrome is characterized by a port-wine stain (capillary malformation) on the face of vascular malformations in the pia mater and choroid of the trigeminal nerve region in the brain.

Reference: Nozaki T, et al. Syndromes associated with vascular tumors and malformations: a pictorial review. *Radiographics* 2013;33(1):175–195.

2a **Answer B.**

2b **Answer B.** Initial chest radiograph demonstrates significant bilateral hilar enlargement. This could be related to either bilateral hilar adenopathy or pulmonary artery enlargement. Although there is a mild degree of mass effect on the trachea from an ectatic aortic arch, there is no significant stenosis. Additionally, there are no findings of pneumothorax such as a pleural line, absence of peripheral lung markings, or a deep sulcus sign.

Contrast-enhanced CT demonstrates significant pulmonary artery enlargement with bilateral eccentric filling defects in the pulmonary arteries. Eccentric defects such as this are much more likely to be subacute or chronic emboli rather than acute. Also notice the partial calcification in the chronic clot on the left. Other arterial manifestations include vessel narrowing, intimal irregularity, and web formation. Secondary signs may include bronchial artery collateralization or other transpleural collateral vessel development. Fat emboli typically manifests as airspace disease including ground glass and consolidation as the fat particles are too small to occlude central arteries like this. Likewise, septic emboli are more highly associated with cavitating nodules, especially peripheral nodules.

Reference: Castañer E, Gallardo X, Ballesteros E, et al. CT Diagnosis of chronic pulmonary thromboembolism. *Radiographics* 2009;29(1):31–50.

3 **Answer B.** Mosaic attenuation is caused by either hyperinflation or decreased blood perfusion to a focal area of lung. Hyperinflation would result in air trapping on expiratory imaging and be consistent with causes of small airway disease such as obliterative bronchiolitis or asthma. Although emphysema is related to hyperinflation, there is no actual parenchymal destruction in this case to form the "black holes" seen in emphysema.

Mosaic attenuation related to decreased blood perfusion to the lung is most frequently related to pulmonary emboli or less likely vasculitis. Additional review of the image above demonstrates a subtle decrease in size and number of pulmonary vessels in the regions of hypoattenuation, which is seen in the setting of vascular causes of mosaic attenuation. There is also striking main pulmonary artery enlargement (3.0 cm is the upper limit of normal and this far main pulmonary artery exceeds the size of the adjacent aorta). Other pulmonary parenchymal signs of chronic thromboembolic disease include peripheral parenchymal bands, wedge-shaped opacities, or linear opacities related to scarring from prior infarcts. These abnormalities may be associated with adjacent focal pleural thickening as well.

Reference: Castañer E, Gallardo X, Ballesteros E, et al. CT diagnosis of chronic pulmonary thromboembolism. *Radiographics* 2009;29(1):31–50.

4a **Answer C.**

4b **Answer B.** Lemierre syndrome is a relatively rare clinical entity consisting of a primary oropharyngeal infection resulting in internal jugular vein thrombophlebitis. Distal septic emboli are frequently seen, and the lungs are most frequently involved as that is the first capillary bed encountered during normal blood flow from the jugular veins. However, any distal site can be affected. Diagnosis is frequently delayed as the initial infection can be indolent and chest complaints, such as cough or pleuritic pain, may be the first presenting symptom with chest imaging performed prior to imaging of the neck. Pulmonary involvement is typical of septic emboli with randomly distributed peripheral cavitating and noncavitating nodules and a risk of effusions and empyema.

Leriche syndrome refers to aortoiliac occlusive disease with a triad of symptoms including buttock claudication, absent femoral pulses, and impotence. Lhermitte-Duclos is a dysplastic gangliocytoma of the cerebellum. Lambert-Eaton syndrome is an autoimmune myasthenic syndrome.

Reference: O'Brien WT, Lattin GE, Thompson AK. Lemierre syndrome: an all-but-forgotten disease. *Am J Roentgen* 2006;187:W324–W324.

5 **Answer D.** Both pulmonary capillary hemangiomatosis and pulmonary venoocclusive disease (PVOD) are rare causes of pulmonary arterial hypertension and typically affect young adults. They are both characterized by postcapillary vein obliteration resulting in variable degrees of interlobular septal thickening (shown here), poorly defined centrilobular ground-glass nodules (also shown here but more subtle), pleural effusions, and lymphadenopathy. Appropriate recognition of this disease by the radiologist is important because these patients are preload dependent and may develop fatal pulmonary edema if treated with the vasodilators frequently used for other causes of pulmonary hypertension. On right heart cath, both capillary hemangiomatosis and PVOD classically demonstrate normal or low capillary wedge pressures instead of the elevated pressures seen in other causes of pulmonary arterial hypertension.

Scleroderma is certainly associated with pulmonary hypertension but more frequently demonstrates a pattern of fibrosing interstitial pneumonia (especially NSIP pattern) rather than the interlobular septal thickening demonstrated here. Lymphangitic carcinomatosis can present as interlobular septal thickening but is typically more nodular, and there is no specific association with pulmonary hypertension. Hepatopulmonary syndrome is related to cirrhosis and liver failure with development of pulmonary vascular shunting. It manifests most frequently as peripheral pulmonary vessel dilatation or, more rarely, discrete AVM formation.

Reference: Pena E, Dennie C, Veinot J, et al. Pulmonary hypertension: how the radiologist can help. *Radiographics* 2012;32(1):9–32.

6a **Answer A.**

6b **Answer B.** The chest x-ray demonstrates mild diffuse left lung hyperlucency relative to the right. Additionally, the left lung pulmonary vessels are diminutive. This is caused by relative oligemia and decreased blood flow to the left lung from an obstructive central pulmonary embolism. This sign is rare and only occasionally seen prospectively. The unilateral hilum may be enlarged due to the embolus as well. On a supine radiograph, an anterior pneumothorax could have a similar appearance or a contralateral layer effusion, but this radiograph is an upright PA film. Occasionally, abrupt truncation of the central pulmonary arteries can also be seen.

Reference: Webb WR, *Higgins CB. Thoracic imaging.* Lippincott Williams & Wilkins, 2010.

7a **Answer A.**

7b **Answer D.** The leading differential considerations for the presence of a "reverse halo" or atoll sign (named after a ring-shaped coral reef) are organizing pneumonia, pulmonary infarct, or infections such as paracoccidioidomycosis (South American blastomycosis). Rare causes include bacterial pneumonia, mucormycosis, tuberculosis, sarcoidosis, radiofrequency ablation, or granulomatosis with polyangiitis (formerly Wegener's). The sign is characterized by central ground-glass attenuation with surrounding ring consolidation, inverse of the more well-known "halo" sign, which is a central nodule or consolidation with surrounding ring of ground glass. Distinction of the central ground glass from cavitation is important to avoid misclassification. Correlation with clinical symptomatology and travel history is important to assist with narrowing the differential.

Reference: Walker C, Mohammed TL, Chung J. Reversed Halo Sign. *J Thorac Imaging* 2011;26:W80.

8a **Answer A.**

8b **Answer B.** Evaluation of the pregnant patient for possible pulmonary embolism is a frequent imaging request. D-dimer result is frequently nonspecific in the setting of pregnancy. Although ultrasound of the femoral vessels is a good initial exam, further evaluation may be required for certain clinical scenarios. In that setting, pulmonary artery CTA and V/Q scans are the typical first-choice imaging modalities. Exact preference for each is generally facility dependent due to conflicting expert opinion. However, CTA does result in a lower overall dose to the fetus as compared to V/Q scanning. However, the hormonally stimulated breast in female patients is particularly radiosensitive and CTA results in a significantly higher breast dose in the setting of pregnancy to the mother. As a general rule, gadolinium is avoided in the setting of pregnancy, which excludes performing a contrast-enhanced MRA. A CT without contrast could potentially provide an alternative diagnosis but is not a first-line choice for specifically evaluating pulmonary embolism.

Reference: Schaefer-Prokop C, Prokop M. CTPA for the diagnosis of acute pulmonary embolism during pregnancy. *Eur Radiol* 2008;18(2):2705–2708.

9 Answer A. The Wells criteria were developed as a more objective method to quantify the risk of pulmonary embolism in the emergency room patient population. Seven factors are assigned points with the total number of points correlating with your relative risk. Criteria include the following:

1. Clinical signs and symptoms of DVT (3 points).
2. PE is the primary clinical diagnosis (3 points).
3. Heart rate > 100 (1.5 points).
4. Immobilization for at least 3 days or surgery in the past 4 weeks (1.5 points).
5. Previous documented PE or DVT (1.5 points).
6. Hemoptysis (1 point).
7. Malignancy with recent treatment (past 6 months) or palliative care (1 point).

The higher the number of points, the higher the risk of pulmonary embolism. Depending on the clinical study, a score of ≤4 correlates with a low risk of pulmonary embolism (3%).

Reference: Wells PS, Anderson DR, Rodger M, et al. Excluding pulmonary embolism at the bedside without diagnostic imaging: management of patients with suspected pulmonary embolism presenting to the emergency department by using a simple clinical model and d-dimer. *Ann Intern Med* 2001;135(2):98–107.

10 Answer C. Radiologic differentiation between a pulmonary artery sarcoma and thromboembolic disease is sometimes difficult and PA sarcomas are rare. Sarcomas tend to present as single large central lesions rather than multiple smaller filling defects. However, a unilateral central filling defect can be seen in either disease as can local expansion of the involved pulmonary arteries (related to pressure overload). Both these findings might suggest the possibility of sarcoma but are not diagnostic of one. Generally, advanced disease can be reliably distinguished due to the presence of tissue invasion and local extension, which would not be present without underlying malignancy. Additionally, PET/CT positivity above the normal background blood pool levels can help distinguish problematic cases and would be the most specific finding of those listed.

Reference: Chong S, Kim TS, Kim BT, et al. Pulmonary artery sarcoma mimicking pulmonary thromboembolism: integrated FDG PET/CT. *AJR Am J Roentgenol* 2007;188(6):1691–1693.

11 Answer A. Behçet disease is a multisystem large- and small-vessel vasculitis. Patients tend to be young adults of Middle Eastern, Mediterranean, or Far East decent with a strong male predominance. There is a classic triad of symptoms including oral ulcers, genital ulcers, and uveitis, but other organ systems can be involved with vascular manifestations present in approximately ⅓ of patients. Upwards of 85% of vascular involvement will relate to the venous system resulting in extrapulmonary venous thrombi. This can include the hepatic veins, IVC, and SVC with causes of Budd-Chiari and SVC stenosis occurring. Behçet disease involving the large vessels is referred to as vasculo-Behçet disease. Pulmonary artery aneurysms (PAA) are the most common pulmonary arterial manifestation in Behçet disease and are frequently accompanied by hemoptysis, which can be life threatening. The other manifestations above can also be seen in the setting of active disease but are less common. Of note, pulmonary emboli are actually less common in this disease despite the high rates of venous thrombi. This is believed to relate to the presence of highly adherent clot to the vessel walls due to active inflammation. Pulmonary parenchymal and pleural involvements are only seen in 1% to 10% of patients.

Reference: Ceylan N, Bayraktaroglu S, Erturk SM, et al. Pulmonary and vascular manifestations of behçet disease: imaging findings. *AJR Am J Roentgenol* 2010;194(2).

12 **Answer D.** Fat embolism syndrome (FES) most frequently affects the lungs, brain, and skin after traumatic long bone or pelvic fracture. Other more rare causes include complications from routine orthopedic procedure or liposuction, sequelae of bone tumor lysis, pancreatitis, or lipid infusion. The chest x-ray and CT findings are frequently nonspecific and manifest as bilateral, multifocal ground-glass opacities that can progress to consolidation. There are not generally visible filling defects in the pulmonary arteries due to the small size of the fat droplets that are embolized. The exact incidence of fat emboli is unknown as many patients are likely asymptomatic. A triad of respiratory distress, cerebral abnormalities, and petechial hemorrhages is the classic description. Severe cases carry a high mortality rate upwards of 20%. A latent period of 24 to 48 hours can help separate FES from typical contusion. Atypical infection would be unusual to develop in such a short time course and would not have a direct relationship to the history of trauma in this patient. Aspiration may present similarly, but the presence of a rash points toward FES.

Reference: Malagari K, Economopoulos N, Stoupis C, et al. High-Resolution CT findings in mild pulmonary fat embolism. *Chest* 2003;123(4):1196–1201.

13 **Answer A.** Ideal catheter position is within 2 cm of the hilum, either left or right sided. Distal location (as demonstrated here) can result in pulmonary artery rupture, occlusion, dissection infarction, pseudoaneurysm, or fistula formation. The pulmonary angiography CT demonstrates a small focal outpouching of a right middle lobe branch pulmonary artery. This is consistent with an iatrogenic pseudoaneurysm.

Reference: Godoy M, Leitman B, Groot P, et al. Chest radiography in the ICU: Part 2, Evaluation of cardiovascular lines and other devices. *AJR Am J Roentgenol* 2012;198:572–581.

14 **Answer C.** All of these vasculitides can affect the thoracic vasculature. However, of those listed, Takayasu and Behçet disease are the only ones that involve large vessels. Interestingly, Behçet disease is more likely to involve the abdominal aorta or pulmonary arteries rather than the thoracic aorta or neck great vessels, making Takayasu's the correct answer.

Takayasu's affects large and medium-sized arteries. There is a predilection for women under the age of 40, who constitute more than 90% of cases. Radiologic manifestations typically reflect aortic or large-vessel involvement with vessel wall thickening, narrowing, dilatation, and premature calcification. This case demonstrates significant aortic wall thickening extending into the neck great vessels. Notice the luminal narrowing of the left internal carotid artery. The pulmonary arteries can be involved in upwards to 50% of cases and result in pulmonary hypertension although severe pulmonary hypertension is rare. Granulomatosis with polyangiitis (GPA, formerly known as Wegener's) can involve the thoracic vessels but is a small-vessel vasculitis. Thoracic manifestations typically center around multiple pulmonary nodules and masses (frequently cavitary), pulmonary hemorrhage, and airway involvement rather than discrete vessel wall inflammation. Goodpasture syndrome manifests in the chest as a pulmonary capillaritis and hemorrhage.

References: Castañer E, Alguersuari A, Gallardo X. When to suspect pulmonary vasculitis: radiologic and clinical clues. *Radiographics* 2010;30(1).

Ceylan N, Bayraktaroglu S, Erturk SM, et al. Pulmonary and vascular manifestations of behçet disease: imaging findings. *AJR Am J Roentgenol* 2010;194(2):W158–W164.

15 **Answer B.** Methyl methacrylate embolization occurs as a sequela of venous leak of cement during vertebroplasty or kyphoplasty into the paravertebral venous plexus. The exact incidence is not well established, but it likely occurs in approximately 5% of cases. Outcomes are also variable with many patients being asymptomatic and others suffering death (although death is very rare). Radiographic and CT demonstrate the MAA cement due to their high density as linear and branching opacities (less frequently nodular). Evidence of prior kyphoplasty on the x-ray or via clinical history confirms the diagnosis. Occasionally, serpentine MAA densities around the spine can also be seen as in this case. Findings of chronic thromboembolic pulmonary hypertension can overlap, but the high density of MAA exceeds that of the calcification sometimes seen in advanced chronic pulmonary emboli. Dendriform pulmonary ossification can be seen on x-ray and CT but is associated with underlying evidence of chronic/recurrent aspiration or pulmonary fibrosis in a majority of cases.

Reference: Pelton WM, Jacobo K, Candocia FJ, et al. Methylmethacrylate pulmonary emboli: radiographic and computed tomographic findings. *J Thorac Imaging* 2009;24(3):241–247.

16   **Answer A.**   Amniotic fluid embolization results from amniotic fluid entering the intravenous system via uterine vein tears. It is an unusual complication from cesarean section with the majority of causes occurring during spontaneous labor (70%). Dyspnea and shock can rapidly progress to cardiopulmonary collapse. Often, no initial imaging is performed as the patient's clinical status rapidly deteriorates to critical. When obtained, radiologic manifestation overlaps with other airspace disease including pulmonary edema, hemorrhage, and aspiration, and as such, accurate diagnosis requires a high degree of clinical suspicion.

Reference: Han D, Lee KS, Franquet T, et al. Thrombotic and nonthrombotic pulmonary arterial embolism: spectrum of imaging findings. *Radiographics* 2003;23:1521–1539.

17a   **Answer A.**

17b   **Answer C.**   The chest x-ray demonstrates left hilar enlargement seen on both the frontal and lateral projections. Note the lateral projection demonstrates the enlargement posterior to the bronchi in a pattern highly suggestive of pulmonary artery enlargement rather than adenopathy. The right hilum is normal. CT is confirmatory that the left pulmonary artery is enlarged and the right pulmonary artery is present and normal in size. Isolated left pulmonary artery enlargement is specifically associated with pulmonary valve stenosis. In cases of long-standing stenosis, often congenital, the pulmonary valve stenotic jet is preferentially directed into the left pulmonary artery, resulting in asymmetric enlargement relative to the right. This can be confirmed with echocardiography or cardiac MRI. Congenital absence of the right pulmonary artery is not possible as the right pulmonary artery is seen in this case. Additionally, both CTEPH and primary pulmonary hypertension would be expected to manifest as pulmonary artery enlargement bilaterally.

Reference: Webb WR, Higgins CB. *Thoracic imaging: Pulmonary and cardiovascular radiology*. North American Edition. Lippincott Williams & Wilkins, 2010.

18   **Answer A.**   Mycotic pulmonary artery aneurysms are rare but are referred to as Rasmussen aneurysms when due to TB (some use the Rasmussen aneurysm more generally for any mycotic aneurysm). Progressive bronchiectasis or cavitation results in vessel wall weakening and eventual possible rupture (which can be life threatening). Approximately 5% of patients with chronic cavitary TB demonstrate evidence of pulmonary artery aneurysm on autopsy. Location is normally peripheral, and involvement of a main pulmonary artery or lobar branch is comparatively unusual.

Reference: Kim HY, Song KS, Goo JM, et al. Thoracic sequelae and complications of tuberculosis. *Radiographics* 2001;21(4):839–858.

19a **Answer A.**

19b **Answer A.** Bland thrombus in the IVC can be seen as sequelae of lower extremity DVT but would be unusual to be a skip lesion as shown (the infrahepatic IVC is patent and contrast enhancing). Similarly, mixing artifact is not possible in this case because the IVC is already opacified indicating that the scan timing was sufficiently delayed to allow circulation of contrast through the abdomen. Several features of tumor thrombus are present including hepatic vein, IVC, and right atrial expansion due to the tumor. Additionally, there is a more subtle heterogeneity to the thrombus suggesting internal enhancement that would not be seen in bland thrombus. Secondary evidence in this case includes peripherally enhancing hepatic lesions as well as at least one more subtle pleural metastatic deposit.

Of the tumors listed, renal cell carcinomas most commonly extend into the IVC. Those tumor thrombi can occasionally reach the right atrium as shown. This case was that of an advanced hepatocellular carcinoma. Adrenocortical carcinomas also demonstrate a predilection for IVC involvement but are less common. Bronchogenic carcinoma involvement of the IVC is relatively rare, but SVC involvement is quite common for advanced disease. IVC thrombus increases the risk of both bland and tumor emboli to the pulmonary arteries. A careful observer may have noticed a nonenhancing left lower lobe artery on the first image indicating such an event in this patient.

References: Kaufman LB, Yeh BM, Breiman RS, et al. Inferior vena cava filling defects on CT and MRI. *AJR Am J Roentgenol* 2005;185(3):717–726.

Sheth S, Fishman EK. Imaging of the inferior vena cava with MDCT. *AJR Am J Roentgenol* 2007;189(5):1243–1251.

20a **Answer C.**

20b **Answer C.** Chest radiography is frequently an initial imaging step for evaluation of pulmonary hypertension, but classic findings are generally not evident until later in the disease course. Central pulmonary artery dilatation on radiograph is most accurately assessed by measuring the right interlobar artery on the frontal projection. The upper limit of normal is 15 mm for women and 16 mm for men. On CT, the main pulmonary artery is more accurately assessed with 30 mm being the cutoff most use for an abnormally enlarged artery suggesting pulmonary arterial hypertension. More specifically, the normal diameter of the main pulmonary artery is approximately 25 mm with the 90th percentile cutoff value being 29 mm in men and 27 mm in women. Note that there is frequent overlap of mild pulmonary hypertension and normal subjects close to this value and the presence of a normal pulmonary artery size does not exclude pulmonary hypertension. Additionally, a main pulmonary artery size larger than the ascending aorta is an easy method to assess size. The more distal pulmonary arteries tend to become "pruned" or smaller in size despite the more central enlargement. Other features commonly assessed on CT include right ventricular hypertrophy (wall thickness >4 mm), interventricular septal straightening, and right ventricular dilatation.

Reference: Peña E, Dennie C, Veinot J, et al. Pulmonary hypertension: how the radiologist can help. *Radiographics* 2012;32(1):9–32.

9 Lung Cancer

QUESTIONS

1 If similar in size, which of the following nodule types would likely have the longest doubling time if malignant?

A. Ground-glass nodule
B. Semisolid nodule
C. Solid nodule
D. Centrally calcified nodule

2 Which of the following patterns of pulmonary nodule calcification has the highest likelihood of malignancy?

A. Central
B. Stippled
C. Lamellated
D. Popcorn

3a Based on the Fleischner Society recommendations for pulmonary nodule follow-up, what recommendation should be made for this low-risk 42-year-old patient with a 7 mm nodule?

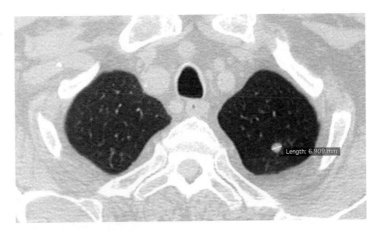

A. Follow-up CT in 3 months
B. PET/CT
C. Follow-up CT in 6 to 12 months
D. CT-guided transthoracic needle biopsy

3b What history would exclude the patient from the Fleischner Society Guidelines for Management of Small Pulmonary Nodules?

A. Malignant disease
B. Recurrent infection
C. HIV
D. 20 pack-years of smoking

4a Chest radiographs are obtained for cough. In what segment is the rounded mass located?

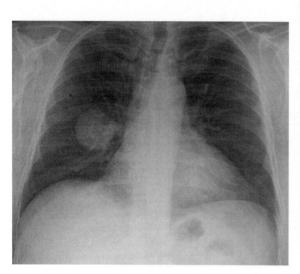
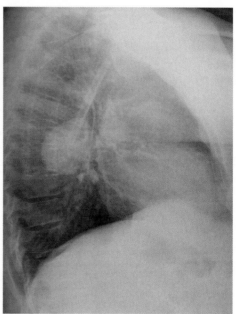

A. Medial segment right middle lobe
B. Lateral segment right middle lobe
C. Superior segment right lower lobe
D. Posterior segment right upper lobe

4b On correlation with CT, what is the diagnosis?

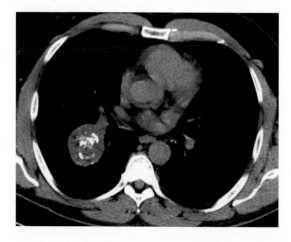

A. Mucinous adenocarcinoma
B. Metastasis
C. Hamartoma
D. Squamous cell carcinoma

4c What percentage of pulmonary hamartomas demonstrate intranodular fat?

    A. 10%
    B. 25%
    C. 50%
    D. 100%

5 A 66-year-old female was treated for pneumonia based on an initial CT (left). On follow-up 3 years later (right), the consolidation in the left lower lobe persists with new development of several nodules such as the one in the right lower lobe. What is the likely diagnosis?

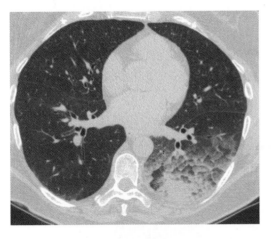 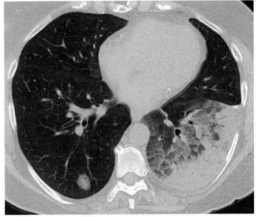

    A. Atypical mycobacterial infection
    B. Chronic fungal infection
    C. Multifocal adenocarcinoma
    D. Organizing pneumonia

6 This is an image from a CT scan performed on a 78-year-old female with a long smoking history. The nodule measures 1.5 cm and has persisted for 3 months. No other abnormalities are identified on the chest CT. Assuming that the patient has an acceptable risk profile for surgery, what would be the best evidence-based course for further evaluation and management?

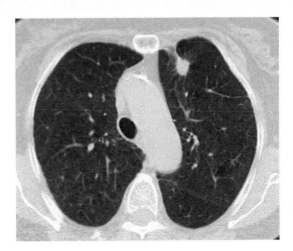

    A. Percutaneous transthoracic biopsy
    B. Thoracotomy, wedge resection of the nodule, and possible completion lobectomy
    C. Preoperative brain MRI
    D. Preoperative brain MRI and PET scan

7a With regard to low-dose CT screening for lung cancer, what value should the dose length product be under for a standard patient?

A. 50 mGy-cm
B. 75 mGy-cm
C. 125 mGy-cm
D. 200 mGy-cm

7b What is the minimum pack-year smoking history recommended for undergoing low-dose CT of the chest for lung cancer screening?

A. 5 pack-years
B. 10 pack-years
C. 15 pack-years
D. 30 pack-years

8 In this patient with a history of malignancy, what accounts for the lesion marked by the white arrows?

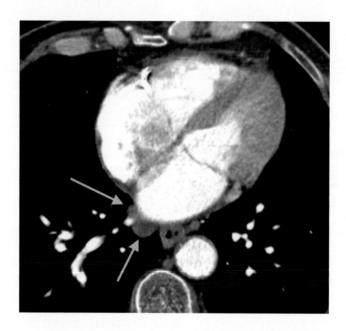

A. Lymphadenopathy
B. Metastatic pulmonary nodule
C. Nonspecific pulmonary nodule
D. Pericardial fluid

9a What is the most common location of a missed lung cancer on chest radiograph?

A. Central and upper lobe
B. Peripheral and lower lobe
C. Central and lower lobe
D. Peripheral and upper lobe

9b What type of observer error is the most common in missed lung cancer?

A. Scanning error
B. Observer error
C. Decision-making error
D. Satisfaction of search error

10a An initial staging CT scan on a 61-year-old female patient with iodine-avid thyroid cancer reveals this lesion in the right lower lobe. An FDG-PET/CT scan performed the following week showed only background activity in this lesion and no lesions elsewhere. What is the next best step?

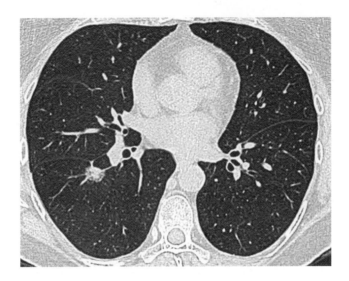

    A. No further follow-up.
    B. Initiate I-131 therapy for metastatic thyroid cancer.
    C. Initiate targeted anti-EGFR therapy for bronchogenic adenocarcinoma.
    D. Three-month follow-up CT.

10b An outside CT scan from 6 years prior has been obtained, shown below with the new CT for comparison (current on left, 6 years prior on right). What is the likely diagnosis?

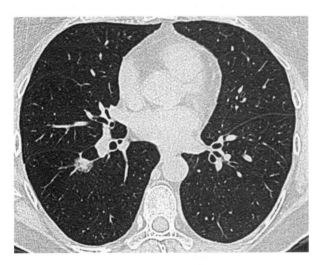
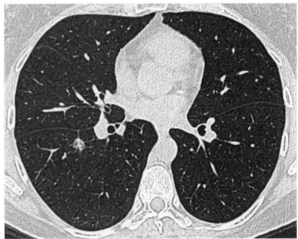

    A. Focal scar
    B. Minimally invasive adenocarcinoma
    C. Thyroid metastasis
    D. Hamartoma

11a This chest radiograph and CT were obtained of a 45-year-old male complaining of shortness of breath and weight loss. In addition to infectious and inflammatory processes, which of the following malignancies should be considered?

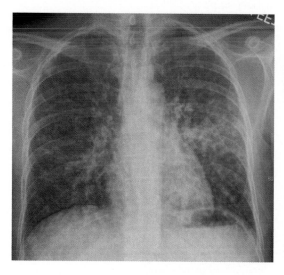
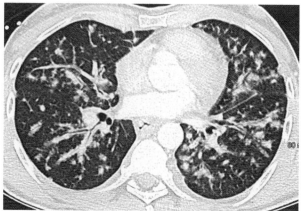

A. Pulmonary lymphoma
B. Intraductal papillary mucinous tumor of the pancreas metastasis
C. Prostate cancer metastasis
D. Epithelioid hemangioendothelioma

11b During this patient's evaluation, it is discovered that he has HIV infection. What additional diagnoses should be considered?

A. None
B. Kaposi sarcoma
C. Pneumocystis infection
D. Cryptococcal pneumonia

12a The following frontal radiograph was obtained in a 67-year-old male with chest pain. In the absence of infectious symptoms, which of the following features on the radiograph is the most worrisome for malignancy?

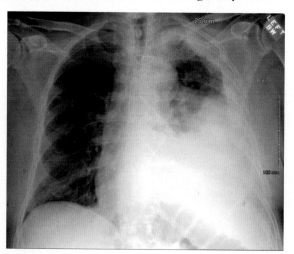

A. Rib destruction
B. Mediastinal shift to the right
C. Large unilateral effusion
D. Prior CABG

12b A CT scan of this patient was performed. Which of the following is the most LIKELY diagnosis?

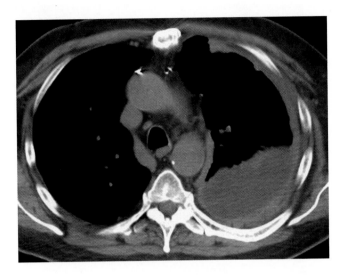

A. Mesothelioma
B. Asbestos-related pleural disease
C. Metastatic adenocarcinoma
D. Chronic fibrothorax

13 An image from a CT scan performed on a 62-year-old female with chest pain is shown. A percutaneous CT-guided biopsy of this lesion has been requested. What is the most important next step prior to biopsy of this lesion?

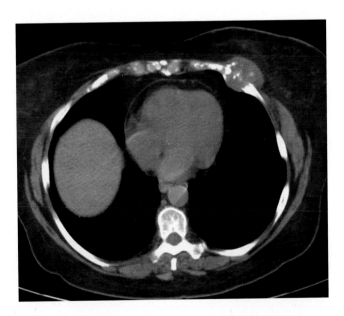

A. Obtain a contrast-enhanced CT, as this may be a highly vascular lesion such as a renal cell carcinoma metastasis.
B. Surgical consultation, as the needle tract will have to be excised.
C. Adrenergic blockage (such as labetalol), as the lesion could be metastatic pheochromocytoma
D. Anesthesia consultation, as this lesion will be very painful to biopsy.

14   A 64-year-old male Complains of shortness of breath and cough. Which of the following entities is demonstrated on his lateral radiograph?

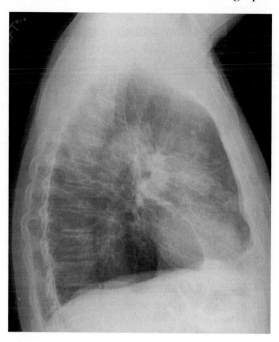

A. Hilar adenopathy
B. Anterior mediastinal mass
C. Lower lobe nodule
D. An expansile sternal lesion

15   A 72-year-old female patient with head and neck squamous cell carcinoma had a diagnostic chest CT and PET/CT performed as part of her pretreatment staging. The chest CT demonstrated multiple bilateral pulmonary nodules. Images shown demonstrate two of the larger nodules. The FDG-PET/CT demonstrated increased uptake in the laryngeal primary but did not demonstrate increased uptake in any of the pulmonary nodules. What is the next best step?

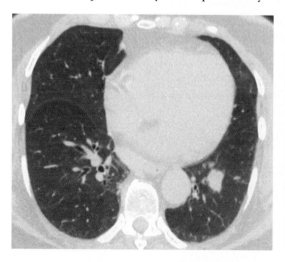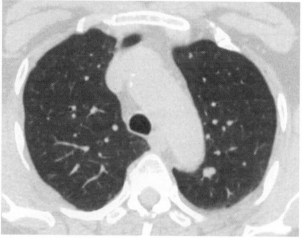

A. No further evaluation, as the lack of PET avidity confirms benignity
B. Repeat PET/CT, as the lack of PET avidity suggests an inadequate study
C. Tissue biopsy, as the nodules are worrisome for metastases
D. Initiation of chemotherapy, as the nodules are definitely metastatic

16a A 76-year-old female presented to her primary physician with chest pain. A PA and lateral chest film was obtained. The PA image is shown. Which of the following findings is present on this radiograph?

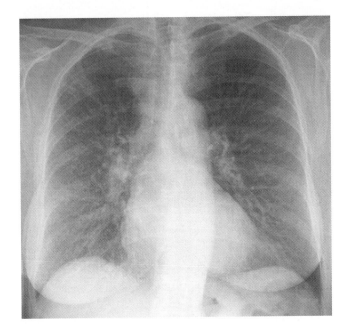

A. Mass lesion projecting behind the right atrium
B. Expansile lesion involving the anterior right second rib
C. Increased interstitial markings only on the right side
D. Diffusely increased interstitial markings, worse on the right

16b A CT was obtained, an image from which is shown. Biopsy demonstrated lymphangitic spread of a previously unsuspected breast cancer. Which of the following findings is most suggestive of lymphangitic spread of cancer on CT imaging?

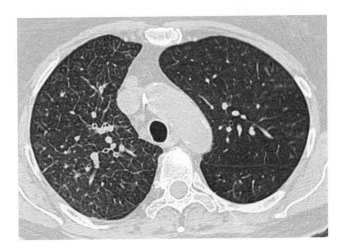

A. Nodular interlobular septal thickening
B. Bronchiectasis
C. Mosaic air trapping
D. Pleural effusion

17a In which nodal zone is the identified lymph node?

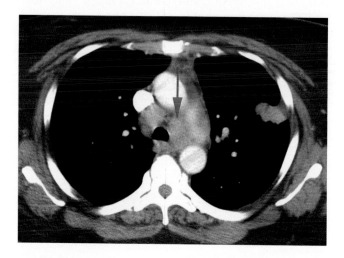

    A. Upper, prevascular
    B. Upper, left paratracheal
    C. Aorticopulmonary
    D. Hilar, interlobar

17b Which of the following techniques is most appropriate for accessing the anterior mediastinum and aortopulmonary window?

    A. Chamberlain procedure
    B. Mediastinoscopy
    C. Transbronchial needle aspiration
    D. Endobronchial ultrasound-guided needle aspiration

17c Following transthoracic needle biopsy which demonstrated adenocarcinoma of the lung in the left upper lobe, PET/CT obtained before further biopsy. The only metabolically active lesions are captured on this single image. What is the suspected radiologic nodal stage?

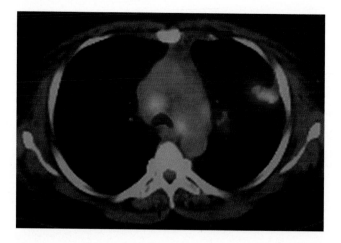

    A. N0
    B. N1
    C. N2
    D. N3

18 Lesion has demonstrated >3 months stability. Approximately what percentage of this type of lesion will end up being adenocarcinoma on surgical resection?

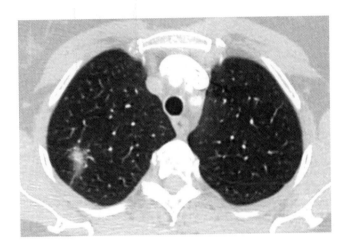

    A. 5%
    B. 25%
    C. 60%
    D. 90%

19a The patient is a 35-year-old nonsmoker. What is the most likely diagnosis?

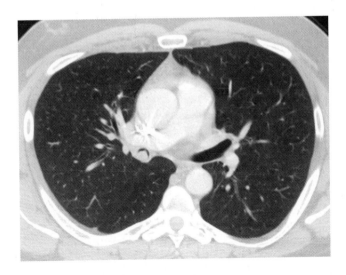

    A. Squamous cell carcinoma
    B. Adenoid cystic carcinoma
    C. Mucoepidermoid carcinoma
    D. Bronchial carcinoid

19b What percentage of bronchial carcinoids cause carcinoid syndrome?

    A. <5%
    B. 10% to 15%
    C. 20% to 25%
    D. More than 30%

20a Portable chest radiograph obtained for suspected pneumonia. What is the best recommendation after initiating antibiotic treatment?

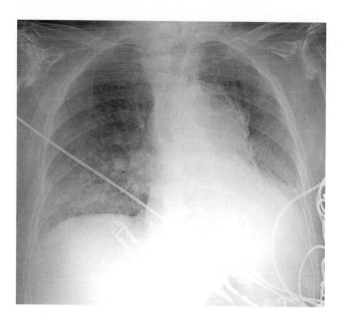

A. No imaging follow-up
B. Follow-up chest radiograph in 6 to 8 weeks
C. Chest computed tomography
D. Bronchoscopy with transbronchial biopsy

20b Biopsy reveals small cell lung cancer. What criteria would make the cancer "limited stage"?

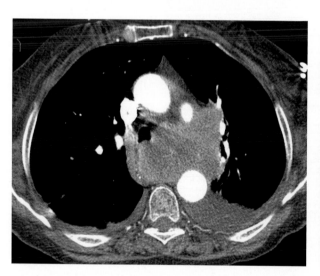 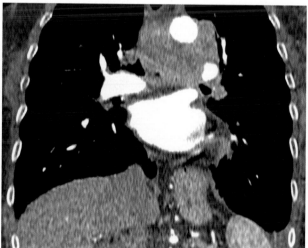

A. Confined to a single radiation port
B. Presence of brain metastases
C. Malignant pleural effusion
D. Extension beyond single radiation port

ANSWERS AND EXPLANATIONS

1 **Answer A.** Of the nodule types listed, the ground-glass nodule has the longest potential doubling time. For malignant solid nodules, the doubling time is generally <100 days. Those with a doubling time more than 400 days are usually benign, and stability over 2 years (730 days) is therefore a reliable indicator of benignity for a majority of solid nodules. A doubling time of <20 days is much more likely infectious although this does not hold true for some aggressive malignancies or malignancy in the immunosuppressed. Comparatively, subsolid nodules can demonstrate a doubling time of more than 1,300 days and still be malignant. As such, follow-up of these nodules is generally longer than for the solid nodules, generally a minimum of 3 years. Semisolid nodules demonstrate doubling ranges between that of subsolid and solid nodules. A centrally calcified nodule is a benign pattern of calcification. In the remarkable small chance that such a lesion were malignant, such as a cancer that enveloped a calcified nodule, the doubling time would be similar to a solid nodule.

References: Naidich DP, Bankier AA, MacMahon H, et al. Recommendations for the management of subsolid pulmonary nodules detected at CT: a statement from the Fleischner Society. *Radiology* 2013;266(1):304–317.

Truong MT, Ko JP, Rossi SE, et al. Update in the evaluation of the solitary pulmonary nodule. *Radiographics* 2014;34(6):1658–1679.

2 **Answer B.** The benign patterns of lung nodule calcification are (1) diffuse, (2) central, (3) lamellated, and (4) popcorn. Presence of one of these patterns is a significant finding indicating a high probability of a benign lesion. Any other pattern of calcification is not a reliable indicator of benignity or malignancy due to calcification being possible in some malignancies including metastasis from GI tumors (mucinous adenocarcinomas), osteogenic malignancies, and even some primary bronchogenic malignancies.

Reference: Khan AN, Al-Jahdali HH, Allen CM, et al. The calcified lung nodule: what does it mean? *Ann Thorac Med* 2010;5(2):67–79.

3a **Answer C.**

3b **Answer A.** The first step in deciding follow-up of incidentally detected solitary pulmonary nodules is characterizing the density of the nodule. In this case, the nodule is solid. Next, measure the nodule in two orthogonal dimensions and calculate the average. In this patient, the nodule is roughly round and therefore, a single measurement suffices. Exclusion criteria for the Fleischner Society "Guidelines for Management of Small Pulmonary Nodules" include age younger than 35 and history of malignancy. Immune status is not a consideration in the recommendations. Finally, the patient is categorized as high or low risk based on smoking history or other risk factors. Taken altogether, the recommended follow-up in this case is repeat CT in 6 to 12 months.

Reference: MacMahon H, Austin JH, Gamsu G, et al. Guidelines for management of small pulmonary nodules detected on CT Scans: a statement from the fleischner society. *Radiology* 2005;237:395–400.

4a **Answer C.**

4b **Answer C.**

4c **Answer C.** On radiographs, the rounded mass projects in the mid right lung; however, on the lateral radiograph, the mass localizes just posterior and inferior to the major fissure. This correlates with the location of the right lower lobe superior segment.

On CT, a well-defined mass is identified with multiple areas of very low attenuation (corresponding with fat, not air), soft tissue attenuation, and high attenuation (popcorn areas of calcification). This pattern of findings is classic for pulmonary hamartoma.

Pulmonary hamartomas constitute the largest portion of benign lung neoplasms. Up to 20% are endobronchial in some studies. The tumors demonstrate disordered growth of cartilage (resulting in the chondroid "popcorn" calcification pattern), fat, fibrous tissue, and epithelial tissue. Symptoms vary depending on location and degree of endobronchial obstruction and include cough, hemoptysis, or fever (such as related to postobstructive infection). Patients are most frequently in their 4th to 7th decade, and there is a male predilection. Intralobular fat (not to be confused with the "bubble-like lucency" of adenocarcinoma or areas of focal necrosis) is the most reliable indicator and can frequently prevent the need for biopsy. Remember that liposarcoma metastases can contain focal fat as can lipoid pneumonia.

Although mucinous adenocarcinomas can demonstrate some calcification, as can some metastases from osteogenic and cartilaginous malignancies (osteosarcomas and chondrosarcomas), the mixed pattern of both macroscopic fat and popcorn calcification would be highly unusual. Squamous cell carcinomas would be expected to be much more irregular than shown here with a frequent predilection to cavitate.

References: Erasmus JJ, Connolly JE, McAdams HP, et al. Solitary pulmonary nodules: Part I. Morphologic evaluation for differentiation of benign and malignant lesions. *Radiographics* 2000;20(1):43–58.

Gaerte SC, Meyer CA, Winer-Muram HT, et al. Fat-containing lesions of the Chest. *Radiographics* 2002;22 Spec No:S61–S78.

5 **Answer C.**   The initial CT demonstrates significant left lower lobe consolidation and some surrounding ground glass. The appearance is nonspecific and could be related to a lobar pneumonia. However, this case highlights why follow-up is important in many cases, especially those with atypical clinical or radiographic features. The most worrisome cause of chronic consolidation is cancer, and this is a case of multifocal mucinous adenocarcinoma. These lesions can be slow growing, as seen here, and frequently can develop multiple sites of disease over time. These could be aerogenous metastases or metasynchronous primaries, and treatment of these lesions remains controversial. There is some evidence for aggressive treatment including surgical resection especially if the nodal stage is N0 or N1. In addition to surgical resection of the primary cancer, the smaller lesions that are accessible and most aggressive appearing should also be considered for resection. Despite the controversial treatment possibilities, it is clear that those with the more diffuse or multifocal forms of adenocarcinoma have a worse prognosis than do those with an isolated nodule.

References: Gu B, Burt BM, Merritt RE, et al. A dominant adenocarcinoma with multifocal ground glass lesions does not behave as advanced disease. *Ann Thorac Surg* 2013;96(2):411–418.

Liu YY, Chen YM, Huang MH, et al. Prognosis and recurrent patterns in bronchioloalveolar carcinoma. *Chest* 2000;118(4):940–947.

Travis WD, Brambilla E, Noguchi M, et al. International association for the study of lung cancer/American thoracic society/European respiratory society international multidisciplinary classification of lung adenocarcinoma. *J Thorac Oncol* 2011;6(2):244–285.

6 **Answer B.**   This is a T1a lesion. We are told that there are no other abnormalities visible on chest CT. In an older patient with a smoking history, it is known that it is more cost-effective and efficient to proceed to surgery, rather than to include the intermediate step of percutaneous biopsy. A spiculated nodule such as this has a >95% chance of being malignant in this patient population. Therefore, answer A is not correct. If the patient was a high surgical risk, and other treatment modalities such as external beam radiation or radiofrequency ablation were being considered, then biopsy would be appropriate.

Preoperative brain MRI is currently recommended in patients with T1b lesions and in all stage II and stage III lesions, but not in patients with T1a N0 disease. Likewise, FDG-PET scans are not currently recommended in this patient population, though they are performed in many centers. Therefore, answers C and D are incorrect.

In patients who are good candidates for potential lobectomy with T1a N0 disease, the sequence of events in answer B corresponds to the current management recommendations. Thoracotomy with wedge resection and immediate evaluation with frozen-section pathology will allow for completion lobectomy in the same setting if proven malignant. Preoperative lymph node sampling, by bronchoscopy or mediastinoscopy, is also not required in this patient population, although lymph node dissection will be performed in conjunction with the lobectomy.

Reference: Ettinger DS, Akerley W, Bepler G, et al; NCCN non-small cell lung cancer panel members. Non-small cell lung cancer. *J Natl Compr Canc Netw* 2010;8:740–801.

7a **Answer B.**

7b **Answer D.** The American Association of Physicists in Medicine (AAPM) does recommend that the dose-length product (DLP) be <75 mGy-cm for a lung cancer screening CT. Remember that this is for the AAPM "standard patient," who is 170 cm tall and weighs 70 kg (BMI = 24). As many of your patients will be larger than this, the actual DLP will be frequently higher than this.

The National Lung Screening Trial population, where a screening benefit was shown, ranged in age from 55 to 74. Some recommendations, including the U.S. Preventive Services Task Force, expand the age of recommended screening to 80, based on evidence from other trials. Some groups advocate for extension of the lower age bound to 50, although there are currently no good data to support this. There are currently no data to support lung cancer screening in patients with a lower pack-year history than 30.

Reference: Aberle DR, Adams AM, Berg CD, et al; National Lung Screening Trial Research Team. Reduced lung-cancer mortality with low-dose computed tomographic screening. *N Engl J Med* 2011;365(5):395–409.

8 **Answer D.** When the pulmonary veins penetrate the pericardium to join the atrium, a "sleeve" of pericardium surrounds the vein. As such, the right pulmonary venous recess or pericardial "sleeve" recess (of which this is an example) is a normal space within the pericardial sac that can occasionally fill with fluid. Knowing this anatomic space is important to avoid misclassifying it as a malignancy or other abnormality. When seen, there is frequently anterior and posterior fluid surrounding the right inferior pulmonary vein with the posterior component generally slightly larger. Superior and inferior components are possible but less frequently seen unless a larger volume of fluid is present. Features to help distinguish from adenopathy in this space include being well circumscribed, a lack of mass effect, and having fluid/water attenuation. Additionally, adenopathy more frequently appears on one side of the vessel.

Reference: Truong MT, Erasmus JJ, Sabloff BS, et al. Pericardial "sleeve" recess of right inferior pulmonary vein mimicking adenopathy: computed tomography findings. *J Comput Assist Tomogr* 2004;28(3):361–365.

9a **Answer D.**

9b **Answer C.**   In a study spanning from 1993 to 2001, non–small cell lung cancers that proved to be evident and missed on prior chest radiograph were reviewed for lesion location. The majority of missed NSCLC lesions were peripheral (85%) and upper lobe (72%). Specifically, the most common lobe for missed lung cancers was the right upper lobe (45%). The average lesion measured 1.9 cm in diameter. Other important lesion characteristics include density and shape.

The body of literature for missed lung cancers on chest radiograph is sizable, but a few landmark studies are commonly quoted. In particular, Kundel et al. performed several studies examining visual tracking with search patterns of radiologists related to missed lung cancers. They described three different observer errors: scanning, recognition, and decision-making errors. While the scanning error (no visual fixation on the lesion) made up 30% of observer errors and recognition error (visual fixation in the region of the lesion, but not on the lesion specifically) made up 30% of observer errors, decision-making error occurred in 45%, where the radiologist visually fixated on the lesion but incorrectly interpreted it as a normal structure. Satisfaction of search is another observer error where lung cancers are more easily recognized with fewer distracting abnormalities. While important to recognize, satisfaction of search is secondary relative to the aforementioned errors.

References: Shah PK, Austin JH, White CS, et al. Missed non-small cell lung cancer: radiographic findings of potentially resectable lesions evident only in retrospect. *Radiology* 2003;226:235–241.

White CS, Salis AI, Meyer CA. Missed lung cancer on chest radiography and computed tomography: imaging and medicolegal issues. *J Thorac Imaging* 1999;14:63–68.

10a **Answer D.**

10b **Answer B.**   Both metastatic and primary neoplasms may elicit sufficient immune response to produce localized fibrosis and scarring, which can produce tethering of the fissure such as this. It is true that thyroid cancer may be negative on FDG-PET, but there are many potential causes for this lesion, and a biopsy proving that this lesion represents metastatic thyroid cancer would be required before initiating therapy. Likewise, while it is true that bronchogenic adenocarcinomas may have this appearance, tissue is required to assess for the appropriate mutation before initiating targeted therapy. Given the semisolid appearance of the lesion, a low-grade adenocarcinoma is the most likely etiology, and comparison with priors if available and obtaining a follow-up CT in 3 months are the next best steps in management.

Many neoplasms may exhibit very slow growth. The FDG activity of this lesion does not actually add any additional information in this case, once the prior CT scan has come to light, as it would be surprising if such a slowly growing lesion had significant metabolic activity and FDG uptake. On the other hand, bronchogenic adenocarcinoma may exhibit very slow growth. In fact, this lesion was resected and was a minimally invasive adenocarcinoma (MIA). MIA is a relatively new pathologic subtype of adenocarcinoma and encompasses the lesions formerly known as bronchioloalveolar cell carcinoma (BAC). These lesions are characteristically slow growing and occur more commonly in nonsmokers than do other types of adenocarcinoma. They are often partly or wholly ground glass in attenuation on CT. For the same reasons, answer C is incorrect. Similarly, although hamartomas can grow, the semisolid nature of this nodule would be extremely atypical for a hamartoma.

It could be argued that, at this growth rate, this lesion would be very unlikely to kill the patient and should therefore be left alone. This can indeed be a reasonable course of action with many patients. There are no good data on the optimal management of these lesions, and the ultimate course of action will be determined by the patient's surgical risk, comorbidities, and the patient's personal preference. As a caveat, the growth rate of such lesions is not necessarily constant. In the absence of good data on the long-term behavior of these lesions, note that in our institution's experience with unresected MIA, roughly 5% will undergo aggressive transformation and become metastatic while they are being monitored.

Reference: Gardiner N, Jogai S, Wallis A. The revised lung adenocarcinoma classification-an imaging guide. *J Thorac Dis* 2014;6:S537–S546.

11a   Answer A.

11b   Answer B.   The findings are those of extensive, and largely confluent, small nodules extending along the bronchovascular bundles, with some subpleural nodules also noted. This is a perilymphatic pattern and could be seen with lymphangitic spread of any tumor. IPMT of the pancreas, prostate cancer, and epithelioid hemangioendothelioma do not commonly produce lymphangitic spread in the lungs. As well, on the chest radiograph, the pattern is very diffuse, and there is no dominant mass lesion. In cases of lymphangitic spread from extrathoracic metastatic disease, the lymphangitic pattern is usually more focal, and there is often a dominant central mass. Therefore, pulmonary lymphoma is correct. Pulmonary lymphoma may be either primary or secondary, and may manifest with a perilymphatic pattern, or may present as one or more airspace opacities.

While it is true that HIV patients are at increased risk for pulmonary lymphoma, certainly other diagnoses could be considered. One such diagnosis would be Kaposi sarcoma. In fact, this particular case proved to be Kaposi sarcoma rather than lymphoma.

HIV patients are at increased risk for pneumocystis and cryptococcal infection but they would not be expected to produce the appearances seen here and are therefore incorrect. Pneumocystis typically produces interstitial and ground-glass opacities, and later in the infection, the eponymous cysts may occur. Cryptococcal pneumonia commonly produces nodules, but a diffuse perilymphatic pattern would not be expected.

Reference: Lambert AA, Merlo CA, Kirk GD. Human immunodeficiency virus-associated lung malignancies. *Clin Chest Med* 2013;34:255–272.

12a   Answer C.

12b   Answer C.   There is no rib destruction present. Obviously, if rib destruction was present, there is a high likelihood of malignancy. Likewise, there is no mediastinal shift—the trachea lines up nicely over the spinous processes. However, if mediastinal shift were present, this would also be a concerning feature, as malignant effusions often behave in an expansile fashion, and a tension hydrothorax can even occur with a malignant effusion. Prior CABG has no particular association with malignancy, although tobacco use is a shared risk factor for both coronary artery disease and lung cancer. A large unilateral effusion has a very high likelihood of being either a malignant effusion or an empyema, so any large unilateral effusion in a patient without infectious symptoms is very worrisome for malignancy.

This is a classic appearance for mesothelioma, with the characteristic feature being the marked thickening of the mediastinal pleura. However, mesothelioma is a rare tumor, and it is actually more common for a malignant effusion from metastatic adenocarcinoma (most commonly breast or lung) to produce this appearance. Asbestos-related pleural disease reliably does not involve the mediastinal pleura, so this is incorrect. A chronic fibrothorax, from prior hemothorax or empyema, nearly always calcifies, and the involved hemithorax is usually smaller, with mediastinal shift toward the pleural abnormality, so answer D is incorrect.

Reference: Truong MT, Viswanathan C, Godoy MB, et al. Malignant pleural mesothelioma: role of CT, MRI, and PET/CT in staging evaluation and treatment considerations. *Semin Roentgenol* 2013;48:323–334.

13 Answer B.   The key to this question is recognizing the presence of calcified matrix within the lesion. Further, the location at a costochondral junction is very typical for this lesion, which is a chondrosarcoma. As chondrosarcomas, like the chondrocytes from which they derive, grow readily in an avascular environment, they may seed the biopsy tract. Management guidelines call for excision of the biopsy tract along with the tumor, so careful planning is required, and answer B is correct. Renal cell carcinoma metastases do not typically contain calcifications, so answer A is not correct. We are given no reason to suspect a metastatic pheochromocytoma, which would require alpha and beta adrenergic blockade, so answer C is incorrect. Malignant tumors are not generally painful to biopsy, as they contain no organized nerves. Any pain is usually derived from the needle path through surrounding normal tissues. Answer D is incorrect.

Reference: Souza FF, de Angelo M, O'Regan K, et al. Malignant primary chest wall neoplasms: a pictorial review of imaging findings. *Clin Imaging* 2013;37:8–17.

14 Answer A.   This lateral radiograph demonstrates one of the classic signs in chest imaging, the doughnut sign, which indicates the presence of hilar adenopathy. The finding is produced by abnormal soft tissue surrounding the left upper lobe bronchus (the doughnut hole). Answer A is correct. The other findings listed in B, C, and D are not present on this radiograph.

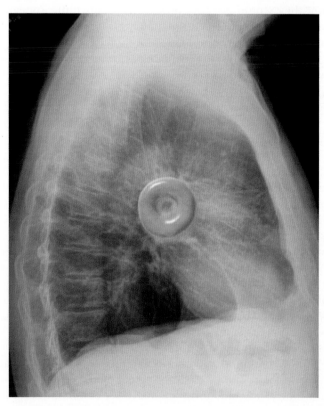

Here are the accompanying frontal radiograph and CT for this patient. The CT image nicely shows the hilar adenopathy surrounding the left upper lobe bronchus. There was an associated central squamous cell carcinoma in this patient.

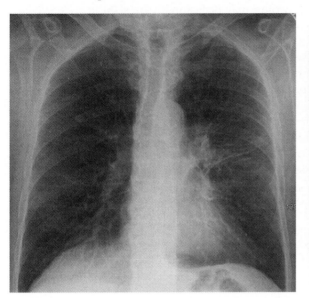
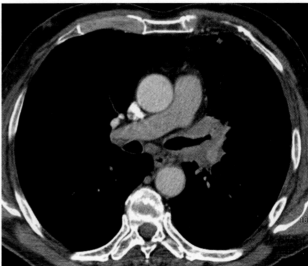

Reference: Feigin DS. Lateral chest radiograph a systematic approach. *Acad Radiol* 2010;17:1560–1566.

15 **Answer C.** Metastases may demonstrate more or less FDG uptake than the primary lesion, as they are often biologically distinct from the primary, with additional mutations. Therefore, answer A is incorrect. It is true that FDG-PET is insensitive to lesions under 8 mm, and this is particularly true in the lungs with the additional consideration of respiratory motion. However, the larger lesion shown in this case exceeds 2 cm in size and should be readily apparent on PET imaging if it takes up FDG. In some cases, depending on the individual clinical situation, a cancer patient who develops new bilateral pulmonary nodules during the course of treatment is assumed to have metastatic disease without tissue proof being obtained. However, this is an initial staging evaluation, and it is never appropriate to make assumptions that alter treatment. Answer C reflects appropriate patient management at initial cancer staging as these are highly worrisome for metastases but this should be proven by pathology.

In this case, in fact, the larger nodule shown above was percutaneously biopsied, and a smaller contralateral nodule was biopsied thoracoscopically. The pathology of both lesions was typical carcinoid, and not metastatic squamous cell carcinoma. Multiple pulmonary carcinoid tumors are not uncommon and may mimic metastatic disease. When they are discovered during evaluation for another malignancy, they often do not have significant impact on the patient's survival or treatment. This patient was able to have curative resection of her head and neck primary.

Reference: Aubry M, Thomas CF, Jett JR, et al. Significance of multiple carcinoid tumors and tumorlets in surgical lung specimens: analysis of 28 patients. *Chest* 2007;131:1635–1643.

16a **Answer C.**

16b **Answer A.** The radiograph demonstrates increased interstitial markings only on the right side. There is no evidence of the other answer choices.

Bronchiectasis is not a feature of lymphangitic spread of tumor. Pleural effusions are often present in patients with lymphangitic spread of tumor, but the vast majority of patients with pleural effusions do not, of course, have lymphangitic spread of tumor, so the presence of a pleural effusion is not suggestive of this entity. Mosaic air trapping may occasionally be seen in lymphangitic spread of tumor, because of the thickening of the walls of the small airways, which contain lymphatics. However, other causes of mosaic air trapping are much more common. Nodular or smooth interlobular septal thickening, almost always focal or asymmetric (as in this case), is almost universally present in lymphangitic spread of tumor. Central lymphadenopathy is also often present in lymphangitic spread of tumor and was present in this case (not shown).

Other causes of nodular interlobular septal thickening are few and include sarcoidosis, pneumoconiosis, and pulmonary alveolar septal amyloidosis. These other causes would not likely be as strikingly asymmetric as in this case.

Reference: Honda O, Johkoh T, Ichikado K, et al. Comparison of high resolution CT findings of sarcoidosis, lymphoma, and lymphangitic carcinoma: is there any difference of involved interstitium? *J Comput Assist Tomogr* 1999;23:374–379.

17a **Answer B.**

17b **Answer A.**

17c **Answer D.** Understanding lymph node stations and non–small cell lung cancer staging is critical in communicating with the treating physicians and for best care of the patient. Nodal zones are further subdivided into nodal stations, but a knowledge of the basic anatomic location is useful for determining the best approach for lymph node sampling. The provided CT demonstrates a left upper lobe nodule with associated mediastinal lymphadenopathy. The specific lymph node identified is immediately adjacent to the left trachea and is medial to the expected ligamentum arteriosum, which is important to anatomic marker to differentiate this from an AP window lymph node.

Various procedures are options for invasive lymph node staging. Of the options provided, they all provide access to the paratracheal lymph nodes with the exception of the Chamberlain procedure. The Chamberlain procedure accesses the anterior mediastinum, primarily for sampling of an aorticopulmonary lymph node. As these lymph nodes are not in the anterior or prevascular mediastinum, they are not accessible by this procedure.

Often, a PET/CT will be obtained following sampling of the primary lesion to determine the extent of disease. The gold standard is surgical/pathologic staging, but PET/CT provides the treating team an overall radiologic stage. In this case, the most important metabolically active lymphadenopathy is in the right lower paratracheal region (station 4R) contralateral to the primary non–small cell lung cancer. Suspected involvement of this node sets the radiologic staging at N3. The sensitivity and specificity for PET in identifying metastatic nodes are 58% to 91% and 78% to 90%, respectively.

References: Greaves SM, Brown K, Garon EB, et al. The new staging system for lung cancer: imaging and clinical implications. *J Thorac Imaging* 2011;26:119–131.

Walker CM, Chung JH, Abbott GF, et al. Mediastinal lymph node staging: from noninvasive to surgical. *AJR Am J Roentgenol* 2012;199:W54–W64.

18 **Answer C.** A semisolid nodule is present in the right upper lobe on CT, meaning that some portions of the nodule are definitely ground glass (less dense than pulmonary vasculature) and some portions are definitely solid (obscures the pulmonary vasculature). The best initial recommendation is a

3-month follow-up to exclude an inflammatory or infectious focus. Since this lesion has demonstrated stability over 3 months, it now falls into the category of a persistent semisolid nodule. In a review of lung cancer screening patients with persistent lung nodules measuring from 2 mm up to 45 mm, Henschke et al. found that 32% of solid nodules, 63% of semisolid nodules (partially solid), and 13% of pure ground-glass nodules (nonsolid) ended up being malignant nodules. When subdividing nodules on the basis of malignancy type, all semisolid nodules were found to be adenocarcinoma. Kim et al. found an even higher percentage (75%) of adenocarcinoma in persistent ground-glass nodules measuring 3 cm or less.

References: Henschke CI, Yankelevitz DF, Mirtcheva R, et al. CT screening for lung cancer: frequency and significance of part-solid and nonsolid nodules. *AJR Am J Roentgenol* 2002;178:1053–1057.

Kim HY, Sim YM, Lee KS, et al. Persistent pulmonary nodular ground-glass opacity at thin-section CT: histopathologic comparisons. *Radiology* 2007;245(1):267–275.

19a **Answer D.**

19b **Answer A.** A nodular filling defect is present in the bronchus intermedius. The most common primary tumor of the bronchi in young adults is carcinoid tumor. Carcinoid tumors can be subdivided into typical and atypical in the spectrum of neuroendocrine tumors along with small cell lung cancer. Carcinoid syndrome is uncommon in bronchial carcinoid (<5%) and generally only in the setting of liver metastases. Approximately 25% of bronchial carcinoids calcify, and evidence of calcification of a nodule with endobronchial component in a young adult is virtually diagnostic. Because it is an endobronchial lesion, patients often present with symptoms related to airway narrowing (cough or wheeze), bleeding (hemoptysis), or obstruction (pneumonia), although approximately a quarter of cases are identified incidentally. Resection of typical carcinoid, as in this case, has an excellent prognosis with a 92% survival rate at 5 years.

References: Jeung M, Gasser B, Gangi A, et al. Bronchial carcinoid tumors of the thorax: spectrum of radiologic findings. *Radiographics* 2002;22:351–365.

Ngo AH, Walker CM, Chung JH, et al. Tumors and tumorlike conditions of the large airways. *AJR Am J Roentgenol* 2013;201:301–313.

20a **Answer C.**

20b **Answer A.** While the portable chest radiograph does demonstrate consolidation in both lung bases, left greater than right, several findings make this more than a typical community-acquired pneumonia. Primarily, a large left mediastinal mass extending into the aortopulmonary window is present. Additionally, there is rightward shift of the trachea from extrinsic compression and leftward cardiac shift due to left lower lobe collapse. No follow-up and follow-up chest radiograph in 6 to 8 weeks after initiation of antibiotic treatment are options for community-acquired pneumonia dependent on patient age. Bronchoscopy is an option here, but the potential for an aortic abnormality as well as guidance for potential biopsy makes CT the best choice before any intervention is performed.

The CT and subsequent biopsy reveal a large middle mediastinal mass from small cell carcinoma. Small cell carcinoma constitutes approximately 15% of all lung cancers but the overall small cell cancer rate has been decreasing since the 1980s. Highly associated with smoking, small cell carcinoma is the most aggressive of the pulmonary neuroendocrine tumors, and at presentation, more than 60% of patients with small cell carcinoma have metastases. More than 10% will have brain metastases at presentation. Small cell carcinoma can be subdivided into limited stage (LS) and extensive stage (ES), primarily based on disease confined to a single radiation port for limited-stage disease. Debate exists over the importance of contralateral mediastinal or supraclavicular lymph node involvement for determining stage.

Reference: Carter BW, Glisson BS, Truong MT, et al. Small cell lung carcinoma: staging, imaging, and treatment considerations. *Radiographics* 2014;34:1707–1721.

10 Trauma

1a What is the diagnosis?

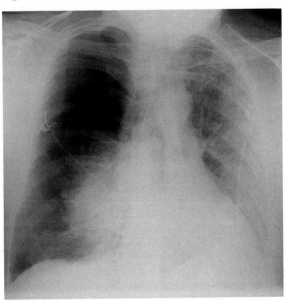

A. Artifact
B. Emphysema
C. Tension pneumothorax
D. Pulmonary contusion

1b What is the reason a tension pneumothorax can quickly become fatal?

A. Rapid blood loss
B. Decreased oxygenation
C. Decreased arterial blood supply to the brain
D. Decreased venous blood return to the heart

1c A small right apical pneumothorax would be easiest to visualize on which chest radiograph?

A. Upright frontal view
B. Lateral view
C. Supine view
D. Right lateral decubitus view

2a A 26-year-old pregnant female is imaged post–motor vehicle collision (MVC). Which of the following is the next best step?

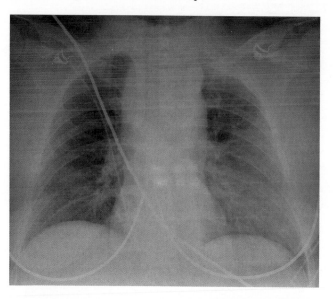

A. CTA of the chest
B. Noncontrast CT of the chest
C. MRA of the chest
D. Direct angiography

2b What is the most likely diagnosis?

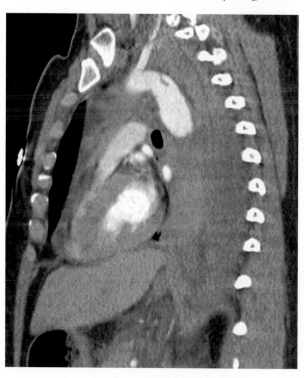

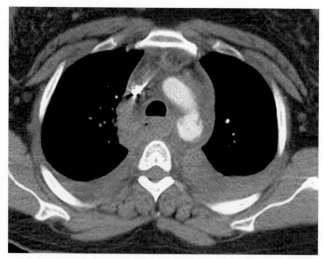

A. Amniotic fluid embolism
B. Traumatic aortic injury
C. Pneumothorax
D. Tension hemothorax

3 Persistent pneumothorax after placement of well-positioned and functioning chest tube should raise the concern for what injury?

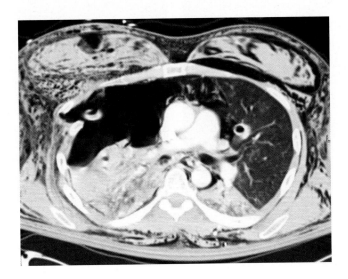

A. Pulmonary laceration
B. Tracheal transection
C. Bronchial tear
D. Diaphragm injury

4 In the setting of blunt trauma, what is the most likely diagnosis for the focus of air posterolateral to the trachea?

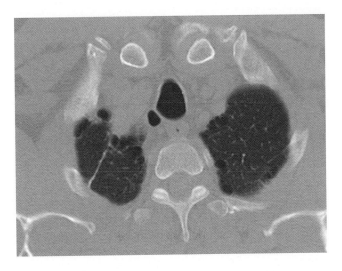

A. Acute esophageal injury
B. Soft tissue gas related to rib fracture
C. Acute tracheal injury
D. Normal variant

5a   What is the diagnosis?

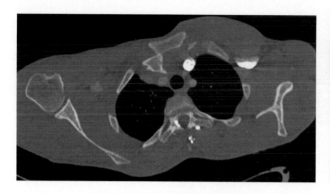 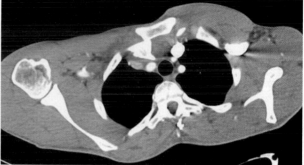

    A. Clavicle fracture
    B. Posterior sternoclavicular dislocation
    C. Manubrial fracture
    D. Sternomanubrial dislocation

5b   What vessel injury is associated with a LEFT posterior sternoclavicular dislocation?

    A. Thoracic aorta
    B. Left carotid artery
    C. Left subclavian vein
    D. Superior vena cava

6   In patients who undergo CT imaging for trauma, what is the most common source of bleeding as seen in this example?

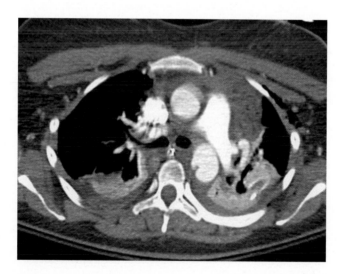

    A. Sternal fracture
    B. SVC rupture
    C. Aortic transection
    D. Small mediastinal venous/arterial injury

7 What is the most immediately life-threatening condition present?

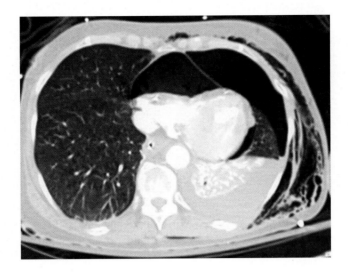

A. Tension pneumopericardium
B. Pulmonary laceration
C. Tension pneumothorax
D. Pericardial effusion

8 A patient presents with acute chest-penetrating trauma with this image from initial ultrasound. What is the diagnosis?

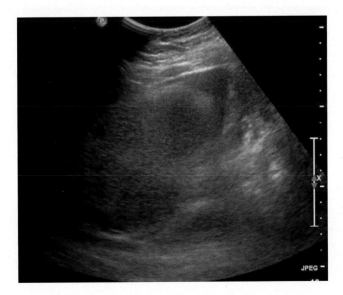

A. Ascites
B. Pleural effusion
C. Pericardial effusion
D. Anterior mediastinal hemorrhage

9 As shown in this example, what is the most common aspirated foreign body in a trauma patient with maxillofacial injury?

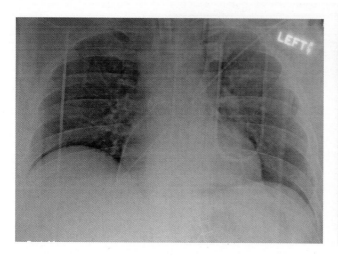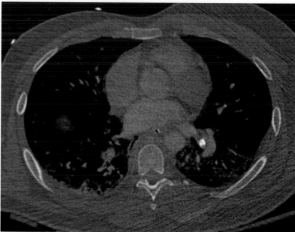

A. Peanut
B. Tooth
C. Food bone (meat/chicken/fish)
D. Windshield glass

10 A patient suffers a gunshot injury to the left chest. What causes the wide path of pulmonary opacity along the bullet pathway?

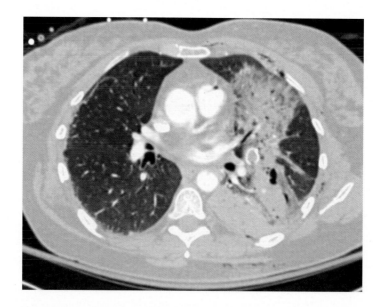

A. Pulmonary contusion from blast cavity effect
B. Aspiration due to mental status changes
C. Direct injury from bullet causing pulmonary laceration
D. Atelectasis related to airway collapse

11a What type of acute traumatic aortic injury is present?

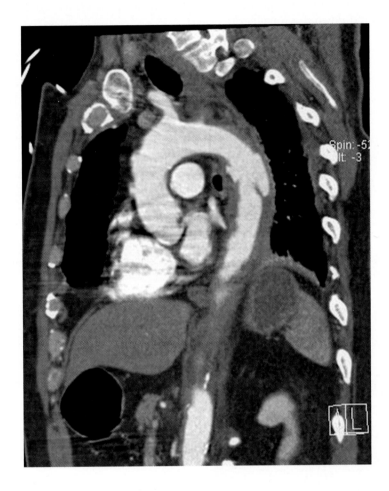

A. Mural thrombus
B. Minimal arterial injury
C. Pseudoaneurysm
D. Complete transection

11b When a traumatic pseudoaneurysm of the thoracic aorta is present, what layer of the vessel wall remains intact?

A. Media
B. Adventitia
C. Intima
D. Vasa vasorum

11c What is the most common site of acute traumatic aortic injury on CT?

A. Aortic isthmus
B. Ascending aorta
C. Aortic arch
D. Distal descending thoracic aorta

12   A 22-year-old female polytrauma patient is post–exploratory laparotomy, splenectomy, and multiple orthopedic injuries with hypoxemia despite intubation and bilateral chest tube placement. What diagnosis could be considered given the images provided?

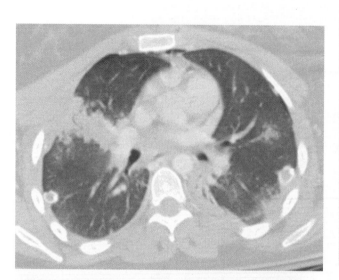

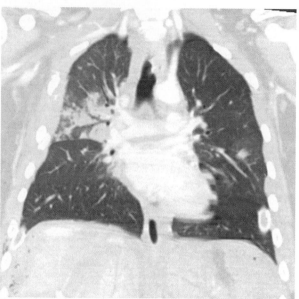

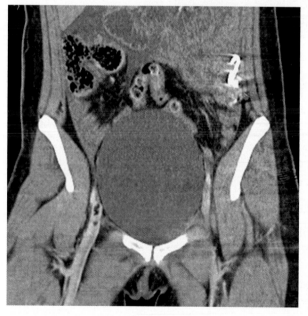

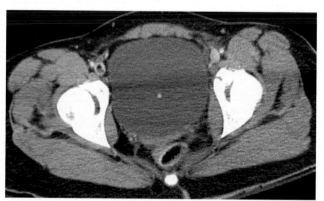

A. Cardiac contusion
B. Abdominal compartment syndrome
C. Tension pneumothorax
D. Fat embolism

13a A 61-year-old patient is post–motor vehicle collision. What radiologic sign is depicted?

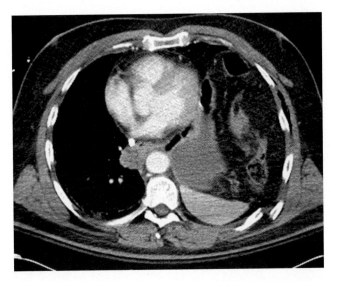

A. Collar sign
B. Dependent viscera sign
C. Bulging fissure sign
D. Colon cutoff sign

13b In a different trauma patient, what radiologic sign is depicted?

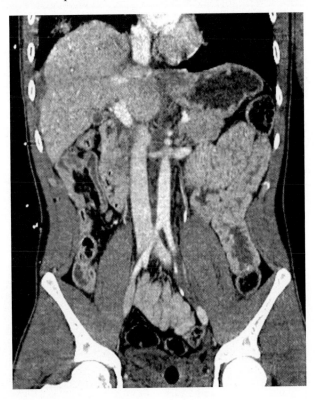

A. Collar sign
B. Dependent viscera sign
C. Bulging fissure sign
D. Colon cutoff sign

14   This patient is a 41-year-old male high-speed blunt trauma victim with multiple extremity and facial fractures. What is the most appropriate next step?

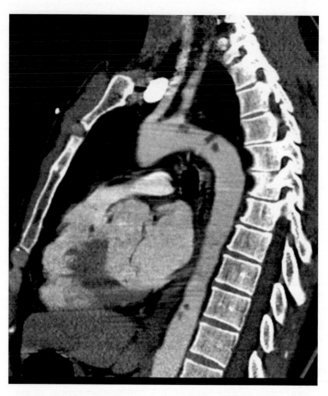

A. Follow up CTA of the chest in 2 to 7 days
B. Vascular interventional radiology consult for diagnostic angiogram and possible stent placement
C. Immediate follow-up cardiac-gated CTA chest
D. No specific follow-up required

15   A 30-year-old male is transferred for evaluation of a cavitary lung mass after a fall. What is the most likely diagnosis?

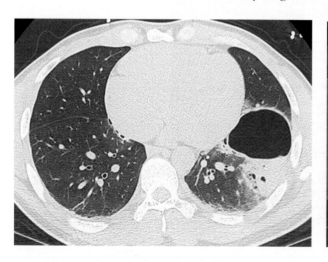
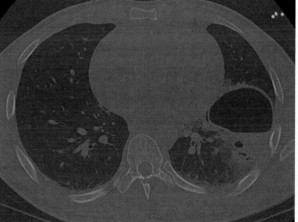

A. Pulmonary laceration
B. Tuberculosis
C. Congenital cystic adenomatoid malformation
D. Cavitary primary neoplasm

16 A 36-year-old male is kicked by a horse. What is the most likely diagnosis?

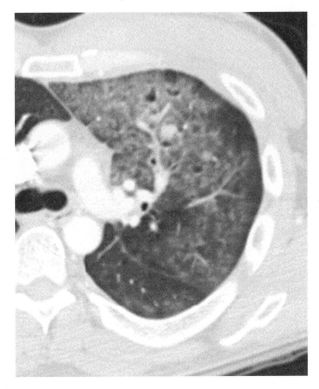

    A. Aspiration
    B. Pulmonary edema
    C. Pulmonary contusion with small lacerations
    D. Atypical pneumonia with cyst formation

17 What pattern of spontaneous respiration is associated with this type of traumatic injury?

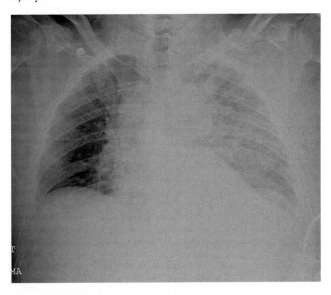

    A. Contralateral paradoxical chest wall motion
    B. Ipsilateral paradoxical chest wall motion
    C. Contralateral paradoxical diaphragmatic motion
    D. Ipsilateral paradoxical diaphragmatic motion

18a Which of the following is the most likely diagnosis given these images?

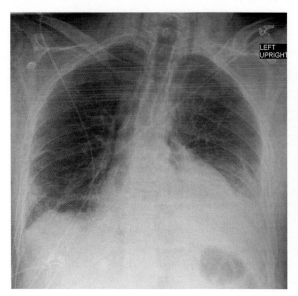

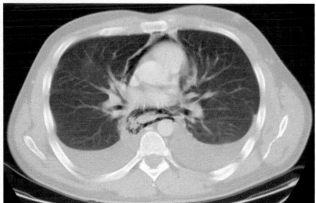

    A. Penetrating trauma
    B. Infectious mediastinitis
    C. Esophageal rupture
    D. Bronchial laceration

18b After this confirmatory esophagram, the most likely cause of injury in this patient is:

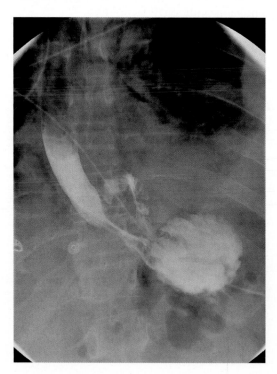

    A. Forceful repetitive vomiting
    B. Blunt trauma
    C. Penetrating trauma
    D. Pressure necrosis secondary to food bolus impaction

19a Which portion of the spinal column has the narrowest central canal?

    A. Cervical
    B. Thoracic
    C. Lumbar
    D. Sacral

19b The fracture above is best classified as which of the following?

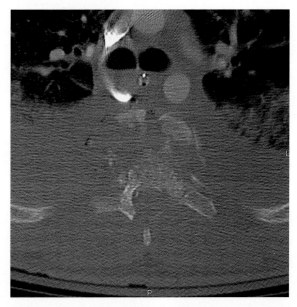

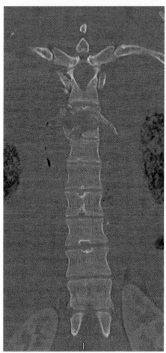
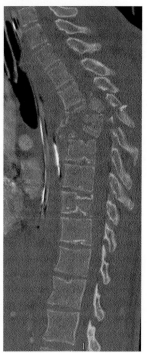

    A. Burst fracture
    B. Compression fracture
    C. Fracture dislocation
    D. Chance fracture

20a What injury is present in this case of blunt force thoracic trauma?

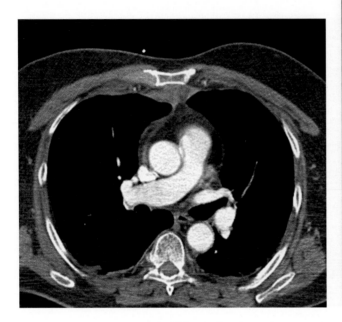
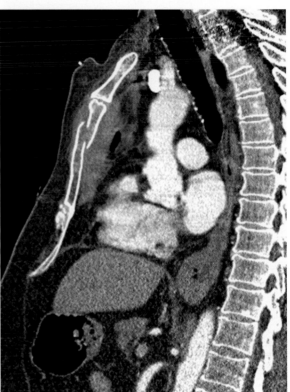

A. Sternal fracture
B. Traumatic aortic injury
C. Cervicothoracic spine burst fracture
D. Esophageal rupture

20b Which of the following diagnostic pitfalls can mimic this type of injury?

A. Aortic pulsation artifact
B. Respiratory motion artifact
C. Streak artifact
D. Surrounding soft tissue injury

ANSWERS AND EXPLANATIONS

1a **Answer C.**

1b **Answer D.**

1c **Answer A.**   Tension pneumothorax is caused by a large volume of air in the pleural space. Often, there is a ball/valve-type mechanism at the site of injury, which allows air in but not out. The entire lung on that side eventually collapses under the pressure, and there can also be a shift of the mediastinal structures to the contralateral side. This shift can cause vascular compromise, and venous structures (being under lower pressure) are the first to be affected causing decreased venous return to the heart and eventually reduced cardiac output. On chest radiograph, if a large pneumothorax is present and there is any shift of mediastinal contents to the contralateral side, a tension pneumothorax should be suggested.

Of the options given, the best radiograph exam to see a pneumothorax on would be an upright frontal view of the chest. For a right-sided pneumothorax, a left lateral decubitus view might also be helpful, or an expiratory view of the chest can often show a smaller pneumothorax better, but those choices were not available.

Reference: Pope TL, Harris JH. *Harris & Harris radiology of emergency medicine*. Lippincott Williams & Wilkins, 2013:522–533.

2a **Answer A.**

2b **Answer B.**   Although the chest radiograph is a diagnostic examination for many blunt traumatic injuries, it is important to remember that it serves only as a screening examination for acute traumatic aortic injury (ATAI). Many radiographic signs are associated with varying degrees of sensitivity and specificity. Widening of the superior mediastinum (>8 cm), enlarged mediastinal to chest width ratio (>0.25), indistinctness of the aortic arch, depression of the left main bronchus, deviation of the trachea to the right, deviation of the nasogastric tube to the right, left apical cap, widening of the paraspinal lines, widening of the right paratracheal stripe, and left hemothorax are all identified in this case except for NG tube deviation (because there is no NG tube).

Computed tomography angiography (CTA) is the standard for evaluation of suspected traumatic aortic injury. The CT appearance varies with location and associated injuries. Mediastinal hematoma nearly always accompanies ATAI. The most common location for ATAI encountered at imaging is the aortic isthmus. A luminal irregularity is usually seen with surrounding hematoma. Pulmonary contusion and laceration, sternal fractures, and rib fractures are commonly associated injuries.

References: Steenburg SD, Ravenel JG, Ikonomidis JS, et al. Acute traumatic aortic injury: imaging evaluation and management. *Radiology* 2008;248:3

Woodring JH, Dillon ML. Radiographic manifestations of mediastinal hemorrhage from blunt chest trauma. *Ann Thorac Surg* 1984;37:171–178

3 **Answer C.**   Persistent pneumothorax after chest tube placement could indicate improper chest tube placement (entire tube or side hole outside of the thoracic cage) or function (clogged or kinked tube). However, if the chest tube is properly positioned, which can be confirmed with imaging, and the chest tube is still functioning (persistent air leak), then air is still entering the pleural space. In trauma, a persistent air leak is most likely from a bronchial tear. The larger the injured bronchus, the more brisk the air leak will be. If the chest tube is not able to clear the air faster than it enters the pleural space, then a persistent pneumothorax will remain.

Reference: Pope TL, Harris JH. *Harris & Harris radiology of emergency medicine.* Lippincott Williams & Wilkins, 2013:533.

4   Answer D.   Tracheal diverticulum or paratracheal air cysts are normal variants that can be seen along the right posterior aspect of the trachea at the level of the upper mediastinum (as seen in this case). When seen in the setting of trauma, these can be confused for mediastinal gas, but awareness of this normal variant can help the radiologist make the correct diagnosis. Some have speculated that this finding is associated with increased pressures in the trachea and a focal weakness in the wall that allows it to develop over time, but others suggest that it is a congenital anomaly. When a small focus of gas is seen in this location adjacent to the trachea, the radiologist should do a diligent search for other foci of potential pneumomediastinum, but in the absence of other signs of injury, the differential should strongly favor tracheal diverticulum.

Reference: Buterbaugh JE, Erly WK. Paratracheal air cysts: a common finding on CT examinations of the cervical spine and neck that may mimic pneumomediastinum in patients with traumatic injuries. *AJNR Am J Neuroradiol* 2008;29(6):1218–1221.

5a   Answer B.

5b   Answer C.   A sternoclavicular (SC) dislocation can be difficult to diagnose on radiograph due to overlying structures, but asymmetry of the clavicles should raise concern for this injury. CT is the best modality to diagnose SC dislocation and might demonstrate anterior or posterior position of the medial clavicle in relation to the manubrium. Posterior SC dislocation on the left should raise concern for left subclavian vein injury because of close proximity and impingement by the displaced clavicle.

References: MacDonald PB, Lapointe P. Acromioclavicular and sternoclavicular joint injuries. *Orthop Clin North Am*; 2008;39(4):535–545.

Pope TL, Harris JH. *Harris & Harris radiology of emergency medicine.* Lippincott Williams & Wilkins, 2013:512.

6   Answer D.   Mediastinal hemorrhage can come from many different sources in the setting of trauma. Direct hemorrhage from the aorta or other large artery/vein is perhaps the most concerning and life threatening, but patients with aortic transection or complete tear rarely live long enough to have a CT scan. In patients that do survive to receive CT imaging, the source of anterior mediastinal hemorrhage is most often from smaller vessels within the mediastinum. Hemorrhage from a sternal fracture is more likely to be directly posterior to the sternum. Any mediastinal hemorrhage, but especially periaortic hemorrhage, should prompt thorough evaluation for large-vessel injury such as the aortic injury shown.

Reference: Pope TL, Harris JH. *Harris & Harris radiology of emergency medicine.* Lippincott Williams & Wilkins, 2013:546.

7   Answer A.   Tension pneumopericardium is a life-threatening event. Small amounts of air in the pericardial sac can be tolerated without symptoms, but once the amount of air is enough to raise the intrapericardial pressures above 265 mm Hg, the heart may experience decreased function. Imaging signs include large volume of air in the pericardial sac, flattening of the anterior border of the heart, and engorgement of IVC/SVC. Treatment is with emergent needle decompression or pericardial drain placement. Trauma is the most common cause of pneumopericardium.

Pulmonary laceration and pericardial effusion are not identified in this case. There is a pneumothorax with no CT findings of tension, but there is evidence of pericardial tension.

Reference: Katabathina VS, Restrepo CS, Martinez-Jimenez S, et al. Nonvascular, nontraumatic mediastinal emergencies in adults: a comprehensive review of imaging findings. *Radiographics* 2011;31(4):1141–1160.

8 **Answer C.** At least one view of the heart should be part of a focused assessment with sonography in trauma (FAST). The heart can be imaged either by a subxiphoid approach or between the ribs just to the left of the sternum. Patient body habitus, lung volume, and current acute injuries might make one location better than the other for viewing the heart. A pericardial effusion in the setting of trauma, especially penetrating chest trauma, should raise concern for cardiac injury. Even a small pericardial effusion might be a sign of bleeding, which can enlarge quickly to cause cardiac tamponade.

Reference: Körner M, Krötz MM, Degenhart C, et al. Current role of emergency US in patients with major trauma. *Radiographics* 2008;28(1):225–242.

9 **Answer B.** While the most common aspirated foreign body in children and adults is food such as a peanut, in the setting of a patient with maxillofacial injury, care should be taken to find any missing teeth to help prevent aspiration of them. Mobile teeth within the oral cavity can be pushed further into the trachea or bronchi during intubation. In the case above, the patient had extensive facial fractures and two missing teeth. One was still in the posterior pharynx, but the second was down in the left lower lobe bronchi as seen on both x-ray and CT. Note enamel is frequently even more dense than is cortical bone.

Reference: Casap N, Alterman M, Leiberman S, et al. Enigma of missing teeth in maxillofacial trauma. *J Oral Maxillofac Surg* 69(5):1421–1429.

10 **Answer A.** The actual bullet path causes direct tissue damage and is often referred to as the permanent cavity. The bullet also causes a pressure wave, which causes tissue damage from outward stretching and shearing forces. The faster the bullet is traveling, the greater kinetic energy it has and thus the larger pressure wave it will generate. This additional area of tissue injury is called a blast cavity or temporary cavity. It is important to find the bullet pathway in a patient with gunshot injury so that you can assess for direct damage from the permanent cavity as well as indirect damage from the adjacent blast cavity.

Reference: University of Utah. Patterns of Tissue Injury. http://library.med.utah.edu/WebPath/TUTORIAL/GUNS/GUNINJ.html

11a **Answer C.**

11b **Answer B.**

11c **Answer A.** Acute traumatic aortic injury (ATAI) includes a wide range of injuries from complete rupture all the way to minimal intimal injuries. Patients with full-thickness tears rarely survive long enough to undergo imaging. A common type of partial-thickness tear is a pseudoaneurysm. In an aortic pseudoaneurysm, the two inner layers (intima and media) are torn but the outer layer (adventitia) remains intact. The adventitia provides approximately 60% of the tensile strength of the aortic wall.

On CT, the most common location of ATAI is at the region of the ligamentum arteriosum, also known as the aortic isthmus. This location accounts for 50% to 71% of ATAI. The reason injuries are common here is because the ligamentum arteriosum acts as a tether point for the otherwise mildly mobile aorta within the thoracic cage. In total, injuries involving the aortic root are actually more common, but initial survival of these is so low that they are much less frequently imaged.

References: Pope TL, Harris JH. *Harris & Harris radiology of emergency medicine.* Lippincott Williams & Wilkins, 2013:542–564.

Soto JA, Lacey BC. *The Requisites: emergency Radiology.* Mosby Inc, 2009:63–64.

12 **Answer D.** Fat embolism syndrome should be considered in polytrauma patients with long bone or pelvic injuries and persistent hypoxemia after initial resuscitation. Imaging features of fat embolism syndrome are nonspecific, and common CT findings include areas of consolidation, ground-glass opacities, and small nodules of various sizes. Fat attenuation filling defects in the pulmonary arteries are not typically seen. The imaging presented shows fat attenuation clot within the right superficial femoral vein (not typically seen).

Reference: Nucifora G, Hysko F, Vit A, et al. Pulmonary fat embolism: common and unusual computed tomography findings. *J Comput Assist Tomogr* 2007;31(5):806–807.

13a **Answer B.**

13b **Answer A.** The sagittal reconstructed image below of case 13A (left) more clearly shows the acute left diaphragmatic hernia. Coronal reconstructed image of case 13B (right) shows further herniation of the liver from the acute right diaphragmatic hernia.

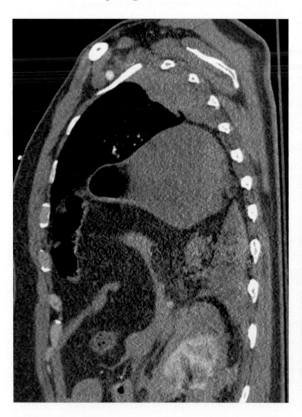 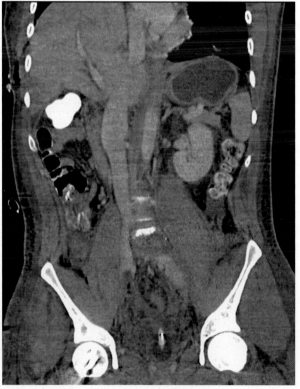

The dependent viscera sign describes abdominal viscera lying directly on the chest wall as an intact diaphragm is no longer present to lift the abdominal contents off the posterior chest wall. In this example, the spleen is lying directly on the dependent chest wall, high in the thoracic cavity. The collar sign describes a collar- or waist-like constriction of abdominal contents as they pass through a tear or defect in the diaphragm. In this case, the liver is constricted by a defect in the right hemidiaphragm. A common pitfall in diagnosis of a diaphragmatic hernia is focal eventration or unilateral paralysis of the diaphragm. Presence of acute traumatic injury (hemothorax, hemoperitoneum, pneumothorax) and the signs described above should aid in the diagnosis of acute diaphragmatic hernias. The bulging fissure sign refers to lobar pneumonia with a particular focus on Klebsiella. The colon cutoff sign refers to an abrupt change in caliber of the colon at the level of the splenic flexure with gaseous distension proximally and nondistension distally and is specifically associated with pancreatitis resulting in focal adynamic ileus.

References: Cantwell CP. The dependent viscera sign. *Radiology* 2006;238(2):752–753.

Killeen KL, Mirvis SE, Shanmuganathan K. Helical CT of diaphragmatic rupture caused by blunt trauma. *AJR Am J Roentgenol* 1999;173(6):1611–1616.

14 **Answer A.**   Minimal aortic injury is a newly recognized entity likely owing to improved spatial and temporal resolution of modern multidetector CT. Injury of the aorta is isolated to the intima. Although there are few data regarding the long-term morbidity associated with minimal aortic injury, many of the injuries resolve or are stable at imaging follow-up. Most experts currently recommend no intervention for minimal aortic injury without progression and would agree that follow-up CTA should be performed to document resolution or stability. This follow-up CTA 48 hours later demonstrates complete resolution of the intimal injuries in this case.

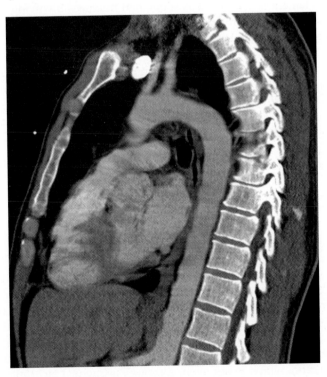

Reference: Steenburg SD, Ravenel JG, Ikonomidis JS, et al. Acute traumatic aortic injury: imaging evaluation and management. *Radiology* 2008;248(3):748–762.

15 **Answer A.** Pulmonary lacerations occur when a tear of the parenchyma results in a cavity in the lung. The surrounding normal lung pulls away from the laceration resulting in a rounded cavity seen at CT. Lacerations are often accompanied by rib fractures, pneumothorax, hemothorax, and surrounding contusion and may be uni- or multilocular. Appearance may also vary depending on contents, for example, air, blood, or both. Treatment is generally supportive with variable degrees of scarring noted after healing.

In this case, the location is atypical for postprimary tuberculosis, which would most commonly involve the apical and posterior upper lobe segments or the superior lower lobe segments. The degree of consolidation and ground glass surrounding the cystic lesion would be unusual for a CCAM/CPAM. As far as cavitary neoplasm, this case demonstrates a very thin, smooth wall, which is much more common in benign etiologies than in malignancy (more frequently >1 to 1.5 cm in thickness and irregular).

Reference: Kaewlai R, Avery LL, Asrani AV, et al. Multidetector CT of blunt thoracic trauma. *Radiographics* 2008;28(6):1555–1570.

16 **Answer C.** Imaging appearance of pulmonary contusions consists of patchy airspace opacities or areas of consolidation adjacent to the region of injury without respect to bronchopulmonary distribution. Subpleural sparing or 1 to 2 mm of clear parenchyma beneath the pleural surface is an imaging sign that is often observed. Contusions are frequently not readily visible on conventional radiography.

References: Kaewlai R, Avery LL, Asrani AV, et al. Multidetector CT of blunt thoracic trauma. *Radiographics* 2008;28(6):1555–1570.

Donnelly LF, Klosterman LA. Subpleural sparing: a CT finding of lung contusion in children. *Radiology* 1997;204(2):385–387.

17 **Answer B.** Flail chest is defined as segmental fractures involving three or more contiguous ribs. The fracture pattern creates a flail segment, which can move paradoxically relative to the remainder of the chest. The diaphragm would move normally unless there is an additional diaphragmatic injury. Flail chest indicates the presence of significant blunt thoracic trauma and is associated with increased morbidity and mortality, prolonged mechanical ventilation, and increased risk of pneumonia. Management depends on each institution's preference and level of expertise. Both surgical management and conservative management have been utilized to manage these physiologically complex injuries.

References: Kaewlai R, Avery LL, Asrani AV, et al. Multidetector CT of blunt thoracic trauma. *Radiographics* 2008;28(6):1555–1570.

Tanaka H, Yukioka T, Yamaguti Y, et al. Surgical stabilization of internal pneumatic stabilization? A prospective randomized study of management of severe flail chest patients. *J Trauma* 2002;52(4):727–732; discussion 32.

18a **Answer C.**

18b **Answer A.** All of the diseases listed can cause pneumomediastinum. However, the pattern of pneumomediastinum in this patient is diffuse with a particular predilection for surrounding the esophagus. In penetrating injury, one would expect to see a focal site of soft tissue emphysema to correlate with the skin entrance site. In the setting of infection and mediastinitis, this degree of pneumomediastinum would be associated with severe mediastinal edema and inflammation, which is not seen. Although a tracheal laceration would be a consideration, a bronchial injury would be expected to be much more asymmetric with a significant component of pulmonary interstitial emphysema or pneumothorax.

Boerhaave syndrome is rupture of the esophagus and most commonly occurs at the gastroesophageal junction after forceful vomiting as this case demonstrates. Pneumomediastinum, pneumothorax, and pleural effusions are commonly seen at imaging. Although the fluoroscopic images above demonstrate extravasation of oral contrast, it is important to know that false-negative examinations have been reported to be as high as 20%. Boerhaave's remains a rare cause of esophageal rupture but should be considered among other pathologic entities when the nonspecific imaging findings are encountered. In this case, blunt trauma sufficient to cause esophageal rupture would almost certainly result in other thoracic injuries, which are not identified. Similarly, there is no penetrating chest wound to correlate with a gunshot or knife wound in penetrating trauma. Impacted food bolus can result in esophageal wall necrosis if untreated, but the esophagram demonstrates no such impaction.

References: Ghanem N, Altehoefer C, Springer O, et al. Radiological findings in Boerhaave's syndrome. *Emerg Radiol* 2003;10(1):8–13.

Backer CL, LoCicero J, III, Hartz RS, et al. Computed tomography in patients with esophageal perforation. *Chest* 1990;98(5):1078–1080.

Bladergroen MR, Lowe JE, Postlethwait RW. Diagnosis and recommended management of esophageal perforation and rupture. *Ann Thorac Surg* 1986;42(3):235–239.

19a **Answer B.**

19b **Answer C.** Discontinuity of the thoracic spine indicates significant blunt traumatic injury. The thoracic spine is relatively rigid and has approximately four times the axial load-bearing capacity compared to the lumbar spine. Much of the increased strength is attributed to the multiple articulations and connection to the sternum via the ribs. Significant injuries of the thoracic spine are usually catastrophic with 50% having neurologic injuries. This at least in part relates to the relatively narrow central canal in the thoracic segments.

The fracture–dislocation patterns of injuries represent a majority of these significant injuries, as shown in the case above. This pattern is associated with significant surrounding soft tissue injury because of the dislocation and frequent rotational component. Chance fractures are a type of flexion–distraction injury most frequently occurring lower in the thoracic spine or in the upper lumbar spine. The Chance fracture injury pattern is that of distraction at a focal point, typically resulting in a three-column injury. It could be similar in appearance to this case, but this case demonstrates an even more significant dislocation than typically seen in those cases without the same degree of posterior column widening. Compression fractures involve the anterior column and do not typically result in neurologic compromise. Burst fractures involve loss of height of the anterior and posterior vertebral bodies, typically from a significant axial loading injury.

References: Patel AA, Vaccaro AR. Thoracolumbar spine trauma classification. *J Am Acad Orthop Surg* 2010;18(2):63–71.

Harris MB, Shi LL, Vacarro AR, et al. Nonsurgical treatment of thoracolumbar spinal fractures. *Instr Course Lect* 2009;58:629–637.

20a **Answer A.**

20b **Answer B.** Sternal fractures are relatively uncommon blunt traumatic injuries and occur at a frequency of approximately 5%. Most of the time, fractures are associated with anterior mediastinal hematoma, which aids in the detection of these injuries. Unfortunately, many trauma CT scans are degraded by respiratory motion artifact, which serves as a pitfall in diagnosis/misdiagnosis.

Conventional radiography can be performed but is of limited utility. It is important to realize sternal fractures are usually accompanied by concomitant injuries (rib fractures, sternoclavicular dislocation, cardiac contusion, pneumothorax, etc.). Management usually depends on these concomitant injuries rather than the sternal fracture itself unless there is severe displacement of the fragments.

A traumatic aortic injury is not seen although there is significant respiratory motion and aortic pulsation artifact resulting in a broken reconstruction of the aorta on the sagittal image. These should not be confused for evidence of aortic injury but do limit the sensitivity of the exam. Similarly, beam hardening at the thoracic inlet frequently occurs resulting in decreased sensitivity for cervicothoracic injury. There is no pneumomediastinum or esophageal wall thickening to suggest esophageal injury. Note, there is an esophageal hernia, but this should not be confused with a traumatic injury.

Reference: Khoriati AA, Rajakulasingam R, Shah R. Sternal fractures and their management. *J Emerg Trauma Shock* 2013;6(2):113–116.

11 Congenital Disease (Adult Presentations)

QUESTIONS

1a What is the diagnosis?

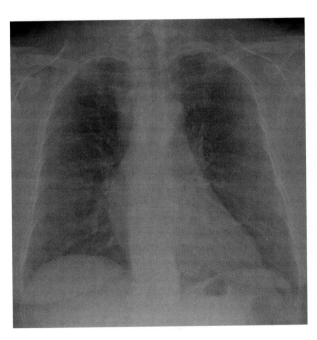

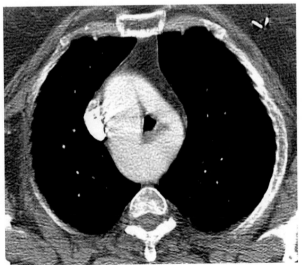

A. Lymphoma
B. Double aortic arch
C. Pulmonary sling
D. Esophageal cancer

1b Double aortic arch is the most common:

A. Cause of rib notching
B. Thoracic congenital aortic arch anomaly
C. Aortic anomaly seen with bicuspid aortic valve
D. Cause of vascular ring

2a The radiographic abnormality is localized to the:

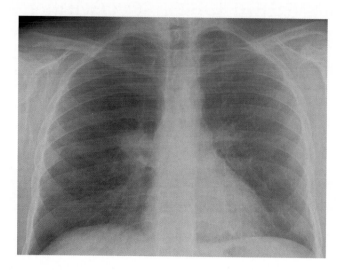

A. Hilar angle
B. Right paratracheal stripe
C. Azygoesophageal line
D. Chest wall

2b Findings are most consistent with which congenital or developmental anomaly?

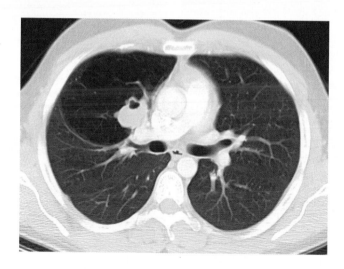

A. Lobar emphysema
B. Pulmonary adenomatoid malformation
C. Bronchial atresia
D. Swyer-James syndrome

3 What is the characteristic vascular supply and drainage associated with extralobar pulmonary sequestration?

A. Pulmonary arteries and systemic veins
B. Systemic arteries and pulmonary veins
C. Systemic arteries and systemic veins
D. Pulmonary arteries and pulmonary veins

4a Disease is localized to which pulmonary lobe?

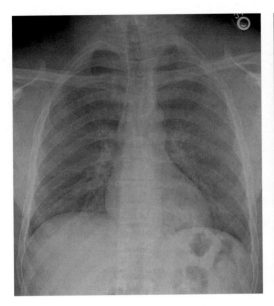 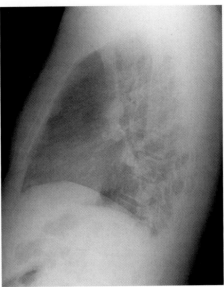

    A. Right upper
    B. Left upper
    C. Right middle
    D. Left lower

4b Which of the following would be most likely in this 28-year-old male with recurrent pneumonias localized to the left lower lobe?

    A. Hypogenetic lung syndrome
    B. Partial anomalous pulmonary venous return
    C. Congenital lobar emphysema
    D. Pulmonary sequestration

4c In this sequestration, the vessel overlying the left hemidiaphragm must:

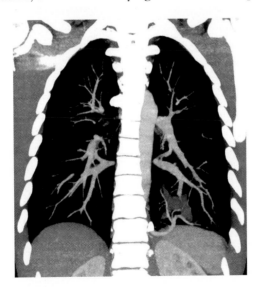

    A. Arise from a pulmonary artery
    B. Drain into a systemic vein
    C. Arise from a systemic artery
    D. Drain into a pulmonary vein

5 The vascular anomaly present:

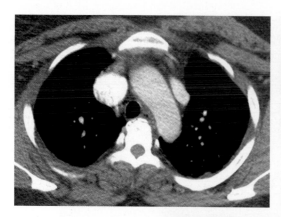
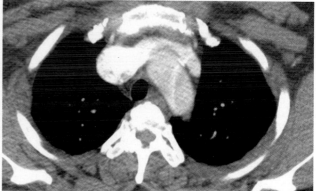
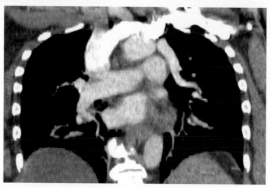

A. Represents a left-to-right shunt
B. Is associated with increased infection
C. Commonly causes dysphagia
D. Most commonly occurs in the left lower lobe

6a Which radiographic shadow is distorted?

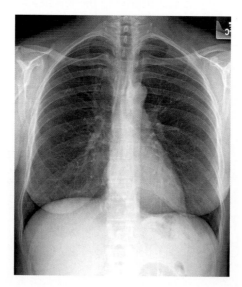

A. Right paratracheal stripe
B. Paraspinal line
C. Azygoesophageal line
D. Anterior junction line

6b What is the most likely cause?

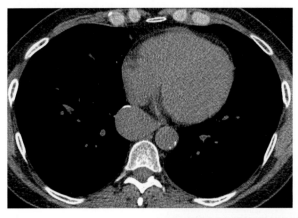
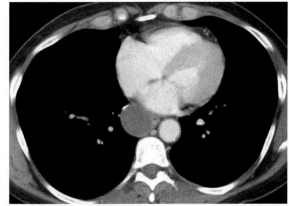

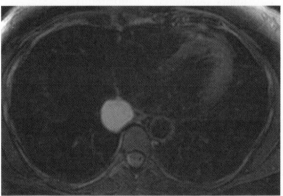

A. Lymphoma
B. Esophageal cancer
C. Foregut duplication cyst
D. Angiosarcoma

7a What imaging pattern is demonstrated on this inspiratory chest CT?

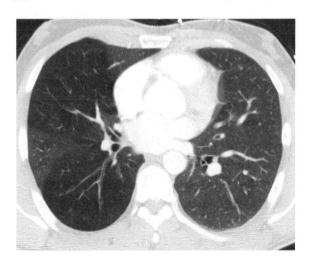

A. Ground-glass opacities
B. Centrilobular nodularity
C. Parahilar nodules
D. Mosaic attenuation

7b What is the most likely cause of the unilateral hyperlucency in this 25-year-old male?

    A. Bronchial atresia

    B. Congenital lobar emphysema

    C. Congenital pulmonary airway malformation

    D. Swyer-James syndrome

7c What is the most common cause of childhood obliterative bronchiolitis (Swyer-James syndrome)?

    A. Human immunodeficiency virus

    B. In utero vascular insult

    C. Toxic fume exposure

    D. Pediatric adenovirus infection

8a Characterize the primary pulmonary abnormality.

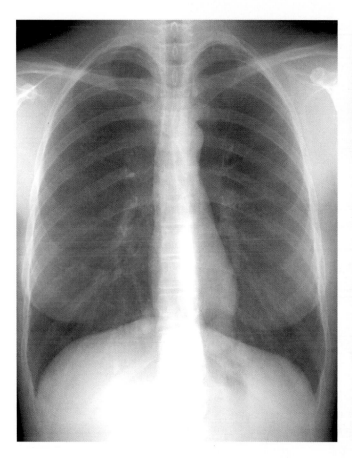 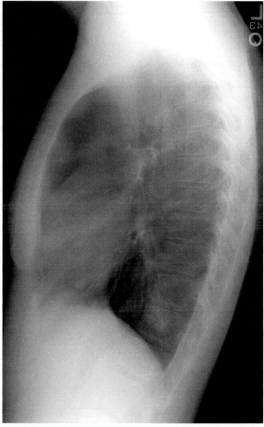

    A. Reticular opacities

    B. Nodules

    C. Consolidation

    D. Pleural effusion

8b These findings represent:

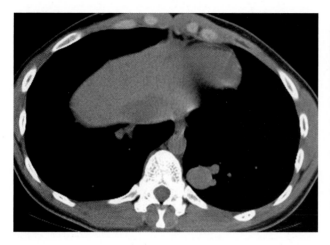 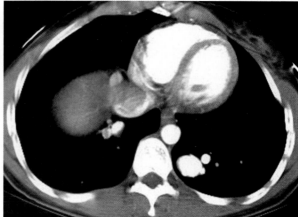

   A. A right-to-left shunt
   B. Malignancy
   C. Carney triad
   D. Prior granulomatous infection

8c Which test has the highest SENSITIVITY for detection of pulmonary AVM in the setting of hereditary hemorrhagic telangiectasia?

   A. Tc-99m macroaggregated albumin pulmonary shunt study
   B. Calculation of abnormal AaPO$_2$ gradient
   C. Transthoracic agitated saline contrast echocardiogram
   D. Anteroposterior chest radiograph

9 What is the most common presentation of the anomaly shown?

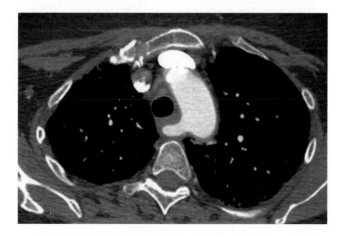

   A. Incidental
   B. Dysphagia lusoria
   C. Aortic dissection
   D. Rib notching

10a What is the diagnosis?

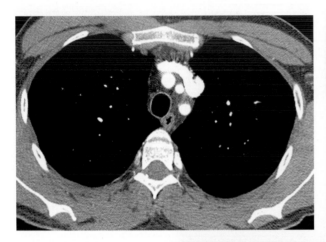
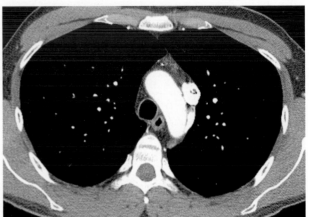

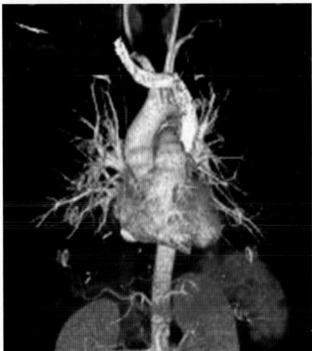

    A. Left-sided superior vena cava

    B. Double aortic arch

    C. Pulmonary sling

    D. Congenital interruption of the inferior vena cava

10b When might this congenital anomaly require surgical correction?

    A. Drainage into the coronary sinus

    B. Drainage into the right atrium

    C. Drainage into the left atrium

    D. Drainage into the hemiazygos vein

11a Localize the radiographic abnormality.

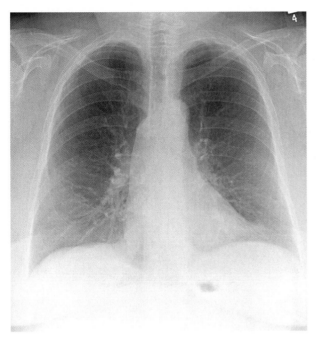 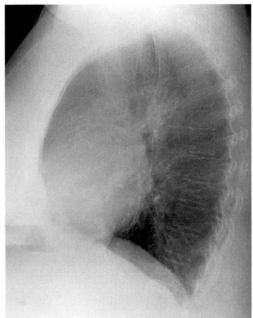

A. Lungs
B. Mediastinum
C. Bones
D. Chest wall

11b The anomalous vessel on the oblique CT image is a:

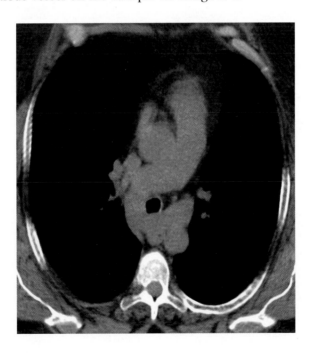

A. Systemic vein
B. Systemic artery
C. Pulmonary vein
D. Pulmonary artery

11c The anomalous left pulmonary artery courses between the:

    A. Esophagus and spine
    B. Esophagus and trachea
    C. Trachea and ascending aorta
    D. Carina and left atrium

12a Based on these CT images, what is the diagnosis?

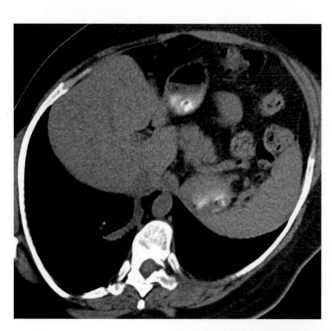
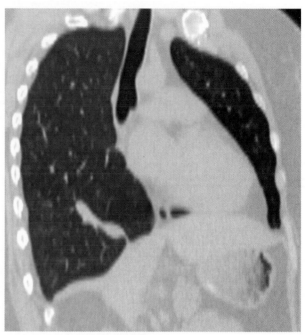
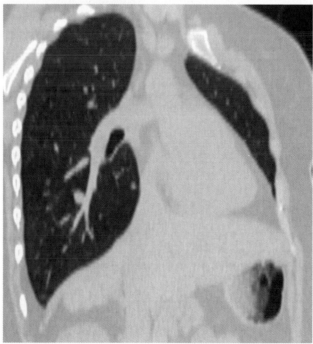

    A. Bronchial atresia
    B. Pulmonary sequestration
    C. Scimitar syndrome
    D. Mucoid impaction syndrome

12b What anomaly associated with scimitar syndrome is present in this patient?

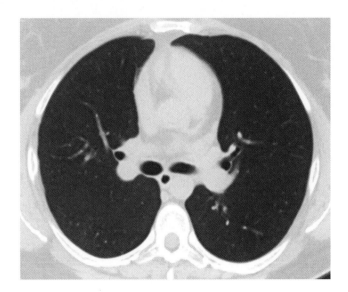

A. Mirror image bronchi
B. Tracheal bronchus
C. Cardiac bronchus
D. Bronchial atresia

13a What chest radiographic finding likely led to obtaining this CT?

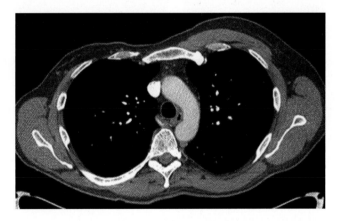

A. Mediastinal widening
B. Hyperinflation of one lung
C. Tracheal narrowing
D. Unilateral hyperlucency

13b What is the diagnosis?

A. Poland syndrome
B. Aortic arch anomaly
C. Foreign body aspiration
D. Left chest wall mass

14a What is the diagnosis based on the CT and V/Q scan?

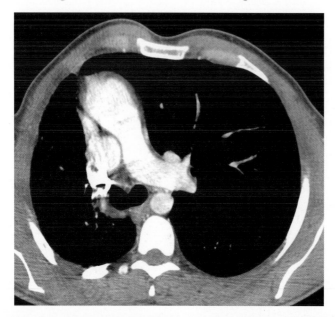

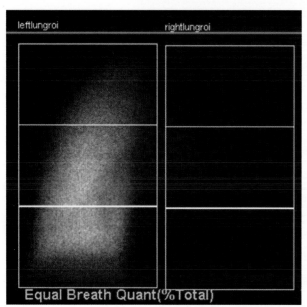

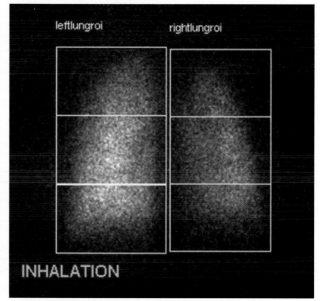

A. Congenital interruption of the right pulmonary artery
B. Congenital atresia of the right mainstem bronchus
C. Congenital absence of the right lung
D. Congenital interruption of the right pulmonary veins

14b What best describes the usual relationship of the interrupted pulmonary artery to the aorta?

A. Occurs opposite the side of the aortic arch
B. Occurs only in the setting of aortic coarctation
C. Occurs on the same side as the aortic arch
D. Occurs with a Kommerell diverticulum

15a What congenital anomaly best accounts for the imaging findings?

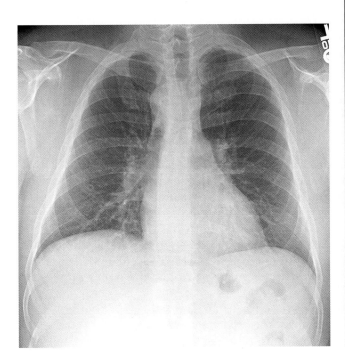 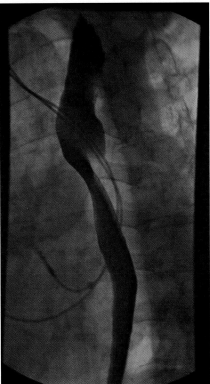

A. Duplicate superior vena cava with left atrial drainage
B. Right-sided aortic arch with mirror image branching
C. Azygos continuation of an interrupted inferior vena cava
D. Right-sided aortic arch with aberrant subclavian artery

15b What is the most likely presentation for the congenital anomaly shown?

A. Paradoxical emboli
B. Pulmonary artery hypertension
C. Dysphagia lusoria
D. Subclavian steal syndrome

ANSWERS AND EXPLANATIONS

1a **Answer B.**

1b **Answer D.** The chest radiograph demonstrates a mild widening of the mediastinum with a well-defined left aortic arch, but a mass impression on the right side of the trachea. Follow-up CT reveals a homogeneous contrast-filled structure surrounding and narrowing the trachea. Taking inventory of the mediastinal structures greatly assists in making the diagnosis, as an image at this level through a normal superior mediastinum needs to contain aorta or arch branch arteries, superior vena cava, esophagus, and trachea. Thoracic lymphoma commonly widens the mediastinum and can compress adjacent structures, but the uniform contrast filling and circumferential distribution around the trachea are inconsistent with a solid tumor of the mediastinum. Pulmonary sling does wrap around the posterior trachea (but in front of the esophagus) but should not arise from or connect to the aortic arch. Additionally, if the axial CT image was at the level of the pulmonary artery, both the ascending and descending portions of the aorta would be visible. Finally, esophageal cancer can certainly surround the esophagus but would not produce this uniform contrast filling consistent with a vascular structure and would be highly unlikely to circumferentially surround the trachea in this way.

Thoracic vascular malformations have particular associations. In double aortic arch, the aorta creates a complete vascular ring, which can cause some compression of the airway and esophagus, resulting in symptoms such as stridor and dysphagia, depending on the degree of compression. Rib notching and bicuspid valve are more closely associated with coarctation of the aorta. Double aortic arch is a relatively rare vascular malformation with a right aortic arch with aberrant left subclavian artery being a much more common congenital anomaly.

Reference: Yilirim A, et al. Congenital thoracic arterial anomalies in adults: a CT overview *Diagn Interv Radiol* 2011;17:352–362.

2a **Answer A.**

2b **Answer C.** Bronchial atresia often manifests on radiograph as a hilar fullness or branching pulmonary opacity from mucoid impaction. In this case, the noncommunicating airway is near completely opacified causing the expected hilar angle, the radiographic right hilar concavity on frontal view at the crossing of the right pulmonary artery and the superior pulmonary vein, to become convex. Lymphadenopathy, hilar mass, and congenital lesions are all considerations and necessitate CT for further evaluation.

The CT image confirms the hilar lesion, which is nonenhancing and of low attenuation and contains a small air component. The associated right upper lobe is hyperexpanded and hyperlucent. Lobar emphysema and Swyer-James syndrome produce varying degrees of hyperlucency and hyperinflation but are not associated with obstructed airway with impaction. Pulmonary adenomatoid malformation generally creates a more bubbly cystic lesion that can look like focal emphysema, again not with the characteristic airway changes.

Occurring most often in the apicoposterior segment of the left upper lobe, the second most common location for bronchial atresia is in the right upper lobe segmental airways. Patients are generally asymptomatic, although some patients may present with recurrent infection. In this latter setting, resection may be required.

Reference: Zylak CJ, et al. Developmental lung anomalies in the adult: radiologic-pathologic correlation. *Radiographics* 2002;22:S25–S43.

3 **Answer C.** Extralobar pulmonary sequestration accounts for approximately 25% of all pulmonary sequestrations with the remaining being intralobar. Nearly all pulmonary sequestrations receive blood supply from the systemic arteries and have variable venous drainage, where the majority of intralobar sequestrations drain to the pulmonary veins and the majority of extralobar sequestrations drain to the systemic veins. Extralobar sequestrations by definition are divided from the normal lung by a pleural investment and most commonly reside between the left lower lobe and hemidiaphragm, although they can occur elsewhere to include the mediastinum, pericardium, diaphragm, and extrathoracic locations. Most commonly identified in infancy, a minority of cases present in adulthood with around 10% of cases incidentally identified in asymptomatic patients. Extralobar sequestrations have a higher rate of associated congenital anomalies compared with intralobar sequestrations, with diaphragmatic hernia being most common. Although these may be asymptomatic, treatment consists of surgical resection.

Reference: Rosado-de-Christenson ML, Frazier AA, Stocker JT, et al. Extralobar sequestration: radiologic-pathologic correlation. *Radiographics* 1993;13:425–441.

4a **Answer D.**

4b **Answer D.**

4c **Answer C.** Positive spine sign on lateral view radiograph supports a lower lobe process, and frontal view correlates with a retrocardiac opacity consistent with a left lower lobe mass-like consolidation. No additional pulmonary parenchymal opacities are present, further confirmed on the follow-up chest CTA.

Recurrent pneumonias isolated to a particular region should raise concern for an underlying lesion or abnormality. In this case, a contrast-filled vessel is seen on coronal MIP CT images extending from the lower mediastinum and diaphragm region to the area of consolidation. In this case, the opacities seen primarily represent mucoid impaction within noncommunicating bronchi. Pulmonary sequestration is defined by systemic arterial supply with rare bronchial connection and variable venous drainage. The affected lung in intralobar sequestration, as seen here, is inseparable from the adjacent normal lung, as opposed to extralobar sequestration, which develops with a pleural boundary separating it from normal lung. Intralobar sequestrations occur most commonly in the left lower lobe. Cases may be discovered incidentally on imaging but can manifest as recurrent infection or massive hemoptysis.

Reference: Zylak CJ, et al. Developmental lung anomalies in the adult: radiologic-pathologic correlation. *Radiographics* 2002;22:S25–S43.

5 **Answer A.** A pulmonary vein is shown draining into the left brachiocephalic vein. By draining a portion of the lung into a systemic vein, the anomaly represents partial anomalous pulmonary venous return (PAPVR). In bypassing the left heart and systemic arterial supply, the oxygenated blood returns to the right heart, increasing the ratio of right heart blood flow consistent with a left-to-right shunt. The majority of PAPVR cases are left upper lobe venous drainage to the left brachiocephalic vein as in this case. Scimitar syndrome is an uncommon variant of PAPVR.

Reference: Rahiah P, Kanne JP. Computed tomography of pulmonary venous variants and anomalies. *J Cardiovasc Comput Tomogr* 2010;4:155–163.

6a **Answer C.**

6b **Answer C.** The azygoesophageal recess represents a portion of the right lower lobe, which extends medially, marginated by the posterior margin of the heart, the anterior margin of the spine, and the right lateral margin of the esophagus. Radiographically, this results in a border that runs vertically over the lower thoracic spine and may deviate a little to the left near the esophageal hiatus. Here, the azygoesophageal border deviates to the right, even extending lateral to the right heart border. The right paratracheal stripe is a line along the right trachea in the superior mediastinum. The anterior junction line is also a superior mediastinal shadow. The paraspinal border by definition will not overlie the spinal column as the azygoesophageal border will.

Noncontrast and contrast-enhanced CT images better demonstrate a low-attenuation nonenhancing right paraesophageal lesion in the lower mediastinum. A small amount of peripheral calcification is present along the anterior aspect, and MR reveals a homogeneous high T2 signal within the lesion all consistent with a foregut duplication cyst. Originating from the embryologic primitive foregut, these mediastinal congenital cysts represent anomalies in the divisions of the foregut from the tracheobronchial tree and neural tube and include bronchogenic cyst, esophageal duplication cyst, and neurenteric cyst.

Reference: Zylak CJ, et al. Developmental lung anomalies in the adult: radiologic-pathologic correlation. *Radiographics* 2002;22:S25–S43.

7a **Answer D.**

7b **Answer D.**

7c **Answer D.** CT image provided in lung window at the level of the aortic root demonstrates relative hyperlucency in regions of the right middle lobe and right lower lobe. This is differentiated from patchy ground-glass opacities by the attenuation of vessels in the hyperlucent lung. While air trapping may be associated with the regions of low attenuation, air trapping is typically an expiratory CT finding, where mosaic attenuation is identified on inspiratory imaging. No significant centrilobular nodularity or parahilar nodules are present on the exams, although normal pulmonary vascular structures may appear as such to the untrained eye.

Each of the pulmonary congenital/developmental abnormalities provided can produce a unilateral hyperlucent lung, but only Swyer-James-(Macleod) syndrome characteristically produces multifocal hyperlucency. In 5 out of 8 patients with Swyer-James syndrome, Moore et al. found multifocal bilateral regions of mosaic attenuation. Congenital lobar emphysema is a consideration for this appearance, but the combination of involvement of the right lower lobe (uncommon) and multifocal nature (rare) makes this diagnosis unlikely. Bronchial atresia is also focal and results from a noncommunicating bronchus often with mucoid impaction, where this case nicely demonstrates patent bronchi in the right lower lobe. Congenital pulmonary airway malformation produces a mass-like or cystic-appearing lesion rather than mosaic attenuation as shown here.

Swyer-James(-Macleod) syndrome is the result of postinfectious obliterative bronchiolitis, due to pediatric pneumonia, particularly adenovirus, but can be seen with other infections such as mycoplasma. Toxic fume exposure can cause obliterative bronchiolitis but is not reported as a significant contributor to childhood obliterative bronchiolitis. HIV had been rarely reported as a cause of obliterative bronchiolitis and not a significant contributor to childhood obliterative bronchiolitis. Outside of infection, follicular bronchiolitis would be a more characteristic small airway manifestation of HIV/AIDS. Finally, while in utero vascular insults may be associated with various pulmonary malformations, it is not a cause of Swyer-James syndrome.

References: Colum AJ, Teper AM, Vollmer WM, et al. Risk factors for the development of bronchiolitis obliterans in children with bronchiolitis. *Thorax* 2006;61:503–506.

Moore ADA, Godwin JD, Dietrich PA, et al. Swyer-James Syndrome: CT findings in eight patients. *AJR Am J Roentgenol* 1992;158:1211–1215.

Wasilewska E, Lee EY, Eisenberg RL. Unilateral hyperlucent lung in children. *AJR Am J Roentgenol* 2012;198:W400–W414.

8a **Answer B.**

8b **Answer A.**

8c **Answer C.** As partial "blind spots" on frontal chest radiograph, the retrocardiac and posterior costophrenic angles are better visualized on lateral exam. If one did not appreciate the large nodular well-defined opacity posterior to the heart projecting over the left diaphragm on the provided frontal chest radiograph, the lateral exam nicely demonstrates a positive spine sign with well-defined margins of a pulmonary nodular opacity. An additional smaller lesion is seen on frontal exam in the medial posterior right lower lobe.

Appropriately, the common concern on the provided chest radiograph is malignancy until proven otherwise. Chest CT with and without contrast demonstrates vascular contrast enhancement of the lesions with dilated feeding arteries and draining veins consistent with pulmonary arteriovenous malformations (AVM) in this case of hereditary hemorrhagic telangiectasia (HHT), also known as Osler-Weber-Rendu disease.

HHT is an autosomal dominant disorder associated with epistaxis, mucocutaneous telangiectasias and visceral AVMs, and (in ~25% of patients with HHT) pulmonary AVMs. The result of pulmonary AVMs is a right-to-left shunt, which potentially allows for paradoxical (systemic) emboli and significant risk of stroke or brain abscess. Due to its high sensitivity and ability for shunt calculation, transthoracic contrast echocardiography is the recommended study for initial screening for pulmonary AVM in the setting of HHT. Tc-99m-labeled macroaggregated serum albumin (MAA), the nuclear medicine "pulmonary shunt study," is highly specific, but less sensitive. The MAA shunt study can semiquantitatively demonstrate degree of shunting with extrapulmonary uptake in the brain and kidneys. Coil embolization is the recommended method of treatment for pulmonary AVMs of significant size.

References: Cottin V, Plauchu H, Bayle J, et al. Pulmonary arteriovenous malformations in patients with hereditary hemorrhagic telangiectasia. *Am J Respir Crit Care Med* 2004;169:994–1000.

Lee EY, Boiselle PM, Cleveland RH. Multidetector CT evaluation of congenital lung anomalies. *Radiology* 2008;247(3):632–648.

9 **Answer A.** While a left aortic arch with aberrant right subclavian artery can occasionally cause dysphagia, this congenital abnormality is generally identified as an incidental finding on imaging. It is the most common aortic arch anomaly. The aberrant right subclavian artery originates as the last arch branch from the aorta with an occasional dilatation of the aorta at its origin, known as Kommerell diverticulum. There is no direct association of the aberrant right subclavian with aortic dissection or rib notching.

Reference: Yildirim A, Karabulut N, Dogan S, et al. Congenital thoracic arterial anomalies in adults: a CT overview. *Diagn Interv Radiol* 2011;17:352–362.

10a **Answer A.**

10b **Answer C.** Despite not seeing the full extent of the anomalous vessel on the provided images, axial CT images demonstrate a contrast-filled structure running vertically along the left lateral aortic arch and connecting to the brachiocephalic veins. The primary differential includes left-sided superior vena cava (the most common superior caval variant) versus partial anomalous pulmonary venous return, but the axial images also reveal an absent right superior vena cava consistent with left-sided SVC. Also, the single projection 3D color reconstruction demonstrates the high density of contrast from the upper extremity intravenous injection confirming the systemic venous flow toward the heart. The majority of persistent left SVC cases drain into systemic veins, particularly the coronary sinus, or directly into the right atrium allowing for the normal flow of blood. A small number of cases will drain into the left atrium, which are often associated with other cardiac anomalies and generally require surgical correction.

Reference: Chung JH, Gunn ML, Godwin JD, et al. Congenital thoracic cardiovascular anomalies presenting in adulthood: a pictorial review. *J Cardiovasc Comput Tomogr* 2009;3(1):S35–S46.

11a **Answer B.**

11b **Answer D.**

11c **Answer B.** The radiographs provided are difficult but do demonstrate changes in the normal mediastinal borders. First, a fullness is seen in the region of the azygos arch with a subtle low origin of the right upper lobe bronchus. Second, the lateral radiograph demonstrates a mass-like opacity posterior to the trachea with a well-defined anterior border. Third, the normal arch of the left pulmonary vein over the top of the left mainstem bronchus is absent. No significant findings are present in the lung, bones, or chest wall.

Pulmonary artery sling can mimic a mediastinal mass posterior to the trachea on chest radiographs. CT definitively characterizes this as an anomalous course of the left pulmonary artery originating from the distal right pulmonary artery and coursing between the trachea and esophagus. While the majority of these cases occur with other congenital anomalies identified in infancy, some isolated cases will present incidentally in adulthood as in this patient.

Reference: Castaner E, Gallardo X, Rimola J, et al. Congenital and acquired pulmonary artery anomalies in the adult: radiologic overview. *Radiographics* 2006;26:349–371.

12a **Answer C.**

12b **Answer A.** Scimitar syndrome has wide breadth of presentations resulting in multiple synonyms to include, but not limited to, venolobar syndrome, hypogenetic lung syndrome, and mirror image lung syndrome. The anomalous draining vein to the inferior vena cava is the primary associated finding although drainage can be into the right atrium or even rarely the left atrium. The anomaly is nearly always right sided, draining a variable portion of the right lung. Pulmonary sequestration is a consideration in this case given the abnormal vessel, but a normal pulmonary arterial supply is shown in the third image. Bronchial atresia can create an abnormal tubular structure in the lung but generally is parahilar or runs parallel to the arteries. Mucoid impaction syndrome is an uncommon condition characterized by bronchial mucoid impactions with rubbery casts that occlude the bronchi and sometimes result in respiratory distress.

The synonyms of scimitar syndrome are useful for remembering the additional findings that can occur. In this case, the patient demonstrates mirror image branching pattern of the bronchi, with the right mainstem bronchus becoming hyparterial and branching into only two lobes. Other cases may demonstrate malformation of the right lung (such as decreased volume correlating with the name hypogenetic lung syndrome), arterial supply, heart, or hemidiaphragm. Usually, the left-to-right shunt is small, with surgical correction reserved for those who are symptomatic.

Reference: Godwin JD, Tarver RD. Scimitar syndrome: four new cases examined with CT. *Radiology* 1986;159:15–20.

13a   Answer D.

13b   Answer A.   Unilateral hyperlucency on chest radiograph has a differential primarily related to pulmonary pathology such as pneumothorax, foreign body aspiration with hyperinflation, and congenital anomalies. It is important to remember the contribution of the chest wall to the apparent density of the hemithorax. Just as a unilateral mastectomy can create hyperlucency, the congenital absence of the pectoral muscle in Poland syndrome results in a decrease in x-ray attenuation. Similarly, asymmetry on chest CT may cause one to question a contralateral chest wall mass, when in fact the asymmetry is normal pectoral muscle on one side (the left in this case) and absent pectoral muscle on the affected side.

Mutlu H, et al. A variant of Poland syndrome associated with dextroposition. *J Thorac Imaging* 2007;22:341–342.

14a   Answer A.

14b   Answer A.   Congenital interruption of the proximal pulmonary artery occurs despite development of the lung and airways. The provided CT demonstrates normal bifurcation of the trachea with a hypoplastic right lung and no associated right pulmonary artery. The subsequent ventilation perfusion scan further demonstrates functional ventilation of the right lung, but an absence of perfusion. Pulmonary vein atresia can occur but would demonstrate a present right pulmonary artery (usually small) with perfusion on ventilation–perfusion scintigraphy.

Interestingly, the interrupted pulmonary artery occurs typically opposite of the aortic arch, meaning that if the left pulmonary artery is interrupted, the patient will also have a right aortic arch. Interruption of the right pulmonary artery, as seen in this case, is more common and occurs with a normal left aortic arch and generally absence of other congenital anomalies. Patients may present incidentally or have associate symptoms from infection, hemorrhage, or general mild dyspnea. Pulmonary arterial hypertension is a common complication.

References: Castaner E, Gallardo X, Rimola J, et al. Congenital and acquired pulmonary artery anomalies in the adult: radiologic overview. *Radiographics* 2006;26:349–371.

Heyneman LE, Nolan RL, Harrison JK, et al. Congenital unilateral pulmonary vein atresia: radiologic findings in three adult patients. *AJR Am J Roentgenol* 2001;177:681–685.

15a   Answer D.

15b   Answer C.   The frontal chest radiograph demonstrates a right-sided aortic arch producing a well-defined round opacity right of the trachea with absence of the expected arch shadow left of the trachea and superior to the left pulmonary artery. The subsequent image is selected from an esophagram demonstrating the impression from the right aortic arch and associated focal narrowing due to the vascular ring from an aberrant right subclavian artery connecting to the left pulmonary artery via the ligamentum arteriosum. The vascular ring results in esophageal narrowing, which causes dysphagia lusoria (related to the Greek phrase lusus naturae and translates to "difficulty swallowing in the freak of nature"), although dysphagia lusoria was originally described in the setting of right aberrant subclavian artery. The other provided clinical presentations are not significantly associated with this congenital anomaly.

A right aortic arch with mirror imaging does not produce a retroesophageal vessel and therefore does not contribute directly to dysphagia or esophageal narrowing, but it does have a high association with congenital heart disease. Duplicate SVC would not explain the absence of a normal aortic arch, would not produce a significant right paratracheal shadow, and would not cause focal narrowing of the esophagus at the level of the aortic arch. Azygos continuation of an interrupted IVC could produce dilatation of the azygos arch and increased opacity in the right paratracheal region, but would not explain the absence of the normal aortic arch nor the esophageal narrowing on esophagram.

Reference: Yilirim A, et al. Congenital thoracic arterial anomalies in adults: a CT overview. *Diagn Interv Radiol* 2011;17:352–362.

Postoperative Thorax

1   A 45-year-old lady has fever and leukocytosis 5 days after a right upper lobectomy. Part of her workup includes the CT scan shown. Findings are most consistent with:

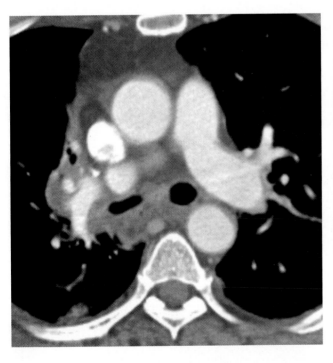 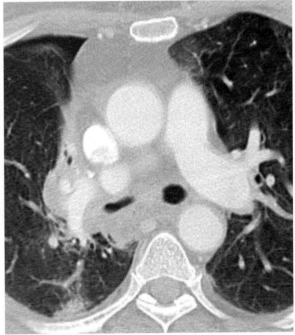

A. Bronchopleural fistula
B. Empyema
C. Lobar torsion
D. Pneumonia

2 A 78-year-old man underwent pneumonectomy for a central squamous cell carcinoma. Six months postoperatively, his follow-up chest CT is shown demonstrating a significant volume of pleural fluid and diffuse pleural thickening. This pleural fluid most likely represents:

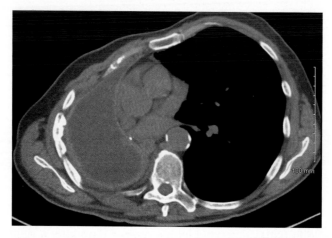

A. Purulent fluid
B. Serous fluid
C. Chylothorax
D. Hemothorax

3 A 24-year-old patient presents for outpatient follow-up after pneumonectomy. Her postoperative course was complicated by bronchial stump dehiscence necessitating reexploration, drainage, and creation of an Eloesser flap. The CT scan above demonstrates an abnormality in the right pleural space, which represents:

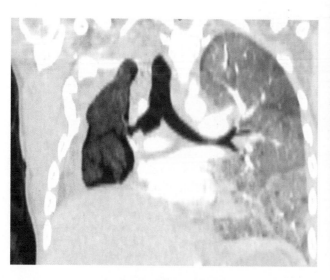
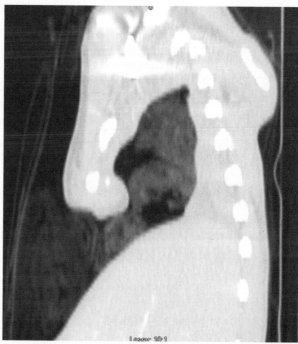

A. Aspergillus infection
B. Retained dressing material
C. Muscle flap
D. Blood clot

4 Five years after pneumonectomy, a 62-year-old lady complains of weight loss, worsening wheeze, dysphagia, and acid reflux. Her symptoms, barium swallow, and chest CT (oblique Maximum Intensity Projection images, MIP) are most suggestive of:

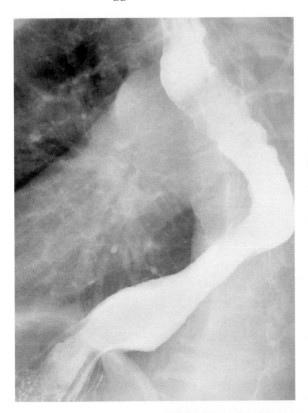
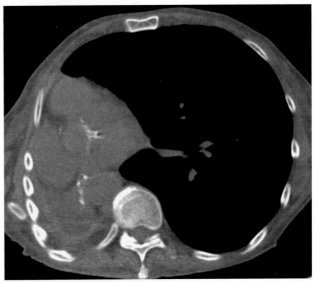
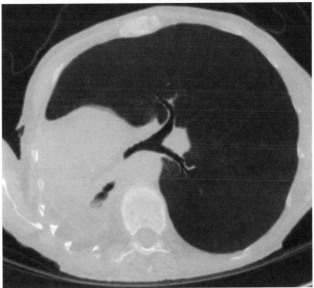

A. Achalasia with aspiration
B. Nutcracker esophagus
C. Postpneumonectomy syndrome
D. Hiatal hernia

5   A tracheal stent has been placed for benign tracheobronchomalacia (TBM) in a patient with COPD. What is the most significant and likely long-term complication of tracheal stent placement in this case?

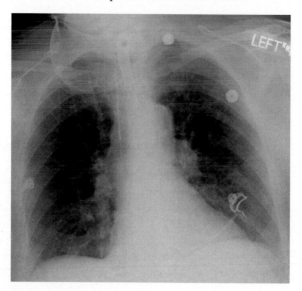

A. Stent migration
B. Malposition of tracheostomy
C. Mucus plug formation
D. Granulation tissue

6   A 66-year-old lady underwent definitive radiation for a central lung tumor. A long-segment stricture has been treated with an esophageal stent as seen in the x-ray. In the following days, what complication is most likely to occur?

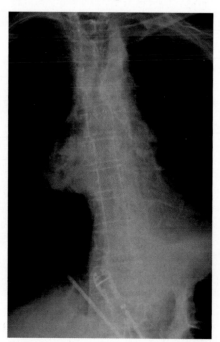

A. Stent migration
B. Stent erosion
C. Stent collapse
D. Stent occlusion

7 These CT scout films are taken 1 year apart (initial on the left, follow-up on the right) and most likely represent which surgical procedure?

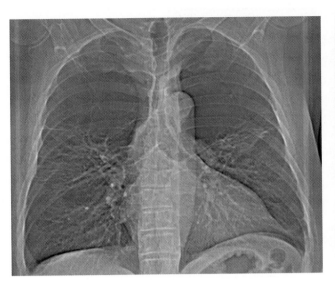 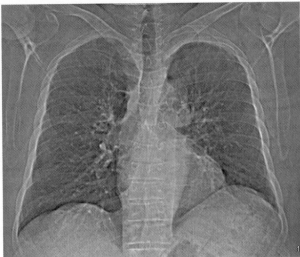

A. Bilateral lung transplant
B. Lung volume reduction surgery
C. Diaphragm plication
D. Pleurodesis

8 A 51-year-old patient returns after surgical treatment for esophageal cancer. He complains of reflux. His CT scan is shown, and findings are suggestive of a(n):

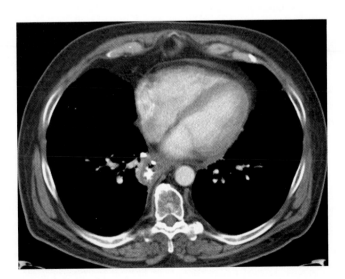

A. Hiatal hernia
B. Normal postoperative appearance
C. Anastomotic stricture
D. Ventral hernia

9 On postoperative day 8, fever and leukocytosis after esophagectomy prompted a CT scan. The image shown is most consistent with:

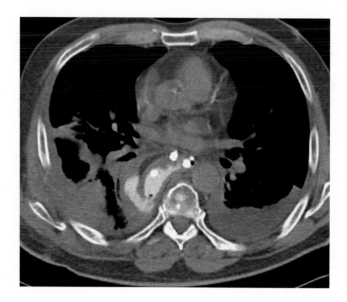

A. Anastomotic leak
B. Pneumonia
C. Gastric tip necrosis
D. Bronchopleural fistula

10 A 60-year-old lady has the provided CT scan with bilateral focal central airway stenoses necessitating endobronchial stents. She most likely is suffering from:

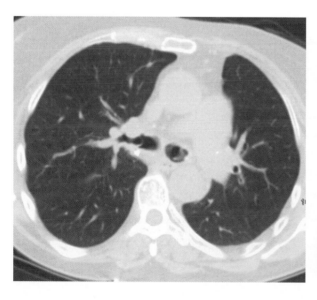 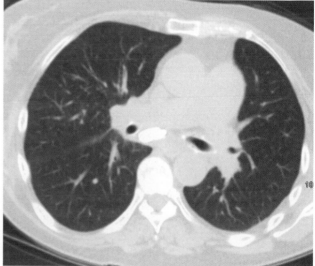

A. Fibrosing mediastinitis
B. Post–lung transplant bronchial stenosis
C. Tracheobronchomalacia
D. Pulmonary fibrosis

11 What do these images most likely represent?

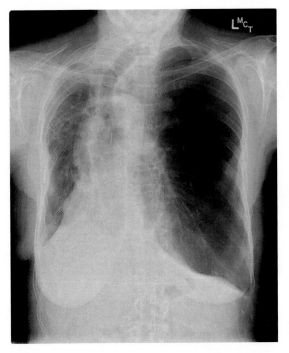

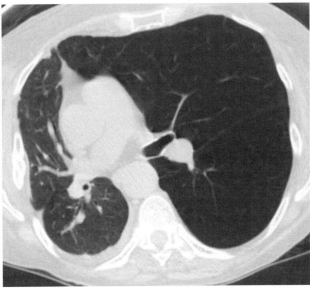

    A. Normal right lung, unilateral bullous disease on the left
    B. Normal left lung, status post lobectomy on the right
    C. Transplanted right lung, hyperinflated native left lung
    D. Transplanted left lung, atrophied native right lung

12 A patient presents with pleuritic chest pain 6 months after a thoracoscopic
    procedure. CT scan is shown and most likely represents:

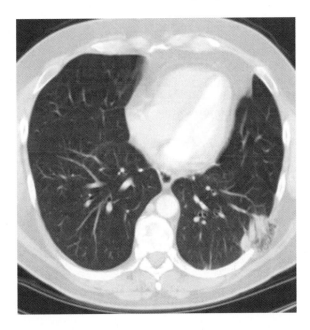

    A. Seroma at the surgical site
    B. Intercostal lung hernia
    C. Osteosarcoma
    D. Empyema necessitans

13 A patient who underwent routine CABG 1 month ago presents with new and worsening chest pain. Imaging shown demonstrates:

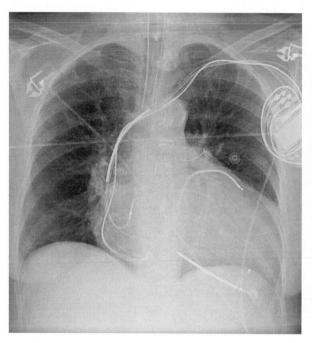 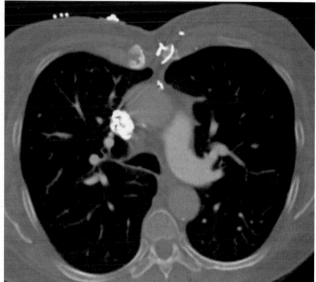

A. Aortic dissection
B. Pulmonary embolus
C. Sternal dehiscence
D. SVC thrombosis

14 Five days after bilateral lung transplant, a patient has worsening mediastinal and subcutaneous emphysema on both exam and chest x-ray. The most likely diagnosis is:

A. Alveolar air leak due to procurement injury
B. Acute rejection
C. Bronchial dehiscence
D. Iatrogenic esophageal injury

15 On each progressive day after bilateral lung transplant, the surgical team is concerned about chest x-rays that show progressive opacification of both lungs with inability to wean the patient from the ventilator. Which imaging test should be performed?

A. Ventilation–perfusion scan
B. Noncontrast chest CT scan
C. Transesophageal echocardiogram
D. Contrast-enhanced chest CT scan

ANSWERS AND EXPLANATIONS

1   **Answer C.**   Contrast chest CT demonstrates narrowing of both the middle lobe pulmonary artery and bronchial obstruction consistent with a partial torsion. In patients with complete fissures, the middle lobe may have a narrow pedicle, which can rotate partially or completely. During upper or lower lobectomy, intraoperative manipulation of the middle lobe may occasionally cause it to become reinflated in a rotated or torsed configuration. This usually presents with venous congestion of the lobe and signs of inflammation/infection, most commonly 5 to 10 days after the primary procedure. Chest x-ray may demonstrate progressive middle lobe opacity; however, a high index of suspicion is required for correct diagnosis. Contrast CT can confirm the diagnosis with either absence/obstruction of venous and/or arterial flow or focal rotation of hilar structures and associated consolidation/collapse. Delayed diagnosis results in necrosis of the affected lobe necessitating resection. Overall incidence is <0.1% of all pulmonary resections.

Reference: Cable DG, et al. Lobar torsion after pulmonary resection: presentation and outcome. *J Thorac Cardiovasc Surg* 2001;122(6):1091–1093.

2   **Answer B.**   After pneumonectomy, the empty pleural space is gradually obliterated by a sequence of normal changes. Initially, the pleural space fills with fluid with expected complete obliteration and opacification of the chest within 4 weeks of surgery. Skeletal changes include contraction of the intercostal spaces, which may be associated with scoliosis in some patients. Hemidiaphragm elevation and mediastinal repositioning allow almost complete obliteration of the pleural space at 6 months. The remaining lung enlarges and commonly herniates anterior to the heart. The heart is displaced to the side of the pneumonectomy. In an asymptomatic patient, fluid within the pleural space is to be expected and, as this is a sterile collection, should not be manipulated. In contrast, a drop in the pleural fluid volume on successive postoperative chest x-rays should raise suspicion for a bronchopleural fistula.

References: Bazwinsky-Wutschke I, et al. Anatomical changes after pneumonectomy. *Ann Anat* 2011;193(2):168–172.

Smulders SA, et al. Cardiac function and position more than 5 years after pneumonectomy. *Ann Thorac Surg* 2007;83(6):1986–1992.

3   **Answer B.**   An Eloesser flap is used as an intermediate step in the management of a postpneumonectomy bronchopleural fistula. Bronchial stump breakdown is associated with contamination of the pleural space and occurs in upwards of 5% of cases, more commonly on the right. The left-sided bronchial stump is naturally reinforced due to its location beneath the aortic arch. Empyema after pneumonectomy is a challenging problem due to the difficulty of clearing infection in such a large cavity. Open thoracotomy allows for daily dressing changes to promote granulation tissue formation, healing by secondary intention, and preparation of the wound bed for additional attempts at closure. In general, ribs are removed allowing for myocutaneous flap to be sewn to the diaphragm, creating a chronic open cavity. The opacity in this patient's film represents packed dressing material.

References: Miller JI Jr. The history of surgery of empyema, thoracoplasty, Eloesser flap, and muscle flap transposition. *Chest Surg Clin N Am* 2000;10(1):45–53.

Thourani VH et al. Twenty-six years of experience with the modified Eloesser flap. *Ann Thorac Surg* 2003;76(2):401–406.

4 **Answer C.** Postpneumonectomy syndrome occurs infrequently in long-term survivors after pneumonectomy and is caused by extreme mediastinal shift after pneumonectomy. The CT scan demonstrates complete rotation of the heart into the right chest and compression of the airway and, in this case esophagus, over the aorta and vertebral column. The most common symptom is progressive central airway obstruction with wheezing. Esophageal obstruction presents with dysphagia as in this case. Mediastinal repositioning is helpful in many of these patients and is generally accomplished with the placement of a silastic implant in the pneumonectomy bed.

Reference: Avgerinos DV, Meisner J, Harris L. Minimally invasive repair of post-pneumonectomy syndrome. *Thorac Cardiovasc Surg* 2009;57(1):60–62.

5 **Answer D.** TBM is seen in adults with COPD and results in dynamic airway collapse. Patients who are appropriate risk for surgery should undergo a posterior stabilization of the membranous trachea (tracheoplasty); however, many patients require palliation with a stent. Although stents provide excellent immediate relief (>75%), and may facilitate wean from a ventilator, they are associated with significant long-term complications. All of the listed complications can occur; however, the most significant and likely to occur in the long term is the formation of granulation tissue, which can obstruct the stent and prohibit its removal. The stent shown is a self-expanding metallic stent. Silicone stents are also available and preferred by some surgeons.

Reference: Wright CD. *Optimal management of malacic airway syndromes. Difficult decisions in thoracic surgery.* London, UK: Springer, 2011:363–366.

6 **Answer A.** Self-expanding esophageal stents are used for both benign and malignant indications. They provide excellent palliation and relief of obstructive symptoms and can restore near-normal ability to swallow for many patients. Unlike the airway, the esophagus in most patients is motile and peristalsis continues to occur. Various design elements have been introduced to minimize migration; however, distal migration remains the most common early problem with esophageal stents. This can easily be detected on daily x-rays and is more likely to occur when the stent is placed for nonmalignant reasons including perforations and leaks. Endoscopy is required to replace, retrieve, or reposition the stent. Small esophageal leaks and injuries can be treated conservatively with stenting: a recent review demonstrated a 76% clinical success rate in carefully selected patients, which can obviate the need to perform an extensive surgery. However, of the above complications, migration is the most common.

Reference: van Boeckel, PG, et al. Fully covered self-expandable metal stents (SEMS), partially covered SEMS and self-expandable plastic stents for the treatment of benign esophageal ruptures and anastomotic leaks. *BMC gastroenterol* 2012;12(1):19.

7 **Answer B.** Although transplant would result in replacement of the diseased parenchyma, this patient still has some evidence of bullae in the right medial lung, and there are no sternal wires that should be seen with a transverse sternotomy (clamshell) as is typically performed for bilateral transplantation. LVRS is a good option for patients such as this who have end-stage lung disease, characterized by nonhomogeneous emphysema and preserved exercise tolerance. The National Emphysema Treatment Trial (NETT) found no advantage to LVRS versus medical therapy in terms of survival in patients with homogeneous emphysema (emphysema distributed diffusely in the craniocaudal plane). However, the risk ratio of death was 0.47 in the surgically treated group with nonhomogeneous emphysema such as this patient (upper lung predominant emphysema). In essence, removal of the hyperinflated, nonperfused, apical segments allows for expansion and recruitment of functionally collapsed basilar segments and can be an effective bridge to transplant in select patients.

Reference: Fishman A, et al. A randomized trial comparing lung-volume-reduction surgery with medical therapy for severe emphysema. *N Engl J Med* 2003;348(21):2059–2073.

8 Answer B. Surgery for esophageal cancer generally consists of esophagectomy and reconstruction with a gastric conduit. The stomach is stapled parallel to the greater curvature to separate this gastric tube from the GE junction and tumor, and the conduit is then passed along the esophageal bed to anastomose with the proximal esophagus. The anastomosis may be performed in the neck or in the chest (commonly referred to as Ivor Lewis). This CT scan demonstrates a contrast-filled gastric tube in the esophageal bed, which is appropriately sized, with no evidence of rotation or hernia. Chest CT is not ideal for evaluation of any anastomotic stricture, which is better visualized with barium swallow or esophagoscopy.

Reference: Gore RM, Levine MS. *Postoperative Esophagus. Textbook of Gastrointestinal Radiology.* Philadelphia, PA: W.B. Saunders, 2000:449–461.

9 Answer C. The scan demonstrates contrast within the gastric conduit; however, the area of leak is posterior and away from the stapled anastomosis, which is visualized close to the left atrium. The blood supply to the gastric conduit is the right gastroepiploic artery. The left and right gastric and short gastric arteries are all divided in mobilizing and tubularizing the stomach. As such, the points of the conduit most distant from this blood supply are the anastomosis and the tip of the conduit. Anastomotic leaks occur with a frequency of approximately 10%; however, conduit failure, characterized by necrosis of the gastric "tip," occurs in <1% of cases. This catastrophic complication generally requires takedown of the anastomosis, esophageal diversion with cervical esophagostomy, and 3 to 6 months of rehabilitation and nutrition before a second attempt with a colon interposition.

Reference: Iannettoni, MD, Whyte RI, Orringer MB. Catastrophic complications of the cervical esophagogastric anastomosis. *J Thorac Cardiovas Surg* 1995;110(5):1493–1501.

10 Answer B. Bilateral central airway obstruction, with healthy-appearing parenchyma, suggests stenosis in a lung transplant recipient. Central airway stenosis can result from technical issues with the anastomosis or local ischemia and is more commonly seen in patients who have had a complex postoperative course including those who have been complicated by a fungal infection. Isolated right-sided issues are also seen in vanishing bronchus intermedius syndrome (VBIS), which is poorly understood. Conventional silicone and expandable metal stents have been used in conjunction with local ablative therapy to manage symptomatic stenosis. Novel biodegradable stents may help overcome the issues of granulation tissue seen with conventional devices.

Fibrosing mediastinitis is most frequently caused by histoplasmosis in the United States, but the case here does not demonstrate the typical hilar and mediastinal distortion seen in those cases. Similarly, the pulmonary parenchyma does not demonstrate any findings of architectural distortion to suggest pulmonary fibrosis, and expiratory imaging is not shown to correlate with bronchomalacia or tracheobronchomalacia.

Reference: Shofer SL, et al. Significance of and risk factors for the development of central airway stenosis after lung transplantation. *Am J Transplant* 2013;13(2):383–389.

11 Answer C. Hyperinflation of the native lung may be seen in COPD patients who receive a single-lung transplant. Mediastinal shift is unlikely after lobectomy, and the different appearance of the parenchyma in both lung fields suggests the presence of a transplant. Unilateral constrictive bronchiolitis such as from prior infection (Swyer-James) is a consideration but considerably less likely given the severity of the abnormality present.

Due to loss of elasticity and destruction of alveoli in the COPD lung, LaPlace law explains the overinflation that occurs from decreased surface tension in the native alveoli versus the transplanted lung. Progressive hyperinflation of the remaining native emphysematous lung can compromise function of the transplanted lung, and some of these patients must undergo a staged sequential transplant as a result. As such, bilateral lung transplant is favored for COPD. Single-lung transplantation is reserved for non-COPD patients or for the occasional older COPD patient who would benefit from transplant but would be less likely to be allocated a double graft based on lung allocation score.

Reference: Motoyama H, et al. Quantitative evaluation of native lung hyperinflation after single lung transplantation for emphysema using three-dimensional computed tomography volumetry. *Transplantation Proceedings* 2014;46(3):941–943. Elsevier.

12 **Answer B.** The image demonstrates herniation of a portion of the lung parenchyma with opacification suggestive of strangulation. Lung hernias are an uncommon complication of thoracic surgery and may be entirely asymptomatic, present as a bulge that moves with respiration, or be associated with pleurisy or signs of infection. Counterintuitively, they may be more likely to occur due to modern minimally invasive techniques as the thoracic ports are not closed with pericostal suture in the same way that a thoracotomy is closed. Management of the majority of cases is purely observational; however, a case of strangulated parenchyma as shown may require revision, resection of involved lung, and patch repair of the defect.

The abnormality shown is not fluid density, and therefore, a seroma is incorrect. Additionally, there is abnormality of opacified lung, not a chest wall mass, making osteosarcoma incorrect. Empyema necessitans refers to a pleural infection that erodes through the parietal pleura and into the chest wall, especially in the setting of tuberculosis empyema.

Reference: Bhamidipati CM, et al. Lung hernia following robotic-assisted mitral valve repair. *J Cardiac Surg* 2012;27(4):460–463.

13 **Answer C.** Sternal dehiscence is a feared complication after cardiac surgery. Routine closure of the sternotomy is performed with sternal wires, and alternative devices are also available such as metallic plates. On chest x-ray, notice the fracture of multiple sternal wires, which are displaced to opposite sides. On CT, the patient appears to have a broken sternal wire with separation of the sternal edges. Fractured sternal wires in isolation are frequently seen as an incidental finding. It is the lateral displacement that is worrisome for dehiscence.

Dehiscence is strongly associated with both diabetes and morbid obesity. One study of this issue in US patients demonstrated a rate of dehiscence of almost 7% in morbidly obese patients (BMI > 30) compared with 1.6% in nonobese patients. The occurrence of dehiscence was associated with infection and mediastinitis in 96% of patients and carried a 40% mortality. Management generally requires debridement, delayed wound closure, and myocutaneous flap interposition in many cases.

Reference: Molina JE, Lew RS, Hyland KJ. Postoperative sternal dehiscence in obese patients: incidence and prevention. *Ann Thorac Surg* 2004;78(3):912–917.

14 **Answer C.** Although delayed presentation of an intraoperative or perioperative injury to the esophagus or trachea is possible, the most likely explanation for worsening mediastinal air at 5 days is a bronchial dehiscence.

Bronchial anastomotic dehiscence is not common but may be seen in up to 10% of transplants at least in mild severity. It usually presents several days after transplant and is due to ischemia at the bronchial anastomosis with gradual necrosis and ultimately perforation of bronchial tissue. Necrosis seen on bronchoscopy will be the first and most reliable sign, as significant dehiscence has to have occurred to allow for chest x-ray detection of extraluminal air at least initially. Small contained leaks are possible. CT scanning is of particular value to the surgeon and interventional pulmonologist in planning an intervention: fortunately, many of these cases may be managed with placement of an endobronchial stent. However, a minority will require pneumonectomy and possible retransplant, and this carries an expectedly high mortality.

Reference: Porhownik NR. Airway complications post lung transplantation. *Curr Opin Pulm Med* 2013;19(2):174–180.

15 **Answer D.** The differential diagnosis in this case includes acute rejection, pneumonia, congestive cardiac failure, and primary graft dysfunction. Of the studies listed, a contrast-enhanced CT will be the single most useful test. This will allow for demonstration of arterial blood flow to both lungs, evaluation of patency of the venous anastomosis, and assessment for pleural effusions, which are the primary surgical/technical considerations at this point.

Primary graft dysfunction (PGD) is the most likely diagnosis: with an incidence of up to 25% in some form, it represents a spectrum of ischemia–reperfusion. Risk factors for development of PGD include donor smoking, long cold ischemia time, single-lung transplant, and use of cardiopulmonary bypass during implant. As a diagnosis of exclusion, technical issues must first be ruled out. Rejection is ruled out by confirming crossmatch and reviewing pretransplant panel reactive antibody (PRA) testing. Treatment is then primarily supportive with recommendation for early deployment of venovenous extracorporeal membrane oxygenation (ECMO) to allow for extubation and ambulation.

Reference: Diamond JM, et al. Clinical risk factors for primary graft dysfunction after lung transplantation. *Am J Respir Criti Care Med* 2013;187(5):527–534.

"Note: Page numbers followed by f indicate figures"